Breastfeeding and Medication

Sadly, women often feel they have no alternative but to give up breastfeeding, having been prescribed or purchased medication. In many cases, however, this is unnecessary. This book outlines the evidence base for the use of medication during breastfeeding.

Breastfeeding and Medication presents a comprehensive A to Z guide to the most frequently prescribed drugs and their safety for breastfeeding mothers. Evaluating the evidence for interventions and using a simple format for quickly identifying medications that are safe or unsafe to use, it also highlights those drugs where there is inconclusive evidence.

Additional contextual information makes this the most complete text for those practitioners who support and treat breastfeeding women. It:

- provides an overview of the anatomy and physiology of the breast, together with hormonal influences, in order to better understand how complications, such as mastitis, arise and inform the approach to their treatment;
- includes a section on conditions that affect women specifically when they are lactating where prescription of medication may be necessary;
- discusses the importance of breastfeeding and its advantages, as well as its disadvantages; and
- explores how to support breastfeeding mothers, and presents a counselling model approach.

Taking into account the recommendations of NICE Maternal and Child Nutrition guidelines, this is an invaluable reference for all health practitioners and volunteers who work with, support and treat breastfeeding women, including lactation consultants, breastfeeding support workers, health visitors, GPs, practice nurses, pharmacists and midwives.

Wendy Jones is an independent pharmacist prescriber with over 20 years' experience as a breastfeeding support worker for the Breastfeeding Network (BfN). She runs the BfN Drugs in Breastmilk Helpline and has presented widely to healthcare professionals, volunteers and mothers on this subject.

Breastfeeding and Medication

Wendy Jones

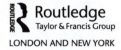
Routledge
Taylor & Francis Group

LONDON AND NEW YORK

First published 2013
by Routledge
2 Park Square, Milton Park, Abingdon, Oxon, OX14 4RN

Simultaneously published in the USA and Canada
by Routledge
711 Third Avenue, New York, NY 10017

Routledge is an imprint of the Taylor & Francis Group, an informa business

British Library Cataloguing in Publication Data
A catalogue record for this book is available from the British Library

Library of Congress Cataloging-in-Publication Data
Jones, Wendy, 1954–
Breastfeeding and medication / Wendy Jones.
p. ; cm.
Includes bibliographical references.
I. Title.
[DNLM: 1. Breast Feeding—Handbooks. 2. Drug Toxicity—Handbooks. 3. Milk,
Human—drug effects—Handbooks. 4. Pharmaceutical Preparations—administration &
dosage—Handbooks. 5. Pharmaceutical Preparations—adverse effects—Handbooks.
WS 39]
649'.33—dc23
2012035634

ISBN: 978-0-415-64105-0 (hbk)
ISBN: 978-0-415-64106-7 (pbk)
ISBN: 978-0-203-08224-9 (ebk)

Typeset in Sabon
by FiSH Books Ltd, Enfield

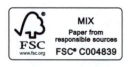

MIX
Paper from
responsible sources
FSC® C004839
www.fsc.org

Printed and bound in Great Britain by
TJ International Ltd, Padstow, Cornwall

Contents

Illustrations

Figures

Tables

Dedication

This book is dedicated to my Mum, Peggy Mary Middleton, who sadly died before it was completed but rejoiced in the news that it was to be written.

It is also written in memory of my Dad, Dennis, who died before he had a chance to know that I would follow in his footsteps to become a pharmacist. I hope he would have been proud of the way I have combined my work and my passionate interest in the support of breastfeeding.

My Mum didn't only breastfeed me, she supported me in breastfeeding my wonderful daughters Kerensa, Bethany and Tara. She gave me the space to spend time with them and have nothing else to worry about. Throughout, she continued to care for me. Without her love and experience, I would never have gone on to work with other mothers who were breastfeeding, nor begin the studies that have culminated in this book.

I'd also like to express my endless thanks to my husband Mike who has always been there to encourage me, to help me with computer glitches, to put science into my 'hobby', and to love and believe in me, however much I have tried his patience.

Last but not least, thank you to my babies who have taught me so much about breastfeeding, each in their own very different way. They have grown into young women who can only be seen as an advert for the benefits of breastfeeding – beautiful, intelligent and a pleasure to be with.

Acknowledgements

I would also like to acknowledge the help of many people who have helped me on the long road to completing the text of this book.

Professor David Brown who taught me so much about academic writing and stopped me writing 'a Sunday afternoon letter to my mum', and who supported me through my PhD studies. Professor Paul Rutter who inspired me to keep writing and helped me look at the evidence behind medicines.

I find it hard to express the extent of my gratitude for the mothers and babies whose photographs I have been allowed to use within the book. To Louise, Bill and baby Amelia who let me share a very special few weeks in their lives: thank you. To the mothers and babies of Portsmouth and the brilliant Breastfeeding Network team who took the photographs, posed so beautifully and were so generous in letting me use the images I can only say you are wonderful. My fabulous cover girls Kelly and Emma (and Rich who took the photograph of them), you have given me something very special.

I would like to thank Grace and James from Routledge who supported me with so much patience, gentle encouragement and understanding, as well as the reviewers whose comments were thought-provoking and challenging but always useful.

I would also like to take the opportunity to acknowledge so many people within the Breastfeeding Network who believed that I would finish this book, who inspired me with their knowledge and mother-centred care as well as providing me with an organisation where I was able to use my skills in looking at the safety of drugs in breastmilk – Magda, Phyll, Lorna, Sarah, Jacqui, Mary and Ruth to name but a few.

Introduction

Breastmilk is best and normal

We know that breastmilk is the ideal form of nutrition for infants: the biological norm. It uniquely caters for each baby. We also know that only a minority of babies receive breastmilk for more than a few weeks (Bolling 2007). Increase in the initiation and duration of exclusive breastfeeding is seen as a priority by the UK Government (Child Health Promotion Programme 2008) and many governments across the world. It has long been established as a goal within the World Health Organization (WHO). The initiatives are built on robust evidence for the improvement of children's health by receiving breastmilk. More recently breastfeeding has also been coupled with a lowering of the risk of obesity both in childhood and in adulthood although evidence for this is less substantial (Off to the Best Start 2007).

So why don't more mothers breastfeed?

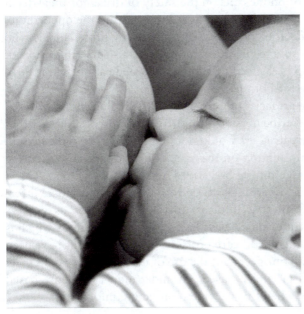

Why are targets for improving breastfeeding incidence and prevalence so difficult to achieve? Why is the experience of breastfeeding so frequently viewed as negative in the media and in the general population? Why is formula feeding regarded as the standard way to feed infants in the UK? Why do 28% of all mothers stop breastfeeding within the first six weeks of their baby's life (Bolling 2007) and why do 29% of mothers find that breastfeeding hurts so much that they have to stop within the first two weeks after they have had their baby (Bolling 2007)?

There are many reasons. Some are embedded in history, others within local cultures and experiences and many related to modern lifestyle and expectations of mothers and healthcare professionals.

For the mothers who have chosen to breastfeed there may have been many barriers to overcome. In addition to the awareness of the positive advantages of breastfeeding for their baby, there is an emotional aspect to breastfeeding that can have a major impact upon the mother's frame of mind as well as the mother–child relationship.

During maternal illness it may be all too easy for the medical professional to ignore these sensitive factors when advising a mother to stop breastfeeding because of the medication about to be prescribed. This recommendation is often founded on information that is neither quantitative nor qualitative, let alone evidence based. This book aims to better inform some of those decisions.

How can this book help?

What does this book offer that is different from other books on breastfeeding? I have written this text not only in the light of my experience as a voluntary breastfeeding worker for the past 25 years, but also as a healthcare professional used to providing evidence based research for interventions. Additionally, I have tried to provide a toolbox for prescribers in the section on medication use during lactation. As a pharmacist I have answered many thousands of phone calls on the safety of drugs for breastfeeding women over the past 16 years. I have been privileged to have had the opportunity to develop an insight into the difficulties experienced, not only by professionals who do not have immediate access to sources of information, but also the confusion of mothers told that they have to stop breastfeeding if they need medication. These difficulties are very real and confusing for both parties.

I qualified as an independent pharmacist prescriber in 2005 and am fully aware of how complex the decision is to prescribe outside of licence. I would not advocate that a medical practitioner prescribe any drug if I would not be happy to prescribe myself. Over the years I have provided information on the safety of drugs and discussed the safest alternatives for mothers to take during breastfeeding.

As a practice support pharmacist, my role has been to research and evaluate information and to present it in a form that informs doctors and nurses as well as pharmacists. On occasions, I present evidence-based information to mothers which is at variance with that supplied by other healthcare professionals. Many of us have been in situations where we disagree with our peers but the use of material to use data from peer-reviewed material wherever possible, based on independent evidence-based research should decrease the times when this becomes conflicting information.

These experiences and statistics are replicated in most other developed countries. Use of my website and social networking site has confirmed that patient and professional needs are the same across the boundaries of countries. There are initiatives in most countries to increase the initiation and prevalence rates of breastfeeding (Amir 2011). Medication has been reported as a barrier to breastfeeding in many countries (Schirm 2004) so the information and theory is transferable across the world.

Babies are precious and vulnerable. We would all do everything in our power to protect them from harm: which is normally best achieved by protecting breastfeeding. Is that possible when prescribing an unlicensed drug? I hope that by the time you have finished reading this book you will be able to make those informed decisions whether you are a mother or a healthcare professional or a member of one of the voluntary organisations supporting breastfeeding.

The safety of drugs in breastmilk

The drug list covered in this book (Drug Reference section) is not exhaustive. In order to provide an easily searchable manuscript, the most common drugs with direct relevance to current practice within the UK are covered. The information presented provides further interpretation beyond that which is given in standard reference sources such as the British National Formulary (BNF) based on studies and information within specialised texts. Other more detailed reference sources are signposted together with options for further information or discussion on multi-drug regimes. The Drugs in Breastmilk Helpline, run on a voluntary basis by the Breastfeeding Network (BfN), is a free service available to discuss less-common drugs or multiple drug regimes. This service is run under my supervision by specially trained breastfeeding supporters who operate on the National Breastfeeding Helpline.

Evidence for breastfeeding and the management of common conditions

I have provided an overview of the anatomy and physiology of the breast together with the hormonal influences on breastmilk production. By understanding how breastfeeding works I hope we may better understand how complications such as mastitis arise and in turn this will inform our approach to treating problems. We can also begin to understand why breastfeeding *is* painful for some women but should not be so.

This book contains a review of the specific biological components of breastmilk. Dependent on these immunological properties, I have provided a brief overview of the evidence base of resultant health benefits for mother and child (WHO 2010). Within the text there is also discussion of when breastfeeding is not appropriate. The management of common conditions that may affect the mother or baby during the period of lactation is also presented.

Implementing an evidence-based approach to all medical interventions is now seen as the gold standard but this is not always easy in breastfeeding. Few of us have received education as undergraduates in the management of 'normal' breastfeeding and any post-graduate information we have picked up will probably have been influenced by our own experiences of babies (Jayawickrama 2010; McFadden 2006; Renfrew 2006).

Counselling breastfeeding mothers

Having trained as a voluntary breastfeeding worker I have always used a counselling model approach with mothers – listening to their concerns, providing information and involving them in decision-making, rather than providing advice and recommendations. So I have included suggestions on how healthcare professionals can implement this, even within the confines of a busy surgery consultation or within a community pharmacy. I have also endeavoured to look at how we can develop a multi-disciplinary team approach to supporting breastfeeding mothers – utilising the individual skills of the team, referring to the specialist in that area.

I hope this book goes some way to making breastfeeding normal even when mothers need medication or have problems with breastfeeding itself.

Part I
Breastfeeding in the wider context

Chapter 1

Breastfeeding in context

The impact of society on breastfeeding

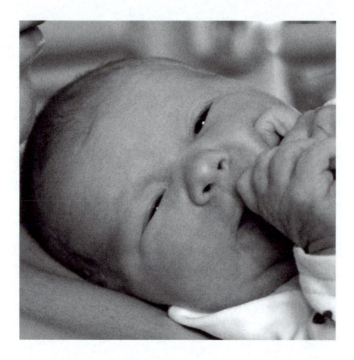

Society has a massive impact on breastfeeding – if we do not see breastfeeding but see only bottle feeding, the latter becomes normal. Breastfeeding reached a low point in 1975 with only 50% of women initiating breastfeeding (Foster 1997). In that era, mothers were instructed to feed their babies no more frequently than every 4 hours and for a maximum of 10 minutes on each side with frequent supplementation with formula milk. A certain way to set the mother up to 'fail' at breastfeeding. Since then the breastfeeding rate has slowly increased, with an early indication of an initiation rate of 82% in 2010 (Infant Feeding Survey 2010). Exclusive, baby-led breastfeeding is now being encouraged (see Figure 1.1).

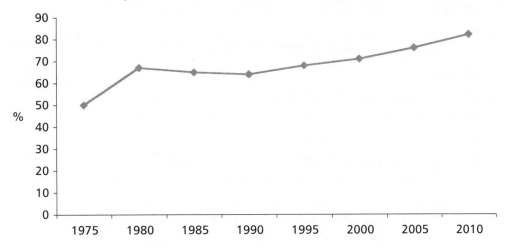

Percentage of mothers initiating breastfeeding in England and Wales

FIGURE **1.1** Initiation of breastfeeding in England and Wales

With the majority of mothers now choosing to breastfeed at least initially, health-care professionals need to consider how they can better protect, promote and support mothers in their chosen method of infant feeding. The intention of this book is not to make women who choose to bottle feed feel guilty or imply that they don't love their babies, merely to support those who have chosen to breastfeed to do so for as long as they wish.

In the USA, the Healthy People 2020 objective is to increase the percentage of the population ever breastfed to 81.9% and those exclusively breastfed to 6 months to 25.5%. Data collected in the Breastfeeding Report Card 2011 showed that, nationally, 74.6% of babies were breastfed at delivery, 44.3% received some breastmilk at 6 months and 14.8% were exclusively breastfed. It is interesting to note that 24.5% of breastfed babies received some formula before they were 48 hours old (see Figure 1.2).

In Australia (ANIFS 2010), 96% of babies were initially breastfed but only 15% continued exclusively at 6 months, although 21% continued to receive some breastmilk. See Figure 1.3 for data in support of this from a different organisation, the Australian Institute of Family Studies (AIFS).

'To increase the percentage of babies who are fully breastfed from birth to six months of age, with continued breastfeeding and complementary foods to twelve months and beyond' was an objective set by the Australian National Breastfeeding Strategy 2010–2015, in line with the view that:

- Australia is a nation in which breastfeeding is protected, promoted, supported and valued by the whole of society.
- Breastfeeding is viewed as the biological and social norm for infant and young child feeding.
- Mothers, families, health professionals and other caregivers are fully informed about the value of breastfeeding.

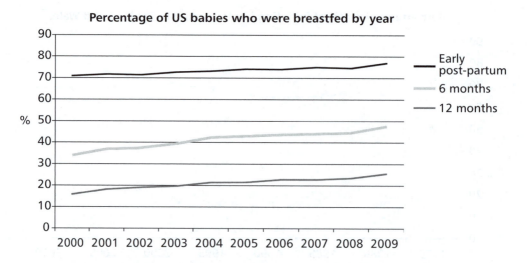

FIGURE 1.2 Breastfeeding rates in children born in USA 2000–2009 (CDC National Immunisation Survey 2011)

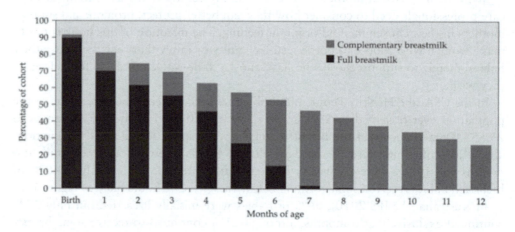

FIGURE 1.3 Breastfeeding rates in Australia 2008 (AIFS)

Health inequalities and the promotion of breastfeeding

Stuart Forsyth noted that breastfeeding is the only health intervention that can lead to better health outcomes for a child from the lowest socio-economic groups compared with an artificially fed counterpart from a more affluent family (Forsyth 2005).

In 1998 Sir Donald Acheson published the *Independent Inquiry into Inequalities in Health* report (Acheson 1998), which is the cornerstone on which many health interventions are founded. He suggested that starting with maternal and child health is likely to bring about the most rapid benefits in improving the health of society. This report drove the strategies to increase the initiation and prevalence of breastfeeding in the UK.

Maternal and Child Nutrition was published by the National Institute for Health and Clinical Excellence (NICE PH11 2008) (updated in 2011), which proposed to help improve the nutrition of pregnant and breastfeeding mothers and children in low-income households. These guidelines aimed to address disparities in the nutrition of low-income and disadvantaged groups compared with the general population.

NICE PH11 recommends that all healthcare professionals should have appropriate knowledge and skills to give advice on:

- the nutritional needs of pregnant women, including use of folic acid and vitamin D;
- promoting and supporting breastfeeding; and
- the nutritional needs of infants and young children.

There is also a recommendation on prescribing for breastfeeding mothers that will be discussed further in the Drug Reference section.

Obesity and infant feeding

The increasing number of children who are obese has become a major concern for the future health of the public in the UK. The role of breastfeeding in reducing the risk of excess weight in later life was highlighted in the white papers *Healthy Weight, Healthy Lives – a cross governmental strategy for England 2008* and *Healthy Lives, Healthy People 2010*. The Government undertook to invest in an information campaign to promote the benefits of breastfeeding as part of wider campaigns on healthy development. It also funded the setting up of a national breastfeeding helpline for mothers.

Breastfeeding in public

The 2005 Infant Feeding Survey (Bolling 2007) noted that although women in the UK are now more likely to breastfeed in public (54% in the UK), more than a quarter reported difficulties in finding a place to breastfeed and 8% had never attempted to feed in public. Interestingly, more than a third of bottle-feeding mothers said that they had never attempted to feed their baby away from home either.

In November 2004 The Breastfeeding (Scotland) Bill became law (Breastfeeding Scotland Bill 2005). This made it an offence in Scotland to stop anyone feeding milk (by whatever means) to children under two in public or in family-friendly licensed premises. The Equality Act became law in England in 2010 (Equality Act 2010). It makes it clear that a woman cannot be discriminated against for breastfeeding her baby in public places such as cafes, shops and buses. For example, a bus driver could not ask a woman to get off the bus just because she is breastfeeding her baby.

A focus group study in the UK (McFadden 2006) found that women feel breastfeeding in public is unacceptable, while bottle feeding was accepted by everybody and in all places. Some women reported breastfeeding in public toilets as the only option and wished that cafes and shops would provide more facilities for breastfeeding.

Influences on breastfeeding initiation

Mothers from the lowest socio-economic groups, who are younger at the time of delivery and who have left full-time education at a younger age, are less likely to breastfeed than their socially more advantaged counterparts (Bolling 2007). In 1995, Jamieson suggested that a tentative breastfeeding mother faced with a professional lacking in skills and encouragement will inevitably fail. Sadly the result is probably still likely to be the same.

Influence of friends and family

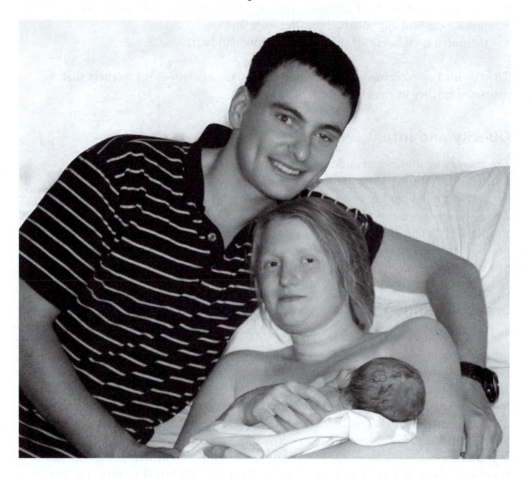

Some women in the McFadden study (McFadden 2006) said that even family and friends found it 'repulsive' to be in the same room when they were breastfeeding and that grandparents, more than fathers, felt excluded if they had no opportunity to feed the baby. It was apparent that the opinion of family and friends was a stronger influence than that of health practitioners input on the advantages of breastfeeding.

Of mothers who were bottle fed themselves as babies, 63% were breastfeeding at 4 weeks compared with 82% of mothers who were entirely breastfed as babies (Bolling 2007). Mothers generally follow the example set by their own mothers (see Figure 1.4).

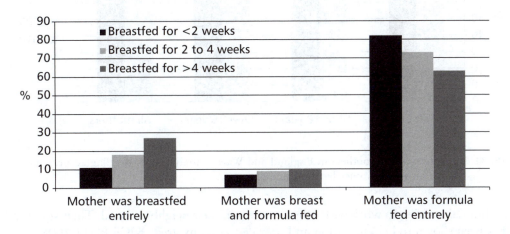

FIGURE 1.4 How mother was fed as a baby affects breastfeeding duration

Similarly, for those mothers whose friends entirely formula fed their children, 59% were still breastfeeding at 4 weeks compared with 85% whose friends entirely breast-fed their babies (Bolling 2007).We are more likely to follow the example of our peers in order to fit into the group.

Impact of education on breastfeeding initiation

In a study (van Rosem 2009) of 2914 women, 95.5% of those educated to the highest level initiated breastfeeding while only 71.3% of those reaching the lowest educational level did. Educational level influenced breastfeeding experiences until the babies were two months of age, but not thereafter (see Figure 1.5).

The Infant Feeding Survey Results (2007, 2010) have shown the same variation in breastfeeding initiation.

Peer support in populations where breastfeeding rates are historically low

Until breastfeeding is seen as normal it will remain difficult for mothers to initiate and sustain breastfeeding while they feel themselves to be acting in a manner which is not common or acceptable within their local society. To influence those mothers, an alternative means of support is required. One of these methods is the introduction of peer support workers. These are mothers who have breastfed and have undertaken

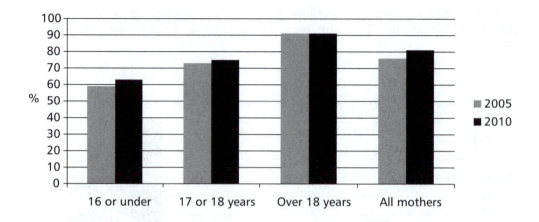

FIGURE 1.5 Percentage of mothers in England and Wales initiating breastfeeding according to age at which mother left full-time education

additional training to work with other mothers in their neighbourhood. Their support has been shown to help initiation and prevalence in any area (NICE PH11 2008)

Difficulties experienced with breastfeeding

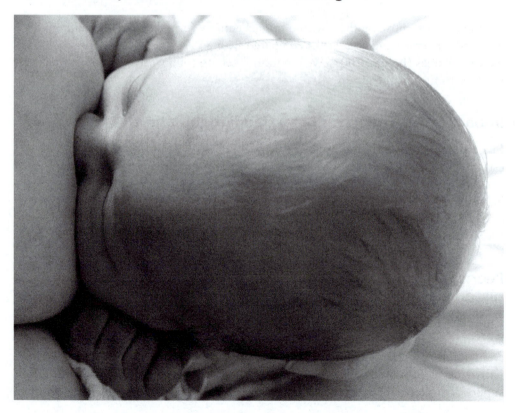

Many women and healthcare professionals perceive breastfeeding to be difficult, painful, messy, restrictive and tiring. However, studies show us that breastfeeding is important for the future health of mothers and children. So why is there this disparity between the importance and the practicality of breastfeeding?

Of mothers who initiated breastfeeding, 39% had stopped because they experienced painful breasts and/or nipples with 26% giving up in the first week (Bolling 2007). A further 14% reported that it took too long or was tiring while 4% were unhappy that the baby could not be fed by others. These mothers fulfilled the expectations that, despite their original commitment to breastfeeding, they had found it to be difficult. The reasons given for stopping breastfeeding continue in a similar vein up to 9 months after birth (see Figure 1.6).

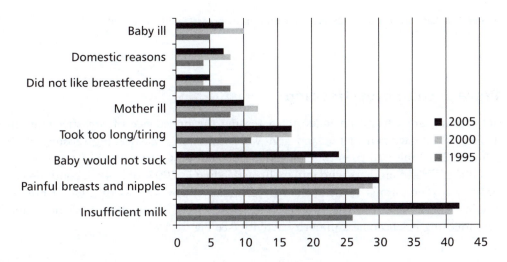

FIGURE 1.6 Reasons given for stopping breastfeeding baby less than 1 week old

However, if we look at how many women would have liked to have fed longer compared to those who have breastfed for as long as they wished very few would probably describe themselves as 'succeeding' in breastfeeding. If we could ensure that all mothers who choose to breastfeed their infants could continue to do so for as long as they wish, the negative picture of breastfeeding might be addressed.

The purpose of this book is to reduce the number of mothers told to stop breastfeeding because of their need for medication and to add to the knowledge of why breastfeeding may falter and how it can be better supported and therefore maintained (see Figure 1.7).

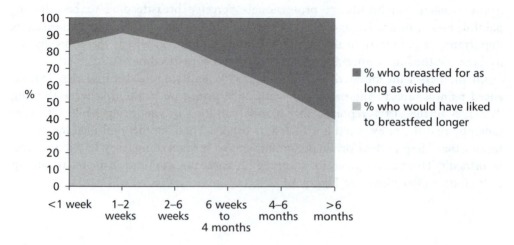

FIGURE 1.7 Satisfaction of mothers with duration of breastfeeding achieved

Prevalence of breastfeeding

So what progress has been made in increasing the prevalence of breastfeeding? In 1975, 50% of women in England and Wales initiated breastfeeding (Foster 1997) while in 2010 this had risen to 82% (NHS Information Centre 2011).

Of the 77% of mothers who initiate breastfeeding in 2005, only 48% continued to provide any breastmilk to their child by 6 weeks of age – a loss of 29% of breast-feeding experiences for the mother and child. In a short period of time and breastfeeding has become a minority activity (see Figure 1.8).

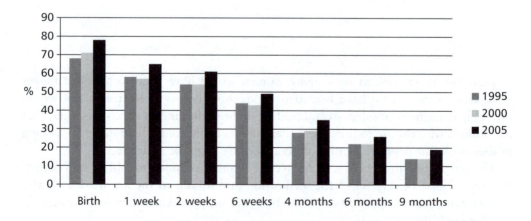

FIGURE 1.8 Percentage of mothers breastfeeding in England and Wales with age of baby

In 2000, 60% of women in manual and routine occupations initiated breastfeeding (Hamlyn *et al.* 2002) compared to 86% of women in managerial and professional occupations. By 2005 (Bolling 2007) the gap had narrowed with 67% manual workers and 89% of professional women beginning to breastfeed their babies (see Figure 1.9).

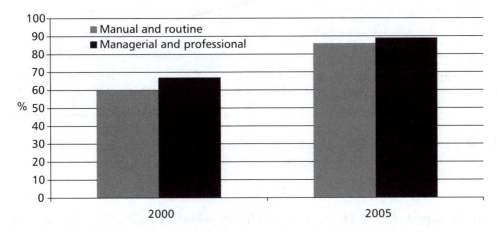

FIGURE 1.9 Percentage of mothers breastfeeding according to occupation

Exclusive breastfeeding rates

The definition of exclusive breastfeeding is that an infant receives 'only breast milk, and no other liquids or solids, with the exception of medicine, vitamins, or mineral supplements'. The UK Department of Health and World Health Organization (WHO) guidelines recommend exclusive breastfeeding for the first six months (Off to the Best Start, WHO 2007).

In 2005 the Infant Feeding Survey for the first time attempted to identify the duration of exclusive feeding (Bolling 2007). Across the UK, approximately two-thirds of mothers (65%) were exclusively breastfeeding at birth. Mothers who gave something other than breastmilk on day 1 were defined as not exclusively breastfeeding at birth. This means that 11% of mothers who initiated breastfeeding lost the exclusivity within the first 24 hours after delivery, generally while still in hospital. By 1 week less than half of all mothers (45%) were exclusively breastfeeding, and this had fallen to around a fifth by 6 weeks. At 6 months, the optimal duration, levels of exclusive breastfeeding were negligible (see Figure 1.10).

So there is a wide gap between what research says is the best way to feed babies and what actually happens. Much work is therefore still needed to meet the recommendations of the Acheson report (Acheson 1998) if we are to improve the health of society by increasing rates of breastfeeding and improving the diet of infants.

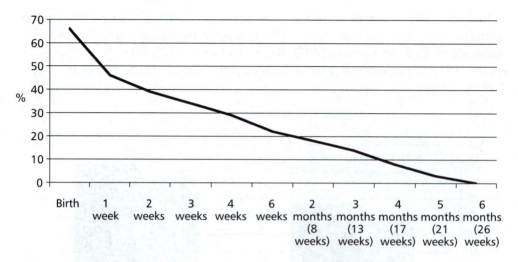

FIGURE 1.10 Percentage of women who initiated breastfeeding who were exclusively breastfeeding at defined age

In January 2012 the Department of Health published *Improving outcomes and supporting transparency*, which included an ongoing indicator to increase breast-feeding initiation and prevalence. The increase 'is expected to reduce illness in young children, which will in turn reduce hospital admissions of the under 1s (and the costs to the NHS that are associated with this'. It also states that:

> in the longer term infants who are not breastfed are more likely to become obese in later childhood, develop type 2 diabetes and tend to have slightly higher levels of blood pressure and blood cholesterol in adulthood.

This paper highlights the importance of breastfeeding as a health promotion matter and the ongoing impetus for all healthcare professionals to protect, promote and support it wherever possible.

Chapter 2

How does breastfeeding work?

This section is included to provide a better understanding of how breastfeeding works. If we understand the anatomy and physiology as well as hormonal influences, it is easier to identify what has gone wrong when mothers experience problems.

It is simple to suggest, as the nineteenth-century 'experts' did, that modern women are no longer equipped to breastfeed their babies without difficultly for more than a limited period of time.

What is currently sadly lacking is the readily available support that enables women to overcome the problems that they encounter, using evidence-based information. Some problems are frequently quoted as reasons for which women feel there is no alternative but to stop breastfeeding e.g. sore and cracked nipples, poor weight gain in the baby.

Breastmilk is a variable product – changing from colostrum at delivery through transitional milk to mature milk. It changes throughout the day and from day to day as the baby grows. The composition of breastmilk exactly matches the nutritional needs of each individual baby at that exact moment in time. It is quite simply one of nature's miracles.

Breastmilk production and supply is initially under the control of two hormones – prolactin and oxytocin. However, ongoing production is in response to the stimulation of the baby suckling and the effectiveness of milk removal, under the influence of a whey protein feedback inhibitor of lactation (FIL).

Anatomy of the lactating breast

To understand how breastfeeding can become challenged, it is useful to understand the anatomy and physiology of the breast and the hormonal influences on it during lactation.

Dr Donna Geddes (née Ramsay) and Professor Peter Hartmann, at the University of Western Australia's Human Lactation Research Group, have recently investigated the lactating breast using sophisticated ultrasound technology (Ramsay 2005). Descriptions and understanding of the anatomy of the human lactating breast had changed little over the last 160 years since Sir Astley Cooper (Cooper 1840) produced diagrams based on dissections of the breasts of lactating cadavers. He poured hot wax down the milk ducts of the breasts of cadavers before eroding the surrounding skin and tissues, leaving a wax model of the duct system (see Figure 2.1).

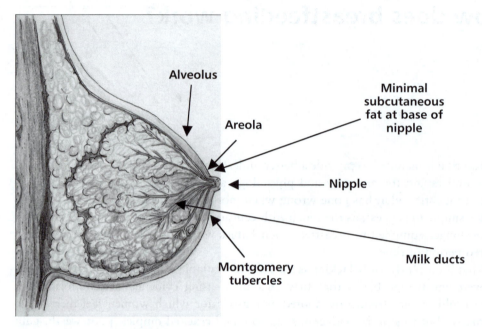

FIGURE 2.1 Structure of the breast
(© J. Richardson)

The size and shape of the breast, nipple and areola vary dramatically between women without affecting the ability to breastfeed. The adipose (fat) tissue determines the size of the breasts but this is independent of quality or quantity of milk produced. Most women are asymmetrical, having one breast larger than the other, with the left often being the largest.

The areola

The areola is a circular pigmented area around the nipple. It turns darker, reddish brown during pregnancy and retains the colour subsequently. However, the colour varies with the general complexion. Montgomery tubercules are small sebaceous glands present in the areola. They become enlarged in pregnancy and appear as small pimples. They are believed to secrete a lubricating substance during pregnancy and lactation to protect the nipple from bacterial infection. Too frequent washing may remove this protection and also make the skin drier with the nipple and areola becoming more prone to soreness and cracking.

Nipples

The nipples generally become more erect in pregnancy and in lactation as does their protractility. Inch (1989), however, reported that there was little if any relationship between protractility and breastfeeding problems as the baby forms a teat from the surrounding areola tissue and not solely the nipple. In a small proportion of women the nipple is inverted rather than erect and protractile, or becomes inverted when the areola is gently compressed.

There are few epidemiological studies of the incidence of inversion of nipples. Park (1999) suggested 3% of Korean women while Alexander and Campbell (1997) found approximately 10% of antenatal mothers in the UK had inverted nipples. As a result they recommended that antenatal examination for poor protractility should be abandoned or delayed until the third trimester. The tissue is held by adhesions at the base of the nipple and these bind the skin to the underlying tissue. While the skin becomes more elastic during the third trimester of pregnancy in preparation for nursing, some of the cells in the nipple and areola may stay attached. The extent of inversion varies greatly, ranging from the nipple that doesn't protrude when stimulated, but can be pulled out manually, to the severely inverted nipple that responds to compressions by disappearing completely.

The Hoffman Technique and the use of breast shells has in the past been recommended ante-natally to break down adhesions but a randomised controlled trial in 1992 did not show that nipple preparation improved breastfeeding success and merely acted to remove the mother's confidence in her ability to breastfeed. The use of such techniques should no longer be recommended (Alexander, Grant and Campbell 1992). Products called Niplette® and Lansinoh Latch Assist® are advertised as drawing out inverted nipples (in pregnant and non-pregnant women) but lack independent research evidence to support use as beneficial for breastfeeding.

Prolactin

During pregnancy, prolactin levels rise steadily, from approximately 10 ng per ml in the non-pregnant state to approximately 200 ng per ml at term (Rigg 1977). Milk secretion is held in check by high circulating plasma concentrations of progesterone and oestrogen originating in the placenta. Stimulation of the nipple causes the hypothalamus to inhibit the release of dopamine, which in turn stimulates the release of prolactin and production of milk (see Figure 2.2). Riordan and Auerbach (2004) reference the possibility that milk production can occur by nipple stimulation alone even in mothers who have never been pregnant.

Prolactin levels approximately double in response to suckling, with levels peaking between fifteen and thirty minutes after initiation of the feed. Efficiency of milk removal henceforth governs the volume of milk produced by each breast. Prolactin levels remain high for 90 minutes after a feed. During the first week after birth, in the absence of nipple stimulation, prolactin levels fall. If the mother does not breastfeed, levels return to the non-pregnant state by 7 days post-delivery. Mothers who smoke are reported to have lower prolactin levels (Baron 1986) while beer is reported to increase prolactin (DeRosa 1981).

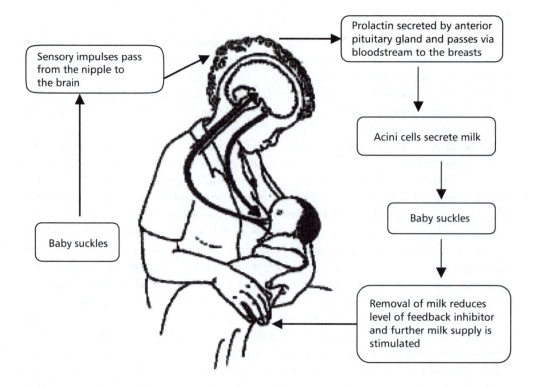

FIGURE 2.2 The prolactin reflex
(taken from UNICEF UK Baby Friendly Initiative Training Pack for GPs)

Lactation is a natural survival mechanism and is not easily disrupted, contrary to nineteenth-century beliefs that it was dependent on relaxation and contentment. However, prolactin is reported to have a relaxing, calming effect that allows a breast-feeding mother to return to sleep easily after feeding her baby. All species of lactating females have lessened responses to stress (Riordan and Auerbach 2004).

Oxytocin

When a baby suckles, oxytocin is released for the posterior pituitary gland within 1 minute. It rapidly enters the circulation and causes the myo-epithelial cells surrounding the alveoli within the breast to contract and expel the milk (see Figure 2.3). This is known as the milk-ejection reflex (MER) or 'let-down'. As well as tactile stimulation of the nipple, release may also be triggered by visual, auditory and olfactory senses. A woman hearing her baby cry, or seeing a photograph of her child, may release her milk in anticipation of the feed. Some women report a tingling sensation in their breasts which heralds the dripping of their milk, others a more vigorous let down accompanied by sharp needle-like pains, while a proportion of women are unaware of any sensation. The release of milk does not rely on what the mother feels and lack of sensation does not imply poor let down or supply.

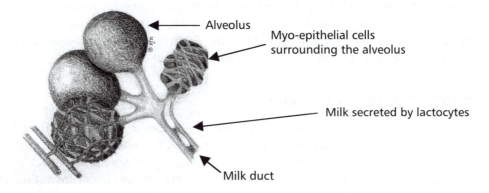

Alveolus

Myo-epithelial cells surrounding the alveolus

Milk secreted by lactocytes

Milk duct

FIGURE 2.3 Structure of myo-epithelial cell
(© J. Richardson)

Oxytocin also causes the uterus to contract which helps to control post-partum bleeding and more rapid involution of the uterus to the pre-pregnant state (see Figure 2.4). Uterine cramps may be experienced as period-like pains at each feed during the first few days after delivery. These become more pronounced after each delivery and a multi-parous mother may need to take regular analgesics in anticipation of this discomfort. The uterus continues to contract for 20 minutes after feeds finish although secretion of oxytocin returns to normal levels 6 minutes after nipple stimulation ceases.

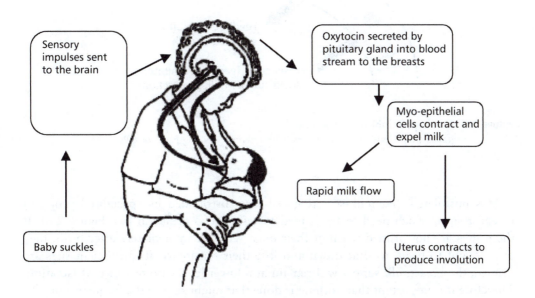

Sensory impulses sent to the brain

Oxytocin secreted by pituitary gland into blood stream to the breasts

Myo-epithelial cells contract and expel milk

Rapid milk flow

Baby suckles

Uterus contracts to produce involution

FIGURE 2.4 The oxytocin reflex
(taken from UNICEF UK Baby Friendly Initiative Training Pack for GPs)

The MER can be inhibited by embarrassment, pain, tension, fatigue or anxiety. Milk continues to be produced under the influence of prolactin, but ejection is slower and may cause the baby to pull away from the breast in frustration. Relaxation and reassurance may help the mother continue to breastfeed.

Inhibition of milk production

In established lactation, continued breastmilk production is controlled primarily by the infant's demands via suckling and ongoing, effective milk removal. Breastmilk contains a whey protein, which inhibits milk synthesis by a negative feedback mechanism (see Figure 2.5). Removing milk from the breast removes the protein (FIL) and allows more milk to be produced. Decreased removal of the protein reduces the supply. Thus cutting down on the frequency of feeds, the addition of supplementary bottles (with consequential reduction in the demands of the baby for breastmilk) or accumulation of milk in the breast because of poor attachment lowers milk production. Retained fragments of placenta may also inhibit milk production by preventing the decline in oestrogen and progesterone levels. Therefore, if the milk is not effectively removed, frequently the mother may perceive a poor milk supply, which demonstrates the link between poor attachment and the reason so many women give up breastfeeding.

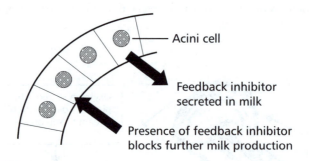

Figure 2.5 Feedback Inhibitor of Lactation
(taken from UNICEF UK Baby Friendly Initiative Training Pack for GPs)

It is postulated that milk-secreting cells are surrounded by specialised prolactin receptor sites, which need to be primed to respond to prolactin (see Figure 2.6). If these sites are not primed when at their most sensitive immediately after birth, they are thought to begin to shut down and lose their sensitivity. If insufficient sites are primed, the breastmilk supply will remain at a lower level throughout that lactation. Therefore it is important that nothing is done that might reduce the frequency or efficiency of feeds in the early days, such as giving a dummy or additional fluids (unless clinically indicated), lest it jeopardises future milk production.

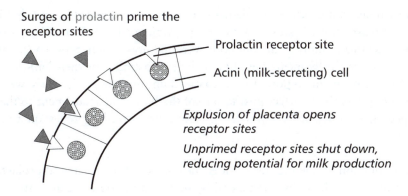

Surges of prolactin prime the receptor sites

Prolactin receptor site

Acini (milk-secreting) cell

Explusion of placenta opens receptor sites

Unprimed receptor sites shut down, reducing potential for milk production

FIGURE 2.6 The Prolactin Receptor Theory
(taken from UNICEF UK Baby Friendly InitiativeTraining Pack for GPs)

Inappropriate use of progesterone contraception during this early, critical period has been thought to be responsible for low supply in some mothers.

Effective breastfeeding

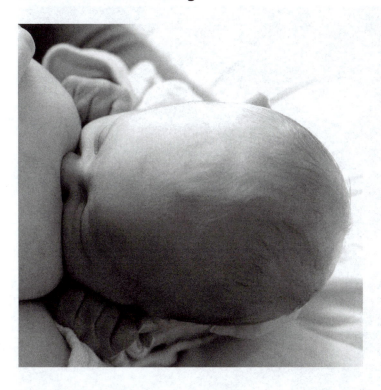

Many breastfeeding 'failures' are due to inappropriate interventions or lack of effective help so it is difficult to determine exactly what percentage of women are truly incapable of producing enough milk to feed their baby. There is good evidence that almost all women can produce an adequate milk supply (Akre 1990) and that in societies where breastfeeding is seen as a natural physiological function and is valued and supported, lactation failure is uncommon. Akre maintains that between 0.2 and 1% of mothers are physically incapable of providing breastmilk for their babies.

Many of the problems reported by breastfeeding mothers in the early weeks may be attributed to less than perfect positioning of the baby and attachment to the breast thus impeding effective milk removal. Effective breastfeeding relies on two inter-related acts:

- milk production by the mother – under the control of oxytocin and prolactin; and
- milk removal by the baby – regulated by hunger and good attachment.

Both processes are needed to ensure that the baby obtains the full volume and nutrient quality of breastmilk. Iatrogenic problems may result following incorrect management of breastfeeding.

How can healthcare professionals support breastfeeding mothers?

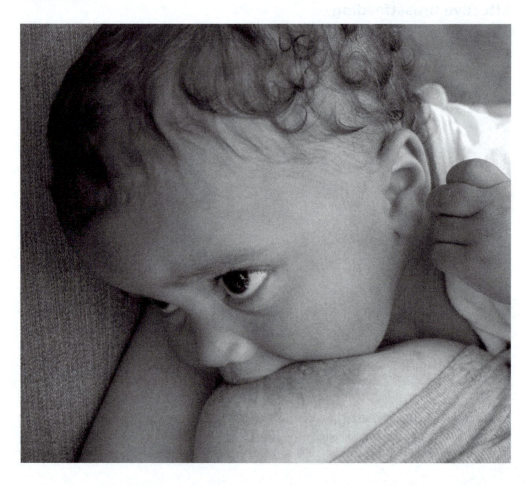

The premise of this book is that healthcare professionals strive to support women in breastfeeding, but lack the time and sometimes expertise in understanding how best to achieve this.

From the data on why women give up breastfeeding before they had intended, it is clear that pain on breastfeeding and perceived lack of milk are major barriers. Our understanding of the physiology of lactation has shown that continued milk production relies on effective drainage of the breast by the baby achieving good attachment. In addition, good attachment achieves pain-free breastfeeding. Therefore if we can help mothers to achieve good attachment then ongoing lactation should be 'problem-free' although it may still be subject to a variety of social pressures which are outside of the control of healthcare practitioners.

Assessing attachment and drainage of the breast

NICE Postnatal Care Guidelines (NICE CG37 2008) suggest the following checklist to assess effective attachment and drainage:

- baby's mouth wide open;
- less areola visible underneath the chin than above the nipple;
- chin touching the breast, lower lip rolled down and nose free;
- mother experiences no pain on latch or during the feed;
- audible and visible swallowing of milk;
- sustained rhythmic suck;
- baby's arms and hands relaxed;
- baby has moist mouth indicating it is well hydrated;
- regular soaked/heavy nappies;
- mother's breast softens after feeds;
- no change in shape of the nipple after feeds indicating lack of compression; and
- woman feels relaxed and sleepy during and after feeds.

Assessment of infant stools as an indicator of good milk transfer

In the first few days after birth, the baby's bowel motions are dark and tarry, due to the passage of meconium. The latter is composed of materials ingested during the time before the birth. Colostrum is a natural laxative and helps the infant to pass the first stool.

As the mother's milk volume increases, the baby's stool colour and consistency changes. An exclusively breastfed baby will produce loose and unformed motions of a dark-green colour that changes gradually to a mustard-yellow, sweet-smelling motion. Breastfed babies normally produce frequent bowel movements in the early days. The bowel motions of a breastfed baby are very different from those of a bottle-fed baby, which are much more formed and smell less sweet (see Figure 2.7).

Much information can be gleaned from the appearance of baby bowel motions.

how do i know that my baby is getting enough milk?

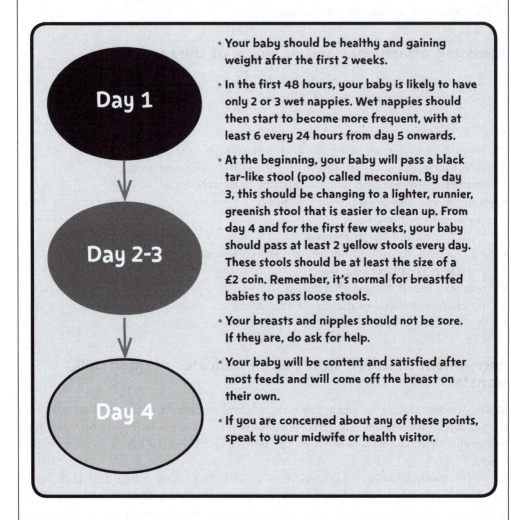

- Day 1
- Day 2-3
- Day 4

- Your baby should be healthy and gaining weight after the first 2 weeks.

- In the first 48 hours, your baby is likely to have only 2 or 3 wet nappies. Wet nappies should then start to become more frequent, with at least 6 every 24 hours from day 5 onwards.

- At the beginning, your baby will pass a black tar-like stool (poo) called meconium. By day 3, this should be changing to a lighter, runnier, greenish stool that is easier to clean up. From day 4 and for the first few weeks, your baby should pass at least 2 yellow stools every day. These stools should be at least the size of a £2 coin. Remember, it's normal for breastfed babies to pass loose stools.

- Your breasts and nipples should not be sore. If they are, do ask for help.

- Your baby will be content and satisfied after most feeds and will come off the breast on their own.

- If you are concerned about any of these points, speak to your midwife or health visitor.

FIGURE 2.7 'Off to a good start'

- Lack of stools/infrequent stools in the early days is usually a sign that a baby is not receiving enough milk.
- The change to yellow motions is a sign that milk production has commenced and that the baby is feeding well.
- Green and frothy motions may be a sign that the baby is receiving too much lactose, which has a rapid gut transit time. This may be due to an excess of the early less-fatty milk or switching the baby between breasts before emptying one breast first.
- Green nappies can also be a sign of not enough milk.

The National Childbirth Trust (NCT) produce a leaflet called 'What's in a nappy?'.

Pain on breastfeeding

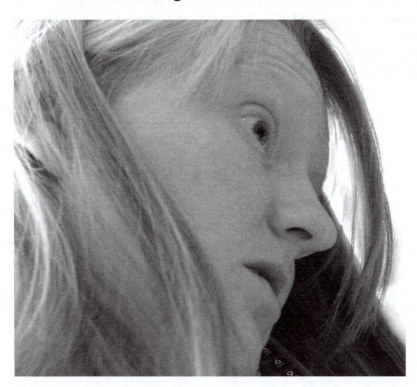

If a mother reports pain on breastfeeding in the first few weeks after delivery it is likely that the baby is not optimally attached and the mother will benefit from referral to a breastfeeding expert, such as midwife, health visitor, local breastfeeding advisor, breastfeeding peer support group or to one of the voluntary breastfeeding organisations.

Multi-disciplinary team working will provide her with other points of access to support her while she is breastfeeding and later weaning her baby, leaving the medical professionals to deal with physical symptoms of illness.

By developing a team approach, each healthcare professional can utilise their own expertise – the infant feeding specialists to help the mother achieve effective attachment and the GP to diagnose and treat any medical conditions.

By using the evidence-based information within training schemes equivalent to the Baby Friendly Initiative, as recommended by NICE Guidelines (NICE PH11 2008), mothers will be given consistent advice and support by all members of the multi-disciplinary team be they professional or voluntary.

By concentrating breastfeeding support on women who have chosen to breastfeed rather than attempting to pressurise those who feel uncomfortable with the idea, breastfeeding will become less of a contentious matter within society.

Key points

- Understanding how breastfeeding works may facilitate problem solving.
- Breastmilk production is controlled by the release of oxytocin and prolactin.
- Breastmilk removal sustains supply.
- Most breastfeeding problems resulting in mothers stopping breastfeeding relate to problems with attaching the baby to the breast and effective breastmilk removal.

Chapter 3

Constituents of breastmilk and formula milk

Breastmilk – a remarkable liquid

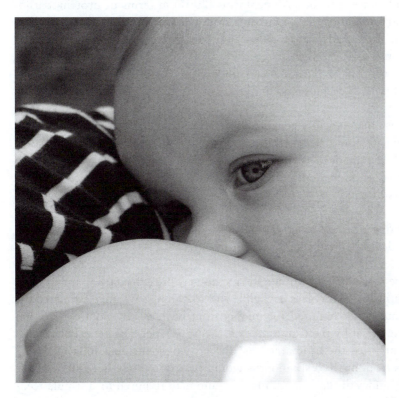

Over 200 constituents of breastmilk have been identified. There is variation in the content of breastmilk depending on the stage of lactation, the time of day and the interval since the preceding feed. These factors are specific to meet the nutritional needs of the individual infant at that time.

Formula milk is modified cow's milk (with the exception of some specialised milks necessary for infants with cow's milk protein intolerance). Manufacturers have an impossibly difficult task in developing and marketing their product. They have to produce a standardised, heavily regulated product at an affordable price. Each company seeks to achieve a proportion of the sales market by the power of advertising and perceived advantages of their brand over their competitors. Brand loyalty is encouraged although there is no evidence that any brand of formula is superior to any other. Similarly there is no evidence to support the recommendation to switch from whey to casein dominant milk if the baby is thriving, or the introduction of follow-on milks or to specially designed toddler milks if the weaning diets of babies over 6 months of age are adequate.

However, the manufacturer's main difficulty stems from the problems in identifying and reproducing the immunological components of breastmilk. Even if the chemical structures can be replicated, it may be difficult to associate chemicals with the transport mechanisms within the body to enable them to be absorbed, i.e. bioavailability.

Formula milk is a nutritionally adequate fluid, the content of which is controlled by the internationally agreed Codex Alimentarius (2007) in terms of protein, carbohydrate, vitamin and mineral content. Outcome studies on the benefits of adding these ingredients are limited by study size, data on individuals lost to the study and long-term patient orientated data.

In a response to the Infant Formula and Follow-on Formula Draft Regulations 2007 (SACN 2007), SACN commented that:

> If an ingredient is unequivocally beneficial as demonstrated by independent review of scientific data it would be unethical to withhold it for commercial reasons. Rather it should be made a required ingredient of infant formula in order to reduce existing risks associated with artificial feeding. To do otherwise is not in the best interests of children.

In a written answer to the House of Commons in June 2009, Gillian Merron (Minister of State for Public Health) stated that:

> Breast milk is the best nutrition for infants. Exclusively breastfeeding an infant from birth to six months of age involves negligible cost to parents. We have estimated the amount of formula milk required for infants from birth to six months based on energy requirements set by the Committee on Medical Aspects of Food Policy.
>
> At the current price the estimated cost for providing formula milk as a sole food for infants from birth to six months would be approximately £180 to £210. This estimate excludes the cost of additional equipment required for formula feeding such as the feeding bottles, teats and sterilisation equipment.
>
> (Hansard 2009)

The feeding of neonates makes a critical contribution to their short- and long-term health. At no other period in human life is there total dependence on one food to meet all nutritional needs to secure optimal growth and development.

Breastmilk contains important constituents that promote active immunity. Contamination and infection can occur at many stages in the preparation of artificial milks: the vessel used to feed the milk to the baby may not be sterilised, the water used to dilute the powder may not be sterile, the standard of storage may be inadequate, etc. The NICE background briefing paper on the Promotion of breastfeeding initiation and duration (Public Health Collaborating Centre 2006) states that there is incontrovertible evidence that use of breastmilk substitutes results in increased risks to infant and maternal health in developed as well as developing countries.

Ip's meta-analysis (Ip 2007) showed that:

- Infants not breastfed show an increased incidence of morbidity due to infections including otitis media, gastro-enteritis, urinary tract infection and pneumonia as well as increased risks of childhood obesity, Type 1 and 2 diabetes, leukaemia and sudden infant death syndrome.
- Premature infants who are not breastfed are at an increased risk of necrotising enterocolitis (NEC) with associated increased risk of mortality.
- Mothers who do not breastfeed show an increased risk of breast cancer, particularly pre-menopausal ovarian cancer, Type 2 diabetes and the metabolic syndrome as a result of failure to lose excess weight gained during pregnancy.

Stuebe (2009) suggests that infant feeding is an important modifiable risk factor for disease in mothers and children.

So what is it that is in breastmilk that provides the baby with better health outcomes than those who are formula fed? How do these immunological factors protect the infant?

Lactoferrin

- Lactoferrin is a protein that binds to iron, thus facilitating absorption
- Lactoferrin has antimicrobial properties – by binding to iron it reduces levels available for bacterial growth
- Lactoferrin binds to receptor sites on the surfaces of bacterial cell membranes causing lysis (breakdown)
- Lactoferrin suppresses viral replication
- Lactoferrin promotes the growth of gut intestinal epithelium

Lactoferrin accounts for 10–15% of the total protein content of breastmilk. Human milk is lower in protein content than the milk of many other mammals. Lactoferrin and secretory immunoglobulin A (SigA) are as concerned with immunoprotection as they are with nutrition. Lactoferrin is resistant to digestion by gut enzymes and is found in the stools of breastfed infants.

It is an iron-binding protein which mediates the absorption of iron by the baby from breastmilk, thereby reducing the levels of free iron in the blood. It is one of the main components of the immune system as in addition to iron transport it also has promotes antimicrobial activity by depriving bacterial flora from the iron, which is necessary for growth. Breastmilk has relatively low levels of iron but the presence of lactoferrin increases bio-availability. In comparison, artificial formula has five to six times as much iron but as it is in free form it is far less bio-available to the infant and its presence supports the growth of bacteria and raises the risk of gastro-intestinal infections.

Micro-organisms have specific receptor sites on their cell surfaces to which lactoferrin binds. This disrupts the membrane's permeability and results in cell lysis. Only 10% of lactoferrin is saturated with iron, which leaves the remaining 90% free to exert this bactericidal activity. Administration of supplementary iron to a breastfed infant interferes with this level of saturation resulting in decreased bactericidal activity. However, iron supplements given to anaemic breastfeeding mothers do not interfere with the levels of lactoferrin in her breastmilk (Zavaleta 1995).

In vitro studies have shown that lactoferrin also acts on the herpes simplex virus, hepatitis C, human respiratory syncytial virus and *Candida albicans*. Many viruses bind to lipoproteins in cell membranes and penetrate cells. As with bactericidal activity, lactoferrin preferentially binds onto these sites consequently repelling viral fragments. It also suppresses viral replication which follows cell penetration, thereby increasing protection against these micro-organisms.

Lactoferrin is also an essential growth factor for beta cell lymphocytes and T cell lymphocytes. It is believed to promote the growth of gut intestinal epithelium in association with epidermal growth factor and also to enhance the growth of bifidobacteria.

The concentration of lactoferrin is highest in colostrum (5–7 g per litre) and declines gradually over the following 5 months before it reaches a steady state (1–3 g per litre). Taking into account the differences in the volume of colostrum consumed and the volume of milk taken by an exclusively breastfed baby the reduction is less pronounced in absolute terms.

Oligosaccharides

- Oligosaccharides block the attachment of microbes and toxins in the gastro-intestinal tract
- Oligosaccharides produce a protective coating through the gut
- Oligosaccharides produce a protective coating through the urinary tract

Oligosaccharides are a combination of five monosaccharides produced by the epithelium of the mammary glands. Ninety different types have been identified in human milk. Levels are ten times lower in bovine milk.

They block the attachment of microbes and toxins to receptors on the mucosal epithelium of the gastro-intestinal tract. As they remain intact during their passage through the intestine they line the gut with a protective layer. Additionally about 1% is excreted intact in the urine so oligosaccharides are able to block urinary pathogens as well as intestinal ones. Reduction in microbial adhesions to the mucosal epithelium has also been shown for *Streptococcus pneumonia*, which is responsible for otitis.

Artificially fed infants have fewer oligosaccharides in their stools and they are of a different composition to those found in breastfed babies.

Lysozyme

- Lysozyme is bactericidal
- Lysozyme has anti-inflammatory activity
- Lysozyme causes lysis of bacterial cell walls
- Lysozyme is a non-specific antimicrobial protein factor. It is stable to temperature and acidity. It is found in large concentrations in the stools of breastfed infants but not those who are artificially fed
- Lysozyme levels increase during lactation, peaking at around 6 months. It has been hypothesised that this is to protect the gut during the introduction of weaning foods to the diet
- Lysozyme contributes to the lysis of Gram-positive bacterial cell walls, while in vitro studies have shown that it can penetrate Gram-negative bacteria in the presence of lactoferrin and SigA

When cow's milk is added to human milk the effect of lysozyme is reduced. There are currently no studies to confirm the importance of Lysozyme in breastfeeding, but there is research into genetically programming cows to produce it for addition to formula milk.

Epidermal growth factor

- Epidermal growth factor (EGF) seals the intestine preventing the absorption of undigested protein and reducing the risk of allergy
- EGF increases the production of lactase which breaks down lactose
- EGF promotes the expansion and maturation of gut epithelial cells and strengthens the formation of DNA
- EGF is a small polypeptide containing 53 amino acids.

Dvorak (2003) showed that levels of EGF are higher in many mothers who deliver extremely prematurely compared with those who deliver prematurely or at term and that it may be involved in protecting the baby against Necrotising Enterocolitis (NEC).

Undigested cow's milk protein can pass through the immature infant gut producing intolerance and allergy. EGF seals the intestine making absorption of undigested proteins more difficult and thus reducing the risk of allergy. EGF also increases the production of lactase, which is the enzyme involved in the breakdown of lactose into glucose and galactose.

Secretory immunoglobulin A

Stoliar *et al.* (1976) hypothesised that IgA antibodies to the enterotoxin produced by *Escherichia coli* are present in breastmilk and transfer to the infant which may explain why breastmilk prevents *Escherichia coli* diarrhœa in the neonate. It is believed to coat the gut making it impermeable to pathogens and thereby protecting the baby. Concentrations are particularly high in colostrum. The tight junctions close over a few days after delivery to allow free passage of all the immunoglobulins which protect the baby.

Anti-inflammatory molecules

These molecules dampen down the inflammatory reaction to pathogens in the gut. It may account for the lowered incidence of inflammatory bowel disease in breastfed babies and the reduction in severity of neonatal enterocolitis (NEC) whose risk factors include prematurity, formula feeding, intestinal ischaemia and bacterial colonisation.

Growth factors

Investigators have identified several growth factors e.g. EGF, transdermal growth factor, inflammatory growth factor and other important antimicrobial and anti-inflammatory molecules including erythropoietin, polyunsaturated fatty acids (PUFAs), IgA, lactoferrin and oligosaccharides which are present in breastmilk but not in formula milk (Frost 2008).

Bifidus factor

This promotes the growth of *Lactobacillus bifidus*, which inhibits the growth of harmful bacteria by encouraging an acidic environment that is less conducive to pathogenic bacterial growth.

Leukocytes

These white blood cells in breast milk engulf and destroy pathogenic bacteria. They are responsible for the longer time that expressed breastmilk can be stored without curdling.

So how do these factors protect the breastfed infant?

There are hundreds of biologically active factors within breastmilk that provide protection to the infant against infection and auto-immune reactions. Their presence accounts for the benefits of breastfeeding and despite the investment of formula manufacturers to reproduce them, they have largely not been possible to identify the structure of, far less replicate.

Looking at the function of these factors explains why breastfed babies experience fewer gut infections, suffer lower rates of allergic reactions, require less iron in breastmilk and absorb it effectively.

In addition there is the broncho- and entero-mammary pathways which ensure that if a mother inhales or ingests a virus, bacteria or other pathogen her baby is provided with antibodies to the 'germs' that she encountered within a remarkably short time period.

'Instant' protection from infection

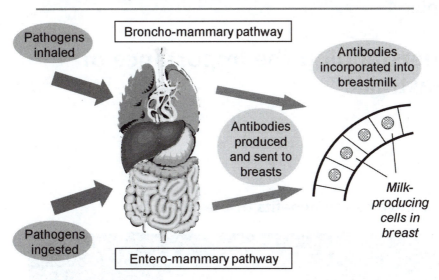

FIGURE 3.1 Entero-mammary and entero-hepatic pathway
(taken from UNICEF UK Baby Friendly Initiative Training Material)

Key points

- There are a large number of immunological factors in breastmilk which protect the infant.
- These factors are specific to the needs of the individual child.
- While formula milk is nutritionally adequate it is impossible to replicate the biologically active components of breastmilk.
- The biochemical factors protect against bacterial and viral infections as well as facilitating transport of other essential molecules and preventing auto-immune reactions.

Chapter 4

Understanding the importance of breastmilk

The positive health benefits of breastfeeding

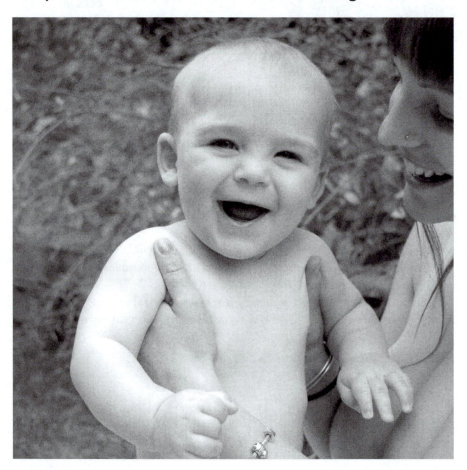

Historically we have always looked at research in terms of studying and quantifying the size of the effect of the advantages to the health of a baby of being breastfed. More recently it has become standard to look at outcomes from the point of view that breastmilk is the natural nutrient for an infant. We should not begin from the point of view that breastfeeding has advantages to the health of mother and baby but that alternatives (formulated from the milk of other mammals) may have risks because they are not bio-specific. So for the baby any change in health is produced by the consumption of artificial formula milk.

The Child and Adolescent Health and Development section of the WHO states that 'breastfeeding is an unequalled way of providing ideal food for the healthy growth and development of infants'. (WHO 2002).

In a clinical review, Hodinott *et al.* (2008) recommended that breastfeeding should be actively supported by all healthcare professionals as an important way to improve child health. They suggest that better implementation of existing evidence is needed to improve the education of all, to address health inequalities and to facilitate breast-feeding outside of the home.

There are many acknowledged and well-researched positive health benefits for infants to support the promotion of exclusive breastfeeding. These will briefly be discussed here with further information being available in the references cited:

- Less risk of gastro-enteritis (Howie *et al.* 1990; Kramer *et al.* 2003; Wilson *et al.* 1998; Quigley 2007; Rebhan *et al.* 2009).
- Fewer middle ear infections (Aniansson *et al.* 1994; Duncan *et al.* 1993).
- Reduction in urinary tract infections (Marild *et al.* 2004; Pisacane *et al.* 1992).
- Fewer lower respiratory tract diseases (Virginia *et al.* 2003; Howie 1990; Ball *et al.* 1999).
- Lower incidence of juvenile onset, insulin dependent diabetes (Alves 2011; Sadauskaite-Kuehne *et al.* 2004; Virtanen *et al.* 1991; Mayer *et al.* 1988).
- Reduced risk of developing Type 2 diabetes in later life if ever breastfed (Liu *et al.* 2010).
- Lowered blood pressure – measurable by the age of 5 but lasting in adulthood (Martin *et al.* 2005).
- Total cholesterol reduced by 0.18–2 mmol per litre if ever breastfed compared with being formula fed as an infant (Owen 2002).
- Normal weight-gain patterns leading to reduction in obesity (Arenz *et al.* 2004; Fewtrell 2004; Gillman *et al.* 2001; Owen *et al.* 2005; von Kries *et al.* 1999; Horta 2007; Li 2010).
- Reduced rates of acute lymphocytic leukaemia and acute myelogenous leukaemia (Kwan 2004).
- Reduced risk of atopic dermatitis in children with a family history of atopy (Burr *et al.* 1989; Fewtrell 2004; Lucas *et al.* 1990; Saarinen and Kajosaari 1995; Host 1991; Rothenbacher 2005).
- Reduced risk for infants without a family history of asthma in children. The evidence in families with a family history of asthma is less clear (Oddy 1999; Ip 2007).
- A reduction in sudden infant death with any breastfeeding compared to exclusive formula feeding (McVea 2000; Ip 2007).

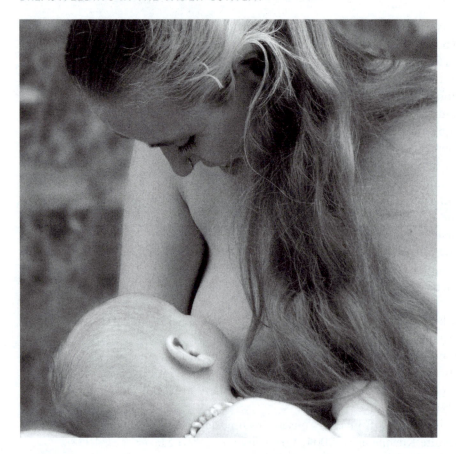

Mothers who do not breastfeed at all show an increased risk of breast cancer, particularly pre-menopausal – a reduced risk of 4.3% for each year of breastfeeding (Ip 2007); ovarian cancer risk reduced with any breastfeeding (Ip 2007); and the metabolic syndrome as a result of failure to lose excess weight gained during pregnancy (Gunderson *et al.* 2009).

Furthermore, there are health benefits for mothers who breastfeed. Compared to women who have not had babies those who do not breastfeed have about a 50% increased risk of Type 2 diabetes in later life (Liu 2010). For women without a history of gestational diabetes, each additional year of breastfeeding was associated with a reduced risk of developing Type 2 diabetes (Ip 2007).

Three studies found an association between early cessation of breastfeeding or not breastfeeding and an increased risk of post-natal depression cause and effect cannot be determined. However, the studies were not of the highest quality and did not screen for depression as a baseline (Ip 2007).

Women who have breastfed are at lower risk of hip fractures and reduced bone density (Paton 2003; Polatti 1999). Delay in return of menstruation leads to less depletion of iron stores.

In addition there are health risks from the preparation of formula (Renfrew *et al.* 2003; WHO 2007):

- under or over concentrating the formula;
- the use of formula powder that, due to production cannot be totally sterile, contains high levels of potentially harmful bacteria including *Enterobacter sakazakii* and *Salmonella*, which may multiply if freshly boiled and cooled water is not used to reconstitute it;
- storage of prepared formula milk at room temperature allowing bacteria to multiply; and
- potential contamination of bottles and teats or other feeding vessels.

Implications for the healthcare system

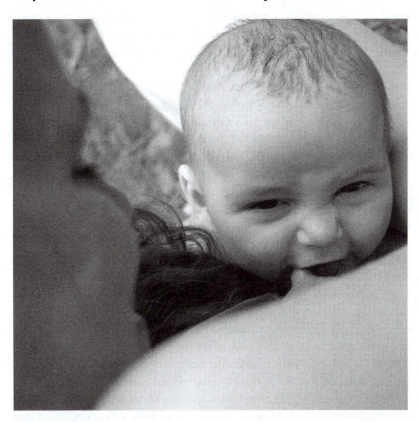

In addition to individual benefits of breastfeeding for mother and child, there are economic savings for the health economy. The NICE Post-natal care guidelines (NICE CG 37 2006) identified potential savings from cases of gastro-enteritis avoided by babies being breastfed. These savings are based on the observation from Howie (1990) that the rate of hospital admission for gastro-enteritis of breastfed infants is 1.4% and the rate of hospital admission for gastro-enteritis of bottle-fed infants is 7.8% (Department of Health 1995).

The national tariff cost for an episode of infectious or non-infectious gastro-enteritis (HRG P26) is £662 for an emergency episode (NHS Payment by Results

2010–11). Using these data, the economic evaluation for a 10% increase in breast-feeding suggests 3900 cases of gastro-enteritis would be avoided, at a saving of £2.6 million.

In 1995, it was estimated that the National Health Service would save £35 million per year for every 1% increase in breastfeeding rates, in reduced hospital admission for gastro-enteritis alone (Breastfeeding; good practice guidance to the NHS, Department of Health 1995), which exceeds the estimate from the data above. This is because in 1995 a treatment episode consisted of a 4-day in-patient stay, resulting in a unit cost of around £1300 per case of gastro-enteritis treated. The national tariff for HRG P26 suggests that the average length of stay for treatment of gastro-enteritis is now 2 days.

Babies in the UK who are fed with artificial formula or breastfed for only a short time are five times as likely to be admitted to hospital during their first year of life with gastro-intestinal illness compared with those breastfed for a minimum of 13 weeks

Ball and Wright (1999) showed that there were 2033 more doctor visits, 212 extra days in hospital and 609 additional prescriptions in the first year of life for every 1000 babies who were never breastfed compared with those exclusively breastfed for a minimum of 3 months. These are costs to the health system but also have a heavy impact on babies and their parents in terms of stress and perhaps time away from employment.

Riordan in 1997 estimated that annual healthcare costs in treating diarrhoea, respiratory syncytial virus, insulin-dependent diabetes and otitis media in infants who were not breastfed were US$1 billion each year – this figure will be significantly higher now following inflation over the past 15 years.

Data from the Millennium Cohort Study showed that exclusive breastfeeding, compared with not breastfeeding, protects against hospitalisation for diarrhoea and lower respiratory tract infection. The effect of partial breastfeeding was found to be weaker. Analysis of the data, allowing for confounding variables, suggests that an estimated 53% of diarrhoea hospitalisations could have been prevented each month by exclusive breastfeeding and 31% by partial breastfeeding. Similarly, 27% of hospitalisations for lower respiratory tract infection could have been prevented each month by exclusive breastfeeding and 25% by partial breastfeeding.

However, the protective effect of breastfeeding declines soon after weaning from the breast. The authors conclude that breastfeeding, particularly when exclusive and prolonged, protects against severe morbidity in the UK today. A population-level increase in exclusive, prolonged breastfeeding would be of considerable potential benefit for public health (Quigley 2007). Data collection on hospital admissions was a critical focus of the longitudinal study of 18,819 infants born in the UK in 2000–2002.

The UK Standing Committee on Nutrition (SACN 1994; Williams 1994) issued the following statement in 1994:

The health benefits of breast feeding in industrialised countries are sometimes questioned on the grounds that modern, hygienically prepared infant formulas are safe and nutritionally complete. Uncertainties increase about this view as more is learned about the complex composition of breastmilk. From a teleological perspective, the complexity of breastmilk implies that it possesses numerous functions of biological importance...

However, 33% of breastfed babies included in the data collection in the Infant Feeding Study 2005 received bottles of formula or water during their stay in hospital (Bolling 2007), and very few babies are exclusively breastfed for 6 months.

Table 4.1 shows the estimates of savings produced by the NICE Postnatal care guidelines economic evaluation (NICE CG37 2006b).

TABLE 4.1 Net saving of improvements in breastfeeding

	2006/07	2007/08	2008/09	2009/10	2010/11	2011/12
Additional babies breastfeeding	21,134	31,622	42,478	53,334	59,509	60,416
Cumulative improvement in breastfeeding	3%	5%	7%	9%	10%	10%
	£000s	£000s	£000s	£000s	£000s	£000s
Saving from cases of otitis media avoided	178	266	357	448	500	507
Saving from cases of gastro-enteritis avoided	913	1,366	1,835	2,304	2,571	2,610
Saving from cases of asthma avoided	829	1,263	1,697	2,130	2,377	2,377
Saving from reduced use of formula and teats	36	53	72	90	100	102
Net saving	1,956	2,948	3,961	4,972	5,548	5,596

Maternal beliefs about breastfeeding and its advantages

Virtually all mothers can breastfeed provided that they have accurate information, and support from within their family, within their community and by the healthcare system. Breastfeeding is natural but it does not always happen naturally and without problems. Mothers may need active support from their caregivers to establish breastfeeding.

The Infant Feeding Survey (2007) asked women what had influenced their feeding choice. That breastfeeding was 'best for the baby' was cited by 81% of all mothers with being 'more convenient' the second most popular reason (28%), but less important than in 2000. That breastfeeding is natural and better for the mother's health were mentioned more frequently in 2005 than in 2000. A full list of the reasons given is shown in Figure 4.1.

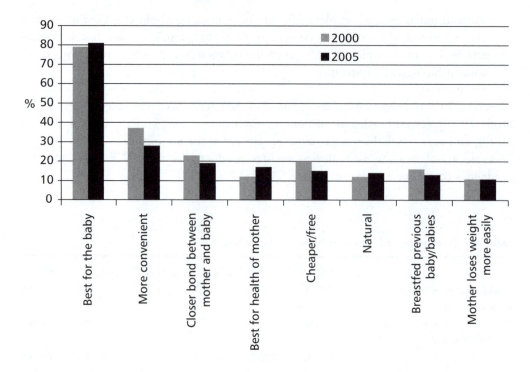

FIGURE 4.1 Reasons cited by mothers for breastfeeding
(Bolling 2007)

Mothers who had breastfed a previous child were more likely to mention 'bonding', 'convenience' and 'cost' as a reason to choose breastfeeding than first-time mothers were. First-time mothers were more likely to concentrate on the health benefits.

When asked why they chose to formula feed from birth, 25% of mothers said that it gave more flexibility with other people being able to feed the baby. However, 32% said that they simply did not like the idea of breastfeeding (this factor was higher in first-time mothers (45%). A further 13% felt that bottle feeding fitted in better with their lifestyle. Perhaps the saddest reason given, and which healthcare professionals can do most about, was the 15% who had been put off by an earlier breastfeeding experience.

The health benefits named by mothers are shown in Figure 4.2.

Disadvantages of breastfeeding

Lawrence (2005) stated that:

Disadvantages of breastfeeding are those factors perceived by the mother as an inconvenience to her since there are no known disadvantages to the normal infant.

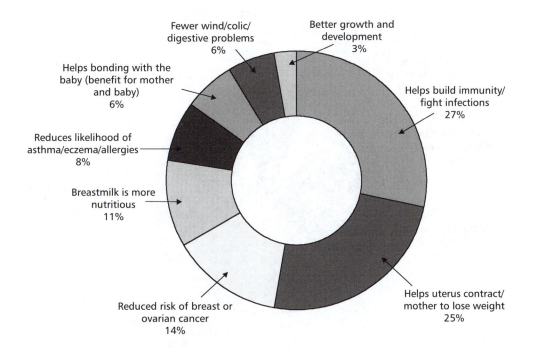

FIGURE 4.2 Named health benefits of breastfeeding cited by mothers
(Bolling 2007)

It has long been claimed that the disadvantages of breastfeeding include:

- the inability to measure the volume of the milk that the baby has consumed;
- that no-one else can care for the baby;
- that breastfeeding can be painful, messy and tiring;
- that breastfeeding may be difficult to establish;
- that breastfed babies wake more often during the night to feed;
- that it is more difficult for mothers to return to work; and
- that the mother may need to modify her diet.

These reasons for choosing to bottle feed exclusively were almost all cited by mothers in the Infant Feeding Study (see Figure 4.3).

In the 2000 Infant Feeding Survey (Hamlyn 2002), 10% of mothers said that they felt pressurised into breastfeeding. Of these, 36% gave up breastfeeding within two weeks compared with 21% of all breastfeeding mothers. The large majority reported that they were subject to pressure from midwives (76%) with 25% feeling pressure from health visitors and 20% from friends.

For the percentage of mothers who reported feeling pressurised into bottle feeding (2%), the pressure was as likely to originate from their mothers (25%) as healthcare professionals (37% midwives; 12% health visitors).

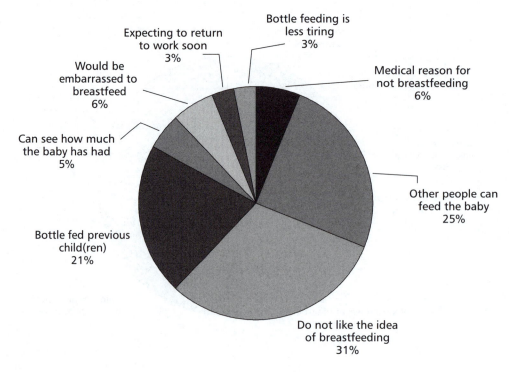

FIGURE 4.3 Reasons cited by mothers for bottle-feeding from birth
(Bolling 2007)

Medical disadvantages of breastfeeding

Medical reasons for not breastfeeding may include very rare, hereditary conditions, which affect the baby's ability to metabolise breastmilk. These conditions include:

Galactosaemia

A hereditary disease affecting carbohydrate metabolism which occurs in approximately one in 60,000 live births (Walker 2006). Symptoms typically include jaundice, enlarged liver, vomiting, poor feeding, lethargy, irritability, convulsions and possibly death. Diagnosis is made by blood screening and a lactose-free formula is generally substituted for breastmilk, although partial breastfeeding may be possible.

Maple syrup urine disease

This is caused by a mutation in at least four genes (Walker 2006). Maple syrup urine disease affects approximately two live births per year. The classic condition is recognised in newborns between 4 and 7 days after birth although breastfeeding may delay the onset until the second week of life. A delay in diagnosis longer than 14 days is invariably associated with mental retardation and cerebral palsy. Treatment relies on dietary restriction of branched-chain amino acids for life.

Phenylketonuria

This is an inherited condition affecting one in 13,500–19,000 live births (Walker 2006). It is due to a deficiency of the enzyme responsible of the metabolism of phenylalanine into tyrosine. Unchecked, the levels of phenylalanine accumulate and interfere with brain development resulting in mental as well as growth retardation. Phenylketonuria is treated by dietary restriction of phenylalanine. Breastfeeding can continue in combination with phenylalanine-free formula while blood levels are monitored.

Chapter 5

Treating conditions related to breastfeeding

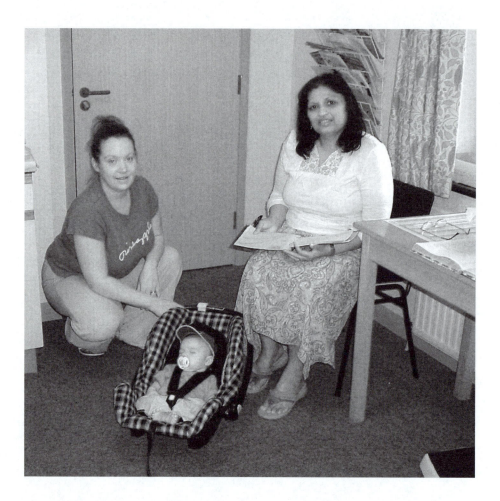

Breastfeeding mothers and their babies may be affected by a variety of conditions which may or may not be related to their feeding method. In the past these may have led to suggestions to stop breastfeeding unnecessarily – often in order to prescribe medication for the mother, e.g. post-natal depression. Conditions specifically related to breastfeeding include engorgement, sore nipples, thrush, mastitis and Raynaud's phenomenon.

Healthcare professionals are often asked for advice or to recommend products for conditions which affect babies who are being breastfed. Many mothers find themselves lacking in confidence in the presence of a baby crying inconsolably or not behaving in the same way as their friend's baby who is bottle fed, e.g. colic and reflux. Mothers may seek to purchase a 'magic solution' or to question their breastfeeding.

Conditions affecting the breastfeeding mother

Engorgement

As well as increased milk production, there is also increased blood flow to the breasts in the first few days after delivery. Some women report symptoms of engorgement as red, swollen, hot breasts. The areola may become hard rather than soft and the skin may appear shiny. The nipple may become flattened which makes latching the baby on more difficult. Engorgement may be associated with a rise in the mother's temperature. This can be managed with simple analgesics, such as paracetamol or ibuprofen. Breastfeeding should be encouraged frequently and be of unrestricted duration, ensuring that the baby is correctly attached at the breast to enable effective removal of the milk. Milk engorgement is almost always iatrogenic and rarely occurs when babies are allowed to feed on demand day and night (Royal College of Midwives 2001).

Engorgement of the breast, accompanied by pathological symptoms (raised temperature, aches and pains), is not normal. It may result from ineffective milk removal or restricted feeds. Treatment involves care with correct attachment (which may be difficult if the breast is overfull), frequent feeds or expression of the milk together with analgesia to reduce the pyrexia.

If the baby is experiencing difficulty attaching to the breast, the removal of some milk by hand expression or gentle application of heat will soften the swollen tissues. This is a period when nipple damage can occur by allowing the baby to feed in order to remove the milk but without paying sufficient attention to correct attachment.

The application of cold compresses after feeding may result in some improvement in symptoms as may taking a shower or bathing before a feed. Heat allows some milk to drip away, reducing some of the pressure. Cold reduces the swelling of the tissues. In the absence of the baby (e.g. due to admission to special/intensive care) mechanical expression using a breast pump or hand expression may be necessary.

Medication should not be routinely used to suppress milk supply. If a mother chooses not to breastfeed she should be supported with simple analgesia while her milk decreases (see Drug Reference section).

If milk is not effectively removed feedback inhibitor of lactation (FIL) may accumulate, leading to decreased milk supply in the long term. Leakage of milk protein into the surrounding tissue may result in symptoms of mastitis with increased pyrexia and discomfort. The resolution of symptoms is most rapidly achieved by frequent removal of the milk from the breast by feeding or if necessary expressing.

Engorgement can also occur at later stages if the mother stops breastfeeding abruptly leading to a build-up of milk. If untreated this can lead to blocked ducts and/or mastitis. If the breast is engorged the mother should feed the baby or express the milk until she is comfortable while the negative feedback of the whey protein reduces the supply.

Mastitis

Mastitis is due to an inflammation of the breast tissue and may or may not be accompanied by an infection. If milk is not removed from the breast, the pressure in the alveoli starts to rise until milk substances are forced out into the surrounding tissues. The breast may feel lumpy and hot to the touch. The mother may also experience flu-like symptoms – increased temperature, shivering, feeling tearful and tired.

The first sign of mastitis is a red, swollen, usually painful area in the breast. The redness and swelling is the body's reaction to the protein in the milk leaking into the surrounding tissue. It is not necessarily associated with a bacterial infection and antibiotics do not need to be prescribed immediately.

Prompt action to increase the efficiency of milk removal, together with an anti-inflammatory medication e.g. ibuprofen if not contra-indicated for the mother, will often halt progress of the symptoms. Efficient milk removal is achieved by good attachment, feeding as frequently as the baby is willing, with additional milk removal either by hand or mechanical expression if necessary.

The true incidence of mastitis is unknown with figures quoted up to 33%. However, it is generally taken to be less than 10% with the vast majority occurring in the second and third week post-partum (WHO 2000).

Non-infective mastitis may result from milk stasis from poor milk removal, from sudden changes in the baby's feeding pattern, trauma from pressure of clothing, from fingers holding the breast or knocks.

Infective mastitis, which is less common, is caused by infections either in the outer skin of the breast or within the glandular tissue. Unless treated effectively this may result in abscess formation requiring surgical drainage.

Research shows that even with antibiotic treatment, resolution of symptoms is more rapid if accompanied by help to remove milk optimally (Thomson 1984). The use of ibuprofen as an anti-inflammatory, together with effective milk removal, has been found to be as effective as antibacterial treatment. Inch suggests that the benefit of antibiotics in non-infective mastitis is due to their anti-inflammatory action rather than antibacterial properties (Inch 1995). Referral to the health visitor or voluntary group may help the mother achieve better attachment and drainage.

If the symptoms continue to develop despite increased improved milk removal or the mother feels worse, oral antibiotic treatment may be necessary. The WHO recommendation (WHO 2000) is the use of flucloxacillin 250–500 mg four times a day or amoxicillin 250–500 mg three times a day or, in the case of penicillin allergy, erythromycin 250–500 mg four times a day or cephalexin 250–500 mg four times a day. Frequent milk removal should continue throughout the treatment period and breastfeeding does not need to be interrupted. The safety of antibiotics during breastfeeding is discussed in Drug Reference section.

The UK Clinical Knowledge Summary recommends a slightly different range of antibiotics (Clinical Knowledge Summary 2010).

> Penicillins e.g. flucloxacillin and co-amoxiclav are the antibiotic of choice because they are effective against beta-lactamase-producing organisms (such as *Staphylococcus aureus*) and only trace amounts are found in breast milk.
>
> (Schaefer *et al.* 2007)

> Erythromycin is an alternative where a beta-lactamase-producing organism is the likely cause of infection. Erythromycin should be avoided if the neonate has jaundice. There are case reports of pyloric stenosis in neonates being breastfed by mothers taking erythromycin, but causality has not been established.
>
> (Schaefer *et al.* 2007)

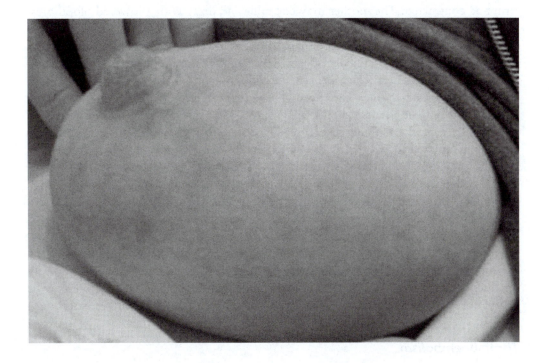

If untreated, mastitis can develop into a breast abscess; these can also develop spontaneously. Abscess should be considered if the mastitis does not respond to frequent drainage plus a course of appropriate antibiotics, and an ultrasound examination undertaken. Breastfeeding can continue after an abscess has been drained even if this has to be undertaken surgically. Abscess exudates should be cultured to ensure that the infection is being treated with an antibiotic to which it is susceptible. Anecdotally there appear to be more cases involving methicillin-resistant *S. aureus* (MRSA) which need microbiology support to choose the appropriate drug (Dixon and Khan 2011).

Bacterial infection of the nipple

It is also possible to develop bacterial infections in the cracks left by attachment difficulties. These are usually obvious as sloughy yellow areas within the crack or a swollen, very red nipple and are best treated with a topical antibiotic such as fusidic acid, rather than systemic antibiotics. The bacterium involved is most commonly *S. aureus* (Livingstone 1996).

Post-partum haemorrhage

Primary post-partum haemorrhage (PPH) is defined as a loss of more than 500 ml of blood in the first 24 hours after delivery. The vast majority of cases are caused by the uterus not contracting efficiently. It is more common after either a very short or very long delivery. Blood may flow freely from the vagina or build up in the uterus. Examination of the fundus height by the midwife may identify it as soft rather than firm and contracted. The mother may feel faint and dizzy with a lowered blood pressure and racing pulse – all signs of shock.

Secondary PPH, occurring more than 24 hours after the birth and up to six weeks later, is usually due to retained placental fragments or the presence of a large, unexpelled uterine blood clot which prevents uterine involution.

In severe cases a mother may need a blood transfusion. In less-severe cases iron supplements may be needed to restore her haemoglobin levels to normal. There is no reason why a mother should cease breastfeeding although anecdotally they may be mistakenly advised to in order to 'restore their strength' and allow others to feed the baby.

Severe bleeding during childbirth can cause tissue death in the pituitary gland, which may cause the gland to lose its ability to function properly (Sheehan syndrome). Symptoms include poor or even absent milk production.

Retained placental fragments are a rare cause of poor lactation, as the placental hormones inhibit the action of prolactin. Treatment is surgical removal followed by antibiotics. Primary PPH may result in low prolactin levels, which may delay milk production. Galactogogues, such as domperidone (see Drug Reference section) may be useful in reversing this situation, along with unrestricted and efficient breastfeeding.

Thromboembolism

Symptoms include unilateral calf pain accompanied by redness and swelling. Risk is higher in obese women and those who are confined to bed for a prolonged period or who have chosen to remain in bed or resting for prolonged periods rather than mobilising normally after delivery. (This may be due to well-meaning advice not to leave the home for a period after delivery). Treatment involves the use of low-molecular-weight heparinoids, including warfarin and aspirin 75 mg, of which none are contraindicated in breastfeeding (see Drug Reference section).

The risk of venous thromboembolism (VTE) rises in women with a baseline body mass index (BMI) greater than 30 (obese). They should be encouraged to mobilise as soon as possible, particularly after caesarean section, and to use of VTE stockings if appropriate (DoH Risk assessment for venous thromboembolism: NICE CG 92 2010).

Post-natal depression

Post-natal depression affects 10–15% of mothers and can lead to behavioural problems in the baby due to lack of stimulation as well as emotional difficulties for the mother. Symptoms of loss of mood should be addressed as soon as possible. Interventions such as encouraging the mother to make social contacts, to take exercise, which may be as simple as pushing the baby in the pram, and talking therapies should be offered before medication (NICE CG45 2007). However, medication or even having depression are not reasons to suggest cessation of breastfeeding, which may be the only thing a mother feels she is able to achieve successfully at that time. See Drug Reference section for options for medication.

Raynaud's phenomenon

Raynaud's phenomenon was first described by Maurice Raynaud in 1862 who referred to 'local asphyxia of the extremities' and 'episodic digital ischaemia provoked by cold and emotion'. Originally it was described as affecting acral parts of the body, mainly fingers and toes, but it can affect ear lobes, nose and lips as well as coronary, gastro-intestinal, penile, placental, ocular and pulmonary vessels.

In 1970, Mavis Gunther referred to psychosomatic sore nipples:

> when the nipples are being examined they blanch, usually the whole face goes white because of the shutting down of the blood supply. Sometimes whilst they are still being inspected the blood supply is restored and the nipples can be watched becoming a mulberry colour. The mother who has this very real trouble usually has some fear or unhappy association connected with breasts or breastfeeding.

The first published study of the impact of Raynaud's phenomenon on breastfeeding was published by Coates (1992). Holmen (2009) presented a case study where a 25-year-old mother took photographs on a camera phone and described extreme bilateral pain lasting 5–15 minutes after feeds that began in the second week after delivery. She had no medical history of poor circulation but suffered sporadic migraines. She did not smoke and had never undergone breast surgery. Nipple pain began in pregnancy (two to three episodes a week in the second trimester increased to two to three a day by the end of the third trimester; resolved immediately after delivery at 38 weeks). The baby weighed 2.8 kg. Breastfeeding technique was checked at 2 weeks post-partum when the unbearable pain began. Prescription of nifedipine produced resolution of the pain totally within a week but it re-occurred when the drug stopped. The mother took nifedipine 30 mg daily for 12 months and breastfed for a total of 18 months.

Lawlor-Smith and Lawlor-Smith (1997) studied five patients with severe, debilitating nipple pain. Three had previously had symptoms during other lactations: one gave up breastfeeding at 6 weeks, another breastfed for 14 months and the third breastfed for 7 months despite the pain. In all women a reduction in environmental temperature precipitated pain. Two out of the five had tri-phasic colour change and 3 bi-phasic. All five exhibited blanching during, after and between feeds. None smoked and two had a history of Raynaud's, two others had parents with Raynaud's. Four mothers had suffered nipple trauma that was difficult to heal.

There are other case reports where women have often been diagnosed with thrush and repeatedly treated with oral medication (see pages 60–5). One study suggested that a mother's stress increased the severity of symptoms which echoes Mavis Gunther's description.

Diagnostic features of Raynaud's phenomenon affecting breastfeeding:

- pain which worsens in the cold e.g. passing fridges in the supermarket or even exposure of the nipple to feed;
- bi- or tri-phasic colour changes immediately after feeds;
- history of circulation problems or close family history of circulation problems;
- history of migraines; and
- early delivery of baby or small baby – due to vasoconstriction of placental blood vessels.

Initial check and optimisation of attachment should occur before suggesting any treatment. It is important that mothers stop smoking and limit caffeine intake (both nicotine and caffeine are vasoconstrictors). Even two cigarettes a day are enough to increase vascular resistance by 100% and cutaneous blood flow is reduced by 40%. Caffeine is not only in tea and coffee but also in soft and energy drinks, as well as some painkillers.

The mother should avoid getting cold, and try moderate aerobic exercise (Cardelli 1989). Diet should be discussed if the BMI is less than 20 and stress should be minimised if this appears to be a trigger for symptoms. Rubbing the nipples gently with warm oil immediately after feeds, covering the breast immediately with a warm, heat-retaining compress can also help reduce symptoms. From a medical point of view medication with decongestants, the contraceptive pill and fluconazole may also exacerbate symptoms.

High doses of vitamin B6 (Newman 2012), magnesium (Smith 1960; Turlapaty 1980; Leppert 1994), calcium (DiGiacomo 1989), fatty acids (Belch 1985) and fish oil supplementation (DiGiacomo 1989) have also been suggested, but take a minimum of 6 weeks to be effective.

Symptoms can be successfully managed by the use of nifedipine 30 mg daily (10 mg capsules three times a day or long-acting tablet 30 mg daily) for two weeks. Some women need ongoing medication but many find symptoms resolve by this stage. However, the drug produces flushing of extremities (particularly the face) and headaches, which some women find intolerable.

Vasospasm

Vasospasm may be confused with Raynaud's phenomenon as the pain is also caused by vasoconstriction but it does not respond to nifedipine. Mothers may describe white nipples after feeds but may also note that the nipple is flattened, creased or pointed after feeds and there may be a white stripe. Symptoms do not get worse with exposure to the cold; there is no history of problems with circulation or migraines.

In Figure 5.1 the nipple is at the back of the baby's mouth, there is no pressure on the base of the nipple and the latch is deep and effective and will not produce vasospasm.

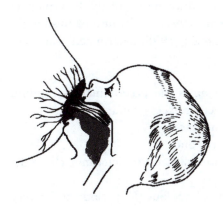

FIGURE 5.1 Baby feeding with deep, effective latch
(taken from UNICEF UK Baby Friendly Initiative Training Material)

Vasospasm is frequently due to poor positioning and attachment with the nipple compressed between the baby's tongue or even gums and roof of the mouth, which cuts off the blood supply temporarily – a shallow latch (see Figure 5.2). It can also occur if the baby is clamping down in order to slow a very fast milk supply or if the baby is tongue tied and unable to extend its tongue over the gum margin (see pages 57–9).

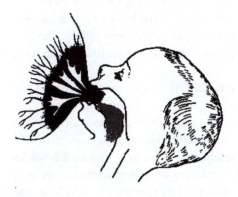

FIGURE 5.2 Baby feeding with a shallow latch
(taken from UNICEF UK Baby Friendly Initiative Training Material)

Conditions affecting the baby

Colic

Colic has been defined as 'spasmodic contraction of smooth muscle causing pain and discomfort'. In studies it has arbitrarily been defined as lasting 3 hours a day on more than 3 days a week for at least 3 weeks (Wessel 1954) although this has been disputed (St James-Roberts 1991). Symptoms are usually described as high-pitched, inconsolable crying accompanied by flushing of the face, drawing up of the legs, passing flatus and difficulty in passing bowel motions (Barr 1991). The cause of this condition remains unclear. In his systematic review Lucassen (1998) determined four main emerging causes:

- problems within the gut where excessive crying is the predominant symptom, caused by cow's milk allergy, lactose intolerance or excess wind;
- behavioural problem resulting from parental interaction;
- excessive crying is at the extreme end of normal; and
- it is a collection of aetiologically different entities difficult to determine clinically.

In most babies, symptoms resolve by 3–5 months of age but the period can be very exhausting for parents who may be frantic to find a 'cure', particularly as symptoms are often worse in the evenings. Incidence is believed to be up to 25%, but is more common in those formula fed (Balon 1997).

Babies of mothers who smoke are twice as likely to experience symptoms of colic as those who do not. Reijneveld *et al.* (2000) also reported that colic is less frequently seen in breastfed babies. There is no evidence that cessation of breastfeeding is beneficial in reduction in colic symptoms. However, observation of feeding technique by a skilled breastfeeding worker may be beneficial to identify any problems associated with an imbalance in milk transfer (Woolridge 1988).

Medication is often used to treat colic based on sparse independent research (The Breastfeeding Network 2002). Information is included here to support healthcare professionals and parents to make appropriate choices in treating babies with colic.

In studies dicycloverine (dicyclomine) proved to be effective but produced adverse effects, including breathing difficulties and apnoea in babies (Williams 1984). The risk of using this drug in a condition, which is self-limiting, is not justified (Lucassen 1998).

Simethicone drops were not shown to be effective although they are popularly recommended to mothers (trade names Dentinox©, Infacol©). The proposed mechanism of action is to bind bubbles of wind together thus aiding dispersion (Garrison 2000). Metcalf (1994) conducted a randomised, double-blind, placebo-controlled study in three GP practices. He studied 83 infants between the ages of 2 and 8 weeks with symptoms of colic and treated them with placebo or simethicone drops in a double-blind crossover methodology. Mothers reported improvements in 54% of the treatment periods, which ranged from 3 to 10 days. Twenty-eight per cent of the infants responded only to simethicone, 37% only to placebo and 20% responded to both. No statistically significant differences were noted. The authors concluded that simethicone is no more effective than placebo in the treatment of infantile colic although it may be perceived as so by parents.

Behavioural interventions ranging from early response to symptoms to reducing stimulation did not provide evidence of benefit although many parents still place children in car seats and drive to settle symptoms (Lucassen 1998).

Eliminating cow's milk protein from the diet can be effective in treating babies with suspected cow's milk protein allergy – in breastfed babies this entails the mother removing dairy products from her diet; in formula-fed babies it involves the use of partially or fully hydrolysed formulas. Most studies have been carried out in formula-fed babies. Permanent dietary restrictions should not be undertaken without professional support and guidance. Lucassen (2000) compared a whey hydrolysate formula with a standard formula. The intervention, it was reported, resulted in a reduction in crying time of 63 minutes per day but the range was 1–127 minutes. Five of the 43 infants did not complete the trial.

NICE (PH11 2008) states that there is insufficient evidence to support the use of hydrolysed formulas to prevent cow's milk protein allergies. NICE Food allergy in children and young people (NICE CG116 2011) recommends that GPs, practice nurses and health visitors diagnose and assess a suspected food allergy using either skin-prick testing or by taking a blood test for immunoglobulin E (IgE) antibodies. The diagnosis should be based on the results of the allergy-focused clinical history undertaken by a suitably trained healthcare professional

Soya milk is not recommended as substitute milk for babies under six months due to phyto-oestrogen and high sugar content. Babies who are cow's milk protein allergic are likely to be allergic to soya protein as well.

In 2007, the Chief Medical Officer reiterated his advice that soya-based infant formulas should not be used as the first choice for the management of infants with proved cow's milk sensitivity, lactose intolerance, galactokinase deficiency and galactosaemia (CMO update 37 soya milk [infant formula], 2007). Soya-based formulas have a high phyto-oestrogen content, which could pose a risk to the long-term reproductive health of infants, according to a 2003 report from the Committee on Toxicity (COT). The Scientific Advisory Committee on Nutrition (SACN 2007) has advised that there is no particular health benefit associated with the consumption of soya-based infant formula by infants who are healthy (no clinically diagnosed conditions). SACN also advised there is no unique clinical condition that particularly requires the use of soya-based infant formulas. As an alternative to soya-based products, more appropriate hydrolysed protein formulas are available and can be prescribed. Soya-based formulas should only be used in exceptional circumstances to ensure adequate nutrition. For example, they may be given to infants of vegan parents who are not breastfeeding or infants who find alternatives unacceptable.'

Goat's milk is not recommended as a milk suitable for babies under one year of age as it is not nutritionally adequate (Department of Health, Infant formula, 2011). Additionally there is no evidence that it produces allergies lower than cow's milk-based formula. Lactose levels are similar to cow's milk.

Bandolier's review in 2000 suggested that at that time there were no evidence-based treatments for colic, merely reassurance that babies do grow out of the symptoms and in the meantime support to develop coping strategies should be made available. A table of the results from the trials found is provided below.

TABLE 5.1 Trials of interventions for colic (Bandolier 2000)

Treatment	Number of trials	Number of infants in studies	Comment
Simethicone	3	272	Three trials with adequate double blinding showed no evidence of efficacy
Dicyclomine	3	134	Dicyclomine better than placebo in three trials. Serious, adverse effects on infants reported. Drug contra-indicated in infants less than 6 months of age
Soy formula	2	158	One study showed good improvement, analysis not possible in larger second study
Increased carrying	2	94	No effect
Hypoallergenic formula	2	72	Indication that hypoallergenic formula has a beneficial effect in two studies
Sucrose	2	72	Sucrose appears to be briefly effective
Lactase enzymes	2	44	No benefit over placebo
Hypoallergenic diet	1	115	Breastfed and bottle-fed infants included. May be a reduction of daily colic symptoms of 25%, but complicated design and inconsistent result reporting
Herbal tea	1	68	Small effect in single study, but no nutritional value and inappropriate in small babies
Fibre-enriched formula	1	54	No effect
Decreased stimulation	1	42	Limited significance in trial with potential for bias
Methylscopolamine	1	40	No benefit and adverse effects
Dairy elimination diet	1	40	No benefit
Car ride simulator	1	32	No effect
Parent training	1	14	No effect in tiny flawed trial

In a review in 2004, Bandolier accepted that there was limited evidence for lactase drops (Colief®) when the milk was pre-incubated. Kanabar *et al.* (2001) conducted a study of 46 children. The drops were added to a bottle of formula milk and left refrigerated for 4 hours before warming to feed to the baby or added to a small amount of expressed breastmilk that was then given to the baby at the end of the feed. Total crying time was reduced in all 46 but reached statistical significance only in the 32 compliant families. In previous studies with lactase there was no pre-incubation of the milk. However, the size of the study and poor compliance leaves the results open to question in terms of the quality of evidence for widespread practice.

Lactose intolerance

Lactose is the sugar within breastmilk. By the action of the enzyme lactase it is broken down into glucose and galactose which can be utilised by the body.

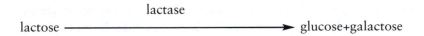

Lactose intolerance is often blamed as being a contributory factor for colic, resulting in cessation of breastfeeding and substitution of lactose-free formula. Primary or congenital lactose intolerance is very rare. It is an inherited metabolic disorder rather than an allergy. It generally manifests within a few days of birth and is characterised by severe diarrhoea, vomiting, dehydration, and discomfort after every feed and failure to thrive.

Some premature babies are temporarily lactose intolerant due to their immaturity. Few infants born at 28 weeks and only 40% born at 34 weeks gestation have significant lactose activity. Secondary lactose intolerance can appear at any age due to damage to the brush borders of gut villae by infection, allergy or inflammation which reduce lactase activity. It is a temporary condition and removal of the cause allows the gut to heal. It may also become apparent in a breastfed baby following maternal use of antibiotics, but resolves without treatment even with continued breastfeeding.

Lactose intolerance in adults is very common. The production of lactase decreases in most humans from the age of 2 years although symptoms of intolerance are rare before the age of six.

Assessment by an experienced breastfeeding worker may be beneficial to ensure optimal milk removal by the baby is taking place before considering lactose-free formulae. Imbalance of milk transfer (caused by less than perfect attachment) can produce similar symptoms i.e. loose bowel motions, which may be green and frothy. This is due to the rapid transit time of large volumes of lower fat milk and consequently an excessive consumption of lactose (Woolridge 1988).

Babies can exhibit excess wind and gastric discomfort, which may be diagnosed as lactose intolerance, but which in fact is transitory lactase deficiency i.e. too much lactose for the available lactase.

Addition of lactase enzymes (Colief®) to breastmilk has been suggested as a treatment for colic as previously discussed.

Tongue tie

Ankyloglossia (tongue tie) is a congenital anomaly characterised by an abnormally short lingual frenulum: the tip of the tongue cannot be protruded beyond the lower incisor teeth. Incidence has been reported to be up to 10% of births. It varies in degree, from a mild form in which the tongue is bound only by a thin mucous membrane to a severe form in which the tongue is completely fused to the floor of the mouth. Breastfeeding difficulties may arise as a result of the inability to use the tongue to suck effectively, causing sore nipples and poor infant weight gain. Where feeding difficulties present in infants, snipping of the frenulum can be carried out painlessly, without sedation or local anaesthesia, using a blunt-ended pair of scissors with immediate resolution of symptoms in many cases (see Figure 5.3). In some cases the tie may be posterior behind a membrane at the back of the tongue. This may be less visible and only apparent on digital examination of the mouth. It should be considered if the mother continues to experience painful breastfeeding despite help to optimise attachment. It appears sore but apparently does not concern the baby (Griffiths 2004; Hogan 2005; Ballard 2002).

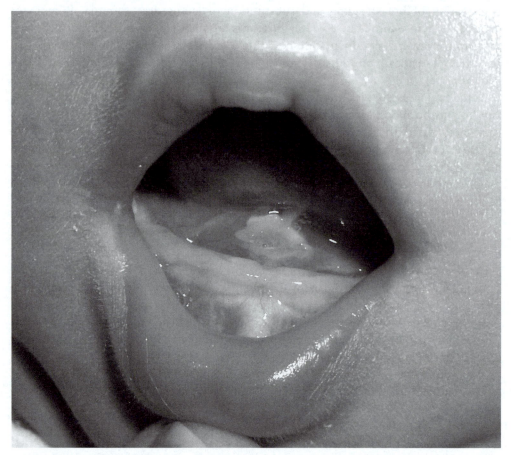

FIGURE 5.3 Diamond scar left immediately after posterior tongue tie has been clipped
(© C Westcott, reproduced with permission)

Geddes (2008) conducted a study in Australia. She used ultrasound to study the efficacy of milk removal and suck before and after tongue tie division in 24 babies.

Milk intake, milk transfer rate and the degree of latch were found to have improved in all babies after the procedure. The mean milk production was measured pre- and post-frenulotomy in six babies by test weighing. It increased from 409 ml to 615 ml per 24-hour period.

NICE (IPG 149 2005) issued guidance that there are no major safety concerns about division of ankyloglossia and limited evidence suggests that this procedure can improve breastfeeding

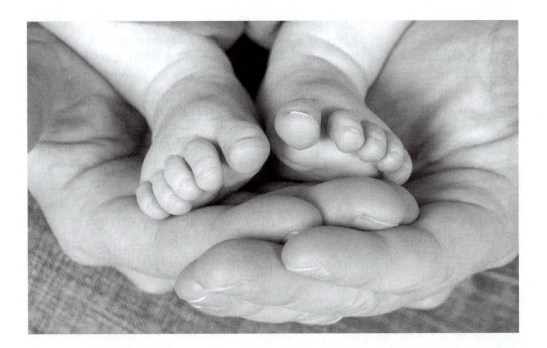

Prematurity

Premature babies may have difficulty in breastfeeding depending on their gestational age. If the baby is unable to tolerate fluids orally he/she may be maintained on intravenous fluids for a period during which time the mother should be encouraged to initiate lactation by expressing either by hand or with an electric pump. Milk can be frozen until such time as the baby is able to receive it either orally or via naso-gastric tube feeding

It is important that the mother expresses frequently, including overnight, in order to maximise her supply. Some women find that sustaining expression over a period over more than 6 weeks leads to a reduction in milk supply. This can be assisted by the use of galactogogues such as domperidone (see pages 261–7).

Skin-to skin-contact can increase milk supply and help the mother to feel part of her baby's care when it is still heavily medically orientated. In kangaroo care (an extension of skin-to-skin contact) the premature baby is carried against the chest of an adult for prolonged periods and may receive all medical care in this position.

Premature babies now receive trophic feeds earlier as trials have shown that it reduces the incidence of sepsis and enables earlier discharge from hospital. Use of human milk reduces the risk of necrotising enterocolitis (NEC) and infection (Williams 2000). If a mother's own milk is not available, premature babies can receive donor breast milk via a local or national milk bank (NICE CG93 2010).

Jaundice

Physiological jaundice is common in neonates due to the breakdown of excess red cells (needed in utero to carry sufficient oxygen), and the accumulation of bilirubin. It begins around the second day of life and resolves around the fifth day. The yellow pigment of bilirubin accumulates in the skin producing a yellowy, sun-tanned effect.

Resolution may be hastened by adequate breastmilk intake which will be provided if the baby is well attached. There is no need for additional non-milk fluids as unconjugated bilirubin is fat soluble and is excreted predominantly in stools, aided by the fats in milk and colostrum rather than aqueous excretion via urine. Treatment with phototherapy may be recommended if levels are significantly raised. Sustained or marked jaundice should be referred for expert evaluation.

Conditions that may affect the mother and baby during breastfeeding

Thrush

Oral Thrush

It is not uncommon for neonates to exhibit a white coating on the tongue, which does not wipe off, as milk curds would do. However, in the majority of cases this clears up without treatment and causes no symptoms in mother or baby. De Vries *et al.* (2006) suggested that oral *Candida* is present in approximately 5% of healthy infants, but commonly resolves spontaneously within a few weeks. White areas can also be confused with Epstein pearls which are normal epithelial cells that become trapped during fusion of the palate and appear as firm white papules on the tongue. Tongue ties can also result in a white tongue as the milk is not thrown to the back of the mouth as effectively and pools at the front of the mouth.

However, if the infant shows problems in feeding **and** a mouth swab cultures for *Candida*, evidence-based treatment may be necessary.

Historically, nystatin has been the first-line treatment for oral *Candida*. However, in a head to head study of miconazole gel with nystatin suspension, miconazole oral gel produced a cure rate of 99% at 10 days compared with 54% with nystatin oral suspension (Hoppe 1996, 1997)

In May 2008, Janssen-Cilag, the manufacturers of Daktarin oral gel®, chose to vary the Summary of Product Characteristics (SPC) to recommend that it is not used in infants under 4 months and only with care below the age of 6 months or in babies born prematurely. This change appears to originate from a published report (De Vries 2006) documenting a 17-day-old baby (born at 36 weeks' gestation) who choked when exposed to miconazole oral gel applied to her mother's nipples before and after feeds on the advice of a pharmacist. The baby suddenly stopped feeding and breathing, became cyanotic and lost consciousness. The mother scooped out the visible miconazole gel and the baby recovered within a few moments. The doctor who was called could find no abnormalities and the baby recovered without further problem. The report mentions nine other cases of babies who suffered some form of difficulty with breathing, one of who was admitted to hospital, but all recovered spontaneously.

The Nederlands Bijwerkingen Centrum Lareb provided information on all the adverse event reports that they have on file (July 2008, personal communication) and all show a latent period to response of a few minutes, confirming a probable link. No serious outcomes are documented. The risk appears to be in response to the method of application of the gel and its viscosity rather than to the active ingredient.

In view of the increased efficacy it would seem reasonable to use miconazole in babies who have a positive mouth swab for oral *Candida* (even though it is outside of its license) with careful information to the parents on the way the gel should be applied. The gel should be applied a small amount at a time and very gently to all surfaces of the mouth, particularly between cheeks and gums four times a day after feeds (Clinical Knowledge Summary 2011).

The Department of Health (Department of Health, Nystatin 2010) made the following statement (last modified in 2010):

> Community Practitioner Nurse Prescribers may exceptionally prescribe nystatin off-label for neonates. Where Community Practitioner Nurse Prescribers are absolutely clear that the diagnosis is one of oral thrush, they may prescribe nystatin at the dose recommended in the British National Formulary (BNF) for Children. An exception for nystatin is allowed on the basis that there is no systemic absorption of the product and the use of the product in treatment of oral thrush is long-established.

This decision is without precedent and there are no other exceptions for off-label prescribing by Community Practitioner Nurse Prescribers.

Topical thrush on the maternal nipples

If a baby shows white plaques in the mouth (which have positive swabs for *Candida*) the mother is likely to develop sore nipples, which do not improve with attention to attachment. Both mother and baby should be treated simultaneously with topical antifungal medication. It is important that careful attention is paid to ruling out problems with tongue tie and compression of the nipple due to poor positioning and attachment before treating for thrush. Failure to do so may result in a delay in achieving resolution of pain and a mother giving up breastfeeding. Thrush is uncommon in babies under 6 weeks of age but anecdotally is commonly diagnosed in this time period when a mother has never achieved pain-free breastfeeding. Using swabs as a diagnostic tool before intervening with medication is suggested.

Thrush of the nipple is characterised by intense pain which begins after a feed has finished and continues for a period up to an hour afterwards (BfN 2009a). The mother may also report nipples which are sensitive to the slightest touch. Thrush is frequently over-diagnosed as symptoms can be mistaken for:

- Poor attachment of the baby at the breast – in which case the pain is severe on latching and continues throughout the feed rather than commencing after the feed has finished.
- Raynaud's phenomenon – mothers have a history of poor circulation at the extremities and notice symptoms are worse in the cold e.g. walking down the frozen food aisle in the supermarket.
- Vasocompression due to restriction of the blood supply to the nipple caused by attachment problems where the nipple is compressed between the baby's tongue and the upper palate. The nipple may change colour becoming white after a feed. This can also occur with an over-abundant milk supply where the baby uses its tongue to slow the milk flow.
- Tongue tie – when damage to the nipple continues until the frenulum is snipped.
- White spot – a blocked outlet on the surface of the nipple behind which milk accumulates. Pain resolves if the overgrowth of skin is removed either by gentle rubbing or by using a sterile needle. Pain is described as pin-point and mothers usually use a single finger to point to the source of the pain rather than an open hand.
- Eczema due to a reaction to breast pads or anything that comes into contact with the nipples e.g. creams.
- *S. aureus* infection of the nipple.

There also appears to be an association between cracked nipples followed by mastitis treated with antibiotics, and the development of thrush in the maternal breast. This can also form a web the underlying cause of which is poor positioning and attachment which if addressed stops the cycle continuing (see Figure 5.4).

It has in the past been assumed that nipple trauma together with antibiotic exposure predisposes overgrowth of *Candida* in the breast. However, this appears to have fuelled the diagnosis of thrush in the first 6 weeks after delivery as many women will be exposed to antibiotics at delivery, e.g. caesarean section or uterine infection, and have had initial nipple trauma. If position and attachment have not been optimised and mothers have been told that their latch 'looks good' even if it hurts, everyone seems to look to the diagnosis of thrush and medication as the perfect solution to a medical rather than basic breastfeeding problem.

Left untreated, breast thrush causes so much pain that very few mothers can continue to breastfeed. However, cracked nipples and mastitis may also be indicative of poor attachment at the breast which can be resolved with expert help without the need for any medication.

The symptoms which allow differential diagnosis are (BfN 2009b):

- shooting pains deep within the breast after a feed has finished which may continue

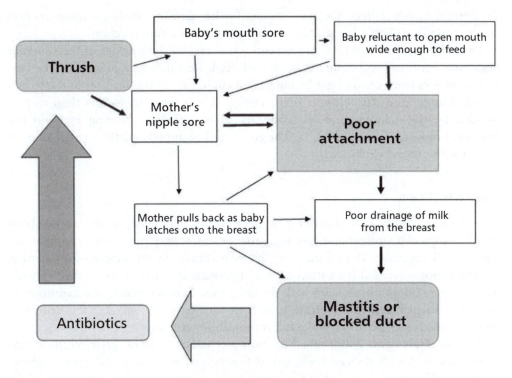

FIGURE 5.4 The web linking poor attachment and drainage of the breast to mastitis and thrush

for an hour. Women may describe extreme feelings of pain right through to the back, the worst pain ever experienced after a period of pain-free feeding;

- pain in both breasts after feeds whether the baby is fed directly or the mother expresses;
- apyrexia;
- absence of red area on the breast; and
- absence of bacterial infection on the nipple.

Breast-fed babies with thrush frequently develop plaques between the cheeks and gums or high in the palate rather than just on the tongue. There is enormous value in swabbing the baby's mouth to ascertain if thrush is present. Babies may also pull away from the breast while continuing to grasp the nipple. This behaviour would suggest that they are experiencing oral discomfort whilst feeding but remain hungry and are therefore reluctant to stop feeding. However, this symptom may also be a sign of the baby not achieving a good latch so should not be used as an isolated diagnostic indication.

Thrush on the surface of the nipple can be treated by applying a **smear** of miconazole cream 2% to the nipple after every feed. Any cream that can be seen should be gently wiped off before the next feed but should not be washed off, as this will remove the natural moisture from the skin causing further damage. If this is necessary too much cream is probably being applied and may lead to a skin reaction.

The baby should be treated concurrently, as there will be transfer of the *Candida* organisms between mother and baby at each feed. Research has shown that the best treatment is miconazole oral gel 24 mg per ml applied to all the surfaces of the baby's mouth four times a day (Hoppe 1996, 1997). This is more frequently than recommended by the manufacturers but appears to be necessary bearing in mind the frequency of feeds in the early days. The gel should be applied gently, a small amount at a time to prevent choking.

Deep breast pain

If the mother continues to describe pain deep within the breast, which has not been cured by topical treatment and care with attachment, it **may** be necessary to treat her with oral fluconazole. Use of this drug to treat thrush on the nipple of a lactating woman is not a licensed indication for oral fluconazole but is being used worldwide to cure the symptoms associated with the diagnosis. In other words, the manufacturers have not included this indication in their application to market the drug and therefore the prescriber has to take full responsibility for use.

A study (Hale *et al.* 2009) failed to show any conclusive link between the symptoms associated with the condition called *Candida* of the breast and growth of the organism. We have assumed that the presence of lactoferrin within breastmilk inhibited growth of *Candida* in microbiological tests making swabs and samples inappropriate. However, using this argument, it is difficult to understand how *Candida* can be said to produce symptoms in the lactating dyad. Hale showed that *Candida* inoculated into breastmilk grew as expected. In my own experience of answering hundreds of calls for the Drugs in Breastmilk Helpline, many apparent cases resolve with good attention to positioning and attachment together with frequent drainage, suggesting this was in fact the cause of the pain.

The dose recommended (Hale 2012 online access) is an initial loading dose of 150–400 mg followed by 100–200 mg daily for 10 days. Anecdotally some mothers find symptoms improve with taking the dose once daily while others report more side effects and prefer to take it on a twice-daily regime. There is currently no research to guide practice. The dose depends on how long the mother has had symptoms and whether she has recently had antibiotics but anecdotally the lower dose is effective and produces fewer side effects for mother and baby. Longer courses **may** be necessary to clear long-standing infection. However, if symptoms are not improving at all after 7 days the diagnosis should be reconsidered rather than continue to expose the mother and baby to unnecessary medication.

- Topical treatment of mother and baby should continue throughout the course of the oral therapy but there is no evidence to continue treatment for longer than this.
- Although fluconazole is not licensed to be given during breastfeeding, it is licensed to be given directly to babies in doses ten times higher than that which passes through breastmilk so is unlikely to produce adverse effects (Hale 2012 online access).

- It has also been studied in premature babies of <1000 g born prematurely and at risk of severe fungal infections, without adverse effects (Kaufman 2001). Thus, the safety profile of the drug may be assumed to be greater than the recommendation that it should not be used during lactation suggests.
- However, fluconazole has a half-life of 30 hours in adults, 88.6 hours in a neonate (Hale 2012 online access). There is a possibility of accumulation within the baby's system particularly if it is given within the first 6 weeks when the hepatic and renal function is not fully developed. The use of the drug without a clear association between the nipple symptoms and *Candida* within this time period should not be encouraged. The level of fluconazole passing into breastmilk is reported as 400 μg per kg per day while the paediatric dose is 6 mg per kg per day to start followed by 3 mg per kg per day (Hale 2012 online access). In premature infants this is given every 72 hours, in the neonate (less than 4 weeks old), every 48 hours due to the extended half life
- The prescriber has to take ultimate responsibility for the prescribing decision outside of license

Side effects of fluconazole for the mother and baby are generally gastro-intestinal symptoms – nausea, diarrhoea and abdominal cramps. The literature (Hale 2012 online access) states that no complications from exposure to breastmilk have been found, although anecdotal reports of abdominal pain, vomiting and rashes in the baby have been highlighted by breastfeeding specialists in the UK particularly at higher doses.

Mothers may report re-occurrence of symptoms soon after completing a course of fluconazole. Depending on the severity, a further course of treatment **may** be justified. However, some women report pain, which is greatly reduced but still present, for up to a month after treatment. It is assumed that this represents ongoing healing of the ducts but this has not been studied. Individual decisions are necessary, taking into account the mother's wishes to receive a further course of treatment and the risk to the baby. Further support with positioning and attachment may also resolve residual pain regardless of the age of the baby.

There is no evidence for the effectiveness of using a single oral over-the-counter treatment of fluconazole and it could lead to resistance. This single dosage should be reserved for vaginal thrush as per the product license.

The diagnosis of thrush of the breast should be a diagnosis of exclusion based on symptoms and microbiological tests rather than assumptions.

Medication for women who may become pregnant

NICE PH11 (2008) made recommendations on the health of mothers pre-conceptually and during pregnancy. Breastfeeding women not actively using adequate contraceptive methods may become pregnant accidentally or the decision may be deliberate. Breastfeeding may continue throughout pregnancy and beyond if the mother chooses. The only reason to stop breastfeeding if the mother becomes pregnant is possibly a history of miscarriages. The uterine contractions produced by oxytocin are unlikely to disturb the pregnancy unless it is already unstable and at risk of spontaneous miscarriage.

Most healthcare professionals come into contact with women who are taking medication that has implications on pregnancy, or who are considering becoming pregnant and taking medication, or find themselves pregnant without planning to be and have taken medication, street drugs or alcohol. They may have information needs but they may also be unaware of those needs. They may need to make changes to protect the health of the unborn child.

Pre-conceptual use of medication

Since the catastrophe of births to mothers who took thalidomide, the medical profession and the general public have become very concerned about the possible exposure of the foetus to any drug. However, many pregnancies are not planned and many women will remember taking medication, recreational drugs or getting drunk in the week immediately after they believe they conceived. Concerns about the use of drugs in lactation may be an extension of the perception of this tragedy.

Pre-conceptual nutrition

Diet is important in the early development of the foetus. Any woman who may become pregnant (because contraception is not being actively used) could benefit from taking the following supplements throughout lactation in case they may become pregnant accidentally (NICE PH11 2008).

Folic acid

The current guidelines on folic acid (Department of Health 2000, 2004; NHS Choices 2011) are that women should begin to take folic acid 400 µg daily before becoming pregnant and should continue for the first 12 weeks of pregnancy in order to reduce the risk of neural tube defects. If the mother is on anti-epileptic medication, is obese (BMI >30), has a history of neural tube defects in a previous pregnancy, has coeliac disease, diabetes, sickle cell anaemia, thalassaemia, she or her partner have spinal cord defects, the dose should be increased to 5 mg daily.

In 2007 the Food Standards Agency (FSA) conducted some research into attitudes and knowledge on folic acid and other dietary changes recommended in pregnancy (Food Standards Agency 2007). They reported that there has, in fact, been no significant change in the rate of neural tube defects in the past 10 years despite health campaigns on the use of folic acid. One reason may be that approximately half of births are unplanned and in the remainder only half of the women took supplements with many presenting for first antenatal contact beyond the first trimester (Healthy Lifestyle in Pregnancy 2007).

Mass media campaigns have been successful in increasing folate awareness but in no study has the post-campaign rate of folic acid use exceeded 50%. It has been recommended that all women of childbearing age should take folic acid regularly on the assumption that they might become pregnant (NICE PH11 2008). Currently neural tube defect affected pregnancies arise in 0.8 per 1000 pregnancies, which translates to 800 pregnancies each year in the UK.

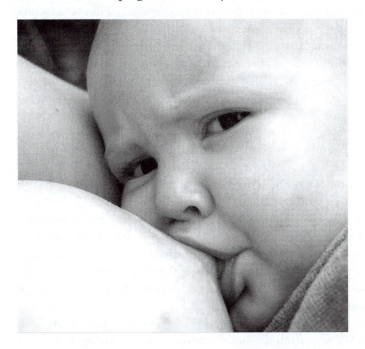

Vitamin D supplements

There has been an unexpected increase over the past 15 years in the number of babies found to be suffering from rickets or symptoms of decreased bone mass which demonstrate poor levels of vitamin D (NICE PH11 2008). Vitamin D deficiency is unusual in babies born at term to mothers with adequate vitamin D status (UNICEF Baby Friendly 2012). Some women enter pregnancy with low vitamin D levels. This may be due to:

- lack of exposure to sunlight due to wearing concealing clothing for cultural reasons;
- inadequate consumption of foods containing vitamin D e.g. oily fish;
- Inadequate consumption of dairy (prevalent particularly in adolescent girls) (Department of Health 2010, SACN 2003);
- BMI greater than 30;
- Women who spend a lot of time indoors or use sun creams limiting the absorption of ultraviolet (UV) light;
- living in the northern hemisphere where levels of UV light are only sufficient to stimulate vitamin D production in the summer months; and
- having dark skin, which prevents absorption of available UV light in the UK climate.

Babies born to mothers with low vitamin D levels may be born deficient. In turn this will be exacerbated by being breastfed as the vitamin D levels in breastmilk will be sub-optimal.

In order to ensure that babies do not develop rickets, mothers at risk of vitamin D deficiency (arguably all mothers in the UK) should take a daily supplement of 10 µg vitamin D daily throughout pregnancy and during breastfeeding. Infants who are exclusively breastfed by mothers in the categories described above should also be given a daily supplement of 7.5 µg per day, beginning soon after delivery. This in no way suggests that the breastmilk of a mother with low levels of vitamin D, does not have all the other health advantages but is a reflection of current awareness of the risk of burning in sunlight balanced with the UK climate and poor levels of sunshine for the majority of the year. Breastfeeding alone cannot redress the deficiency resulting from low levels in pregnancy. Supplementation should be advised for all babies from 6 months receiving breastmilk and appropriate weaning foods (but no infant formula) until 5 years of age.

Vitamin D supplementation for the mother is also beneficial for her own health relating to bone health and many other emerging conditions.

Vitamin D has a reference nutrient intake (RNI) level set as 10 µg per day (400 IU) during pregnancy and lactation (British Nutrition Foundation 2006). The average dietary vitamin D intake of young women in the UK approximates 3 µg per day and less than 1% consume more than the 10 µg (Williams 2007). The National Diet and Nutrition Survey of British adults suggest that if such a threshold were investigated in the UK population data, some 80–90% would be deficient (Henderson *et al.* 2003).

Vitamin D is a fat-soluble vitamin that is found in food and can also be made in the body after exposure to UV rays from the sun. Fortified foods are common sources of vitamin D but without sunshine exposure it is difficult to achieve maximal intake. The American Academy of Paediatrics (AAP) recommends a daily supplement of 200 IU vitamin D for breastfed infants beginning within the first 2 months of life unless they receive at least 500 ml per day of vitamin D-fortified formula (Gartner 2003).

Supplements can be taken as part of multi-vitamin products or with calcium. The correct levels of folic acid and vitamin D are present in Healthy Start vitamins which are available free to some mothers (Healthy Start 2012). Suitable vitamin drops for babies include Healthy Start, Abidec® and Dalavit®.

Sources of vitamin D
- More than 90% of mankind's vitamin D supply is derived from UVB sunlight exposure
- Oily fish including trout, salmon, mackerel, herring, sardines, anchovies, pilchards and fresh tuna
- Cod liver oil and other fish oils
- Egg yolk – 0.5 µg (20 IU) per yolk
- Mushrooms
- Supplemented breakfast cereals, mainly supermarket 'own brands' in the UK. Typically contain between 2 and 8 µg (80–320 IU) per 100 g
- Margarine
- Infant formula milk

In a fair-skinned individual, exposure of the face and forearms to 20–30 minutes of sunlight at midday is estimated to generate the equivalent of 2000 IU vitamin D. Between April and October all of Scandinavia, much of western Europe, including 90% of the UK (roughly north of Birmingham) and 50% of USA is above the latitude where exposure to sufficient UVB is possible (Pearce and Cheetham 2010).

Obesity

Obesity (BMI >30) is a risk factor affecting pregnancy outcomes including increased risk of miscarriage, increased need for caesarean sections and greater risk during the procedure, increased risk of pre-eclampsia and thromboembolism. According to Centre for Maternal and Child Enquiries (CEMACE 2011), 'maternal obesity is now a major and growing risk factor for maternal death' and 49% of the women who died were either overweight or obese and more than 15% were extremely obese'. In 2007, 24% of women in the UK were defined as obese.

Risks to the developing foetus include increased risk of congenital anomalies, macrosomia (large size at birth), stillbirth and perinatal mortality. Potentially there are also long-term obesity risks for the child. A linear association between pre-pregnancy weight and risk of caesarean section has been identified in an observational study (Ahmed *et al.* 2009).

Obese woman should try to lose weight before pregnancy but probably not during pregnancy (NICE PH11 2008; NICE PH27 2010). Actively losing weight would be likely to cause a smaller baby to be born and this may be seen as a less positive outcome of pregnancy. Post-natally women should be encouraged to return to their pre-pregnancy weight as a minimum or ideally to a BMI between 20 and 25 following delivery (NICE PH11 2008) by regular exercise and a low fat healthy diet. Weight loss achieved in this gradual manner will not affect the quantity or quality of milk (NICE PH27 2010).

Smoking

Women planning on embarking on pregnancy should consider smoking cessation before, or as soon as possible after, conception (Department of Health Smokefree 2012). The results of the Infant Feeding Survey (Bolling 2005) showed that 19% of mothers smoked throughout their pregnancy but that 45% gave up either before they became pregnant or during their pregnancy.

Smoking in pregnancy affects the foetus resulting in an increased risk of:

- slow growth of the foetus due to reducing oxygen and increased carbon monoxide in cord blood;
- premature birth;
- stillbirth;
- low birthweight;
- cot death;
- breathing problems; and
- wheezing in the first 6 months of life.

The use of Nicotine Replacement Therapy (NRT) products is now recognised to be less of a risk to the baby than the mother smoking (NICE PH10 2008). Support may be needed to encourage mothers not to resume smoking after the delivery. In the UK, 26% of mothers who had quit smoking before or during pregnancy began to smoke again in the months after the birth of the baby (Bolling 2007). Smoking near children should be actively discouraged. Exposure to secondhand smoke has been linked with an increased risk of colic and perceived low milk supply.

Alcohol

The Department of Health (2011) recommend 'as a general rule, pregnant women or women trying to conceive should avoid drinking alcohol. If they do choose to drink, to protect the baby they should not drink more than 1 to 2 units of alcohol once or twice a week and should not get drunk'.

In the Infant Feeding Survey (Bolling 2007), only 30% of mothers said that they gave up altogether. The majority stated that they had reduced their intake as alcohol could cause damage the baby, 16% because they no longer liked the taste and 15% because it made them feel sick. Only 1% drank more than 14 units per week but in the under 20s the figure rose to 4% providing grounds for concern.

The Patient.co.uk Pregnancy and alcohol study (2012) showed that:

- Pregnant women who drink more than 15 units a week have an increased risk of having a baby with a low birthweight.
- Pregnant women who drink more than 20 units a week have an increased risk of having a baby with some damage to the brain causing impaired intellect.
- Pregnant women who drink very heavily risk having a baby with Foetal Alcohol Syndrome (FAS). Babies with this syndrome have brain damage, a low birthweight and facial malformations.

NICE CG 62 2008 recommends that:

- Pregnant women and women planning a pregnancy should be advised to avoid drinking alcohol in the first 3 months of pregnancy if possible because it may be associated with an increased risk of miscarriage.
- If women choose to drink alcohol during pregnancy they should be advised to drink no more than 1 to 2 UK units once or twice a week (1 unit equals half a pint of ordinary strength lager or beer, or one shot [25 ml] of spirits. One small [125 ml] glass of wine is equal to 1.5 UK units). Although there is uncertainty regarding a safe level of alcohol consumption in pregnancy, at this low level there is no evidence of harm to the unborn baby.
- Women should be informed that getting drunk or binge drinking during pregnancy (defined as more than 5 standard drinks or 7.5 UK units on a single occasion) may be harmful to the unborn baby.

Substance misuse

Many women who are substance misusers are at a greater risk of unplanned pregnancy but where possible they should be counselled prior to conception about the benefits of entering a detoxification programme. Babies born to mothers on heroin undergo a withdrawal period at delivery which entails their admission to neonatal intensive care. Breastfeeding can ease the withdrawal by providing a lower level of medication but this is generally discouraged if the mother continues to use 'street drugs' which may be adulterated with a variety of unknown substances. A detox programme allows the substitution of controlled doses of methadone or buprenorphine to prevent symptoms of withdrawal but without providing the high of drugs of misuse. These drugs, depending on the dose are generally safe to use during breastfeeding (see pages 210–9).

Anecdotally mothers and their partners may make enormous efforts to change their lifestyle for the sake of the unborn baby. For most drug abusers efforts to 'stay clean' involve changing their social groups and, in many cases, moving home to avoid temptation. It is very difficult to provide any set guidelines on management of mothers who are misusers of illegal substances as individual circumstances and drivers to change are hugely variable. These mothers should be provided with information in order to make informed choices for themselves and their children and counselled on an individual, empathetic basis.

Key points

- A variety of physical and mental conditions which affect mother and baby can impact on breastfeeding.
- Mothers may need reassurance and support to overcome difficulties.
- Medication to treat symptoms of colic may not be evidence based.
- Use of lactose-free formula may not be necessary in the presence of symptoms such as diarrhoea. It should not be considered without expert dietetic input.
- Changes to maternal diet or use of hydrolysed formulas to treat suspected cow's milk protein allergy should not be considered without expert dietetic input.
- Problems with positioning and attachment can produce symptoms which may be attributed to other conditions such as thrush, Raynaud's phenomenon, vasospasm and mastitis.
- Medication use in the majority of conditions (including post-natal depression, thromboembolism and PPH) does not preclude continued breastfeeding.
- Pre-conceptual advice may be applicable to any woman not actively using contraception; this may include many breastfeeding mothers who have not recommenced menstruation but may ovulate.
- There are many health promotional messages on pre-conception which can be provided by healthcare professionals on an opportunistic basis.
- There are national recommendations that mothers should be made aware of; the need to take folic acid, vitamin D, to stop smoking, to limit alcohol and to maintain a BMI within the optimum healthy range.

Chapter 6

Decision-making on the safety of drugs in breastmilk

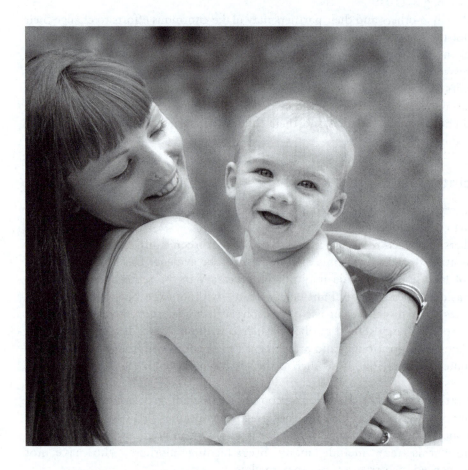

The sheer number of medicines on the market poses dilemmas of prescribing for lactating women. The last time that approximately 80% of women in the UK initiated breastfeeding, was in 1926 to 1939. The difference in prescribing habits since then is enormous. That was an era when antibiotics were being developed; there was no expectation of a 'pill for every ill'. Now we expect that all symptoms can be alleviated by taking a drug. We are aware that prevention and treatment of many more chronic diseases are possible and many women with complex medical needs are able to consider pregnancy and lactation as safe options. Most drugs pass into breastmilk but generally in very low levels and very few drugs are totally contra-indicated for use during breastfeeding.

The dilemma of prescribing

Before prescribing a drug for a lactating woman, the prescriber should be able to make an informed decision on the safety of the drug regime of choice for the mother–baby pair presenting. The prescriber should be able to consider the appropriateness of treatment for the mother while determining the safety of the drug and the likelihood of side effects for the baby. Decisions may need knowledge of pharmacokinetics of the drug. Whether the drug is licensed for paediatric use should also be taken into consideration. If so it is likely to be safe during lactation as levels of drugs passing through breastmilk rarely, if ever, exceed the therapeutic dose.

The licensing application underpins the recommendation in the Summary of Product Characteristics (SPC) and use is restricted in the absence of full clinical data. Use outside of the license application of any drug is the responsibility of the prescriber. Drugs are not tested on lactating mothers – it would be totally unethical to do so; therefore, such use is not included in the licence application. In addition to clinical trials in humans, additional data from animal experiments will also govern the manufacturer's recommendation on safety, although this may not be totally relevant.

The suitability of the drug for the lactating mother and her baby will also depend on:

- the maturity of the baby;
- the age of the baby;
- how often the baby is being breastfed;
- the volume of breastmilk being consumed;
- whether the mother is willing to cease breastfeeding;
- individual susceptibility of the infant to the drug e.g. penicillin sensitivity; and
- concurrent infant disease status e.g. prematurity, respiratory depression, heart failure, renal disease.

Assessment of the transfer of drugs in breastmilk

The measurement of the levels of any drug in breastmilk is complex and rarely undertaken. Often measurements are taken before the drug has reached a steady state in the body and lack detail. Case studies may only present a limited picture. Studies of more than ten women seem to be few and far between.

Anderson (2003) has shown that the absolute incidence of adverse effects on infants of drugs taken by their lactating mothers is low and serious events are rare. He evaluated 100 case reports of adverse reactions presumed to be in infants caused by drugs that had passed through their mother's breastmilk. No reaction was considered definitely linked with the maternal drug, 47 were probably linked and 53 possibly linked. Drugs affecting the central nervous system accounted for half of the reactions, including all three fatalities – although there were additional factors in all of the latter. Sixty-three per cent of the reactions were in neonates and only 4% in babies older than 6 months of age. Of the fatalities, one involved a benzodiazepine drug given to a mother of a child who had already had a near-miss sudden infant death syndrome reaction, phenobarbital given to a mother who was epileptic who overlaid the baby in the parental bed and a 5-week-old baby exposed to methadone but where major signs of neglect and abnormalities of the internal organs were noted at post-mortem examination.

The relatively small number of adverse events published is in contrast to the common belief of the risk of medication given to lactating mothers. Publication bias might be expected to produce more reports than exposure which was not problematic. Anderson suggests that by taking a few simple precautions when prescribing for mothers, breastfeeding rarely needs to be discontinued or discouraged. However, his perception is that medication use shortens the duration of breastfeeding because of overly cautious information from healthcare professionals.

Pharmacokinetic data on the transfer of drugs into breastmilk

Drugs pass into breastmilk in several ways depending on their properties. Intercellular gaps are wide open at delivery and gradually tighten over the days following birth so more of the drug is able to pass into milk on day 1 than on day 3. However, as less volume of 'milk' (colostrum) is produced, so the absolute level of drug transferred remains small (see Figures 6.1 and 6.2).

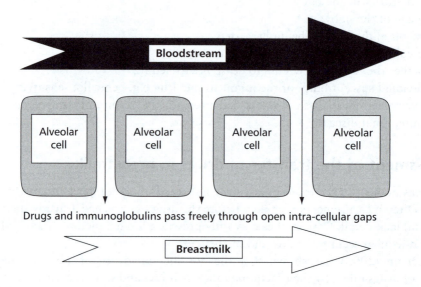

FIGURE 6.1 Passage of drugs into breastmilk in the first few days after delivery when intercellular junctions remain open

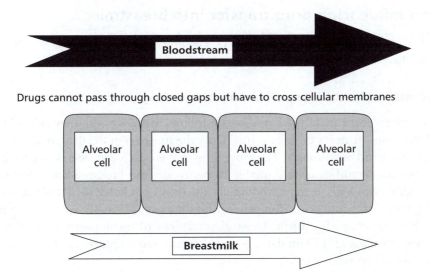

FIGURE 6.2 Passage of drugs into breastmilk when intercellular junctions have closed

Other drugs simply diffuse across the cell membrane and through the body of the cells while others are actively transported through the cell to concentrate in breastmilk. More detailed information is available in Hale and Hartmann (2008) (see Figure 6.3).

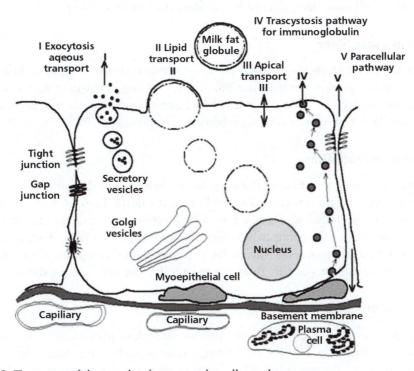

FIGURE 6.3 Transport of drug molecules across the cell membranes

Factors influencing drug transfer into breastmilk

The transfer of drugs into breastmilk depends on a variety of factors, which will be discussed below:

The extent of plasma protein binding of the drug

When drugs enter the maternal bloodstream following absorption, they either become bound to plasma proteins or remain free. Only the free part of the drug is able to penetrate the biological membranes. The more drug that is bound, the less is free to diffuse. Highly protein-bound drugs are unable to penetrate into breastmilk e.g. most penicillins. Drugs with high protein binding are the drugs of choice for administration to lactating mothers. Some drugs compete for binding sites normally occupied by bilirubin in the first week after birth. Drug displacement of unconjugated bilirubin may result in kernicterus and brain damage in the infant and a theoretical risk exists with some drugs e.g. co-trimoxazole.

Milk–plasma ratio

This measurement refers to the concentration of the protein-free fractions in milk and plasma, e.g. fluoxetine has a milk–plasma (m/p) ratio of 0.286, while the m/p ratio of dexamphetamine is quoted as 2.8–7.5, which means that the level in the milk is approximately 3 to 7.5 times that in the plasma i.e. it becomes concentrated in milk. Any ratio over 1 implies that the drug **may** be unsuitable to be prescribed for a lactating mother and other factors need to be taken into consideration.

Oral bio-availability

The oral bio-availability of a drug is the percentage of the drug absorbed into the system having passed through the gut, liver or lungs. First-pass metabolism may reduce the availability. Most drugs given by injection only (i.e. there is no oral formulation available) have poor bio-availability e.g. insulin, heparin.

First-pass metabolism

This may influence the effect of the drug on the mother and the baby. When a drug is absorbed from the gut it is carried to the liver in the portal blood system. There it may be converted into metabolites, which may be inactive and therefore excreted without effect or an active metabolite, which has a therapeutic effect of its own e.g. azathioprine and 6-mercaptopurine. Alternatively, it may pass through the liver unchanged. Drugs which are inactivated by first-pass metabolism are safer for use during lactation.

Drug half-life

The longer the half-life of a drug, the greater the risk of accumulation in the mother and in the infant. The half-life of a drug is defined as the time taken for the serum concentration to decrease by 50%. It is determined by the rate of absorption, metabolism and excretion. A drug with a short half-life has to be taken more frequently than one with a long one. Approximately five half-lives have to elapse before steady state is reached. After this period, timing feeds to avoid peak levels has a minimal effect. Similarly after five half-lives without further medication, almost all (98%) of the drug has been eliminated from the body. Infants, in general, do not metabolise medication as fast as adults due to immaturity of the hepatic system. Thus the infant may begin to accumulate a drug with a long half- life, e.g. the half-life of fluconazole in an adult is 30 hours; in an infant under 4–6 weeks, it is estimated to be 88 hours. Untoward effects may therefore, theoretically, be expected to cause adverse effects in the infant due to accumulation. On this basis, treatment for a lactating mother with drugs with a shorter half-life is preferable particularly in the neonatal period, e.g. ibuprofen rather than naproxen (see Figures 6.4, 6.5 and 6.6).

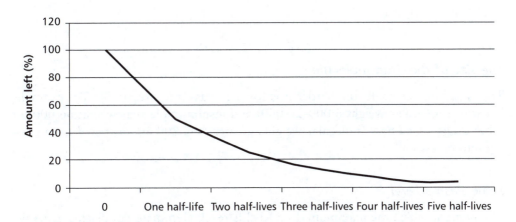

FIGURE 6.4 Percentage of drug left with respect to half-life

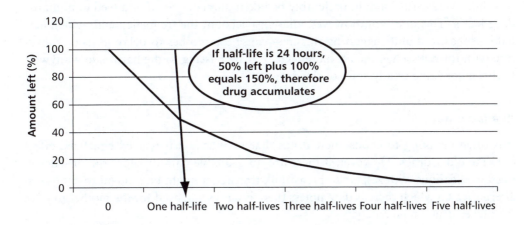

FIGURE 6.5 Percentage of drug left with respect to drug with half-life of 24 hours

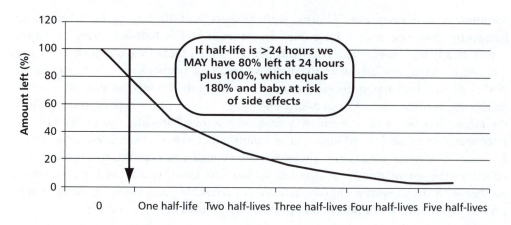

FIGURE 6.6 Percentage of drug left with respect to drug with half-life of more than 24 hours

The size of the drug molecule

The larger the molecule, the harder it is for it to pass into breastmilk. For example, heparins (molecular weight 6,000–20,000) and insulin (molecular weight >6,000) or other drugs which have molecular weights greater than 200 are restricted from passing into breast milk.

Peak plasma level

The point at which the maximum drug level is reached in maternal plasma generally corresponds to the highest rate of entry into milk. This is generally reached 2 hours after an oral dose of non-sustained release medication, or about 20 minutes after an intravenous injection. Ideally the breastfeeding mother should not feed the baby at this time. Medication should preferably be taken immediately after a feed to minimise drug levels. This does not, however, take into account the frequency with which new babies breastfeed and suggesting this may cause the mother to delay feeds or substitute with formula when the absolute level of drug passing to the baby is low anyway. It also ignores the steady state of the drug.

Available data

It is often tempting to choose new drugs that may have a perceived beneficial effect over the older drugs. However, if there are no available data on more recently developed medications with respect to breastmilk transfer, it might be prudent to choose an alternative on which there is data unless there is a pressing need for the mother to have the newer drug immediately.

Fat solubility

Un-ionised drugs which are lipid soluble usually dissolve in, and pass through, the lipid membrane of the alveolar epithelium of the breast. The latter is composed of lipoprotein, glycolipid, phospholipid and free lipids. The average body fat content of infants and neonates is significantly lower than in adults: 3% in premature infants, 12% in term neonates, 30% in 12 month olds and 18% in adults. Because of the relative deficit of fat tissue storage sites, drugs causing central nervous system sedation have a greater effect, even in the relatively low doses found in breastmilk, on neonates than infants of one year old. Many neuroleptic drugs have a high affinity for lipid-rich tissue e.g. benzodiazepines, cocaine and barbiturates. It is particularly important to consider this in premature infants.

Immaturity of the hepatic and renal function of infants

Renal excretion of drugs by infants is lowest in newborns aged 3–9 days but rises quickly within 3 months. Hence, any drug to which a newborn may be exposed should be monitored e.g. pethidine has a half-life in an adult of 3 hours, but in a newborn it may be as long as 32 hours. The premature infant's liver may be overwhelmed by breakdown products of haemoglobin, due to the natural destruction of red blood cells present in the foetus during pregnancy.

Breastmilk production

Unless the drug is highly protein bound, or has a high molecular weight, it will be available to pass into breastmilk by diffusion. If the baby feeds when the mother's plasma level of the drug is high, the exposure via milk will be commensurately higher. The variability of milk composition day to day and during any day will alter the passage of drugs into milk to some degree. As the level of drug in the plasma falls, the reverse passage will permit flow from the milk back into the plasma. Thus the level falls again with time after the peak plasma concentration is passed.

In utero exposure

The foetus receives five- to tenfold higher levels of medication through the placenta than the baby does via breastmilk (Hale 2012 online access). If the infant has been exposed to the medication there may already have been some enzyme induction e.g. phenytoin. It is often assumed that if a drug has been given in pregnancy it must be safe to take during breastfeeding. However, the difference in metabolism in pregnancy and after birth should be borne in mind. During pregnancy the drug is metabolised by the mother's liver and kidneys via placental transfer. Once delivered the infant has to rely on its own systems which are immature and may lead to higher serum levels despite the fact that placental transfer of drugs is higher than breastmilk transfer.

Maturity of the baby

A premature infant may be more vulnerable to any medication consumed, not only because of both its immature hepatic and renal function but also because of its percentage of body fats. An infant over 6 weeks will metabolise drugs more effectively than a newborn while toddlers will rarely be exposed to drugs at a level which exceeds that to which they can be exposed directly.

Age of the baby and volume of milk consumed

The age of the baby influences the volume of milk consumed and the frequency of feeding. During the first few days when colostrum is made, the breast is more permeable to drugs but as the volume of milk consumed is low, the absolute level of drug transferred is low. An older child feeding only once or twice a day will consume less milk and therefore be exposed to a commensurately lower level of drug.

Possible side effects for the baby

For example, if a drug causes the baby to be drowsy, breastfeeding frequency may be reduced and the baby may fail to gain weight. Potential side effects may need to be borne in mind when choosing medication for long-term use. Centrally acting drugs should be avoided if possible with young babies or those at risk of apnoea.

Therapeutic range

If the level of the drug that reaches the baby comes into the therapeutic range it would have the expected effect of that drug on the baby. If the level exceeds the maximum therapeutic concentration side effects would be noted in the baby. However, as in the vast majority of cases the amount of drug passing through breastmilk is below the therapeutic level for that drug, no effect will be seen (see Figure 6.7).

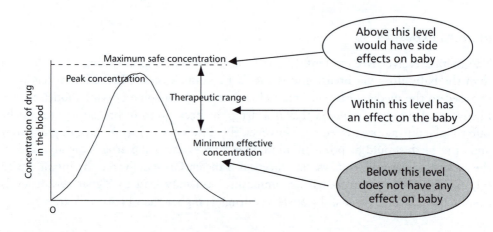

FIGURE 6.7 Potential risk of side effects in the baby according to therapeutic range

Duration of exposure to the drug

A short course of high-dose medication may be acceptable e.g. prednisolone 50 mg.

Relative infant dose

The relative infant dose is being increasingly recognised as a valuable guide to the safety of a drug taken by a breastfeeding woman. Percentages less than 10% are assumed to be the safest options. In order to calculate this, the dose in the infant measured in mg per kg per day is divided by the dose in the mother – also in mg per kg per day, both doses being derived from studies (Hale 2012 online access).

$$\text{Relative infant dose} = \frac{\text{dose in the infant (mg per kg per day)}}{\text{dose in the mother (mg per kg per day)}}$$

Summary of points to determine when a drug is likely to be safe for use during breastfeeding

- relative infant dose – <10%
- m/p ratio – level <1
- plasma protein binding – >90%
- the molecular weight of the drug – >200
- oral bio-availability – poor
- if the drug is licensed for paediatric use

Limitations of the literature on transfer of drugs into breastmilk

Using the drug manufacturer's summary of product characteristics, very few drugs are licensed for use in lactation, so there is no alternative but to cease breastfeeding at least temporarily in the face of no other safety data.

However, using information on the relative infant dose, m/p ratio, protein binding and half-life it is possible to make a decision of relative safety. Unfortunately these details are not available in standard reference texts such as the British National Formulary (BNF). Practitioners need access to specialised literature and websites and to take professional responsibility for clinical judgements for the benefit of mother and child's future health.

Practical application of pharmacological data

Many practitioners may be discouraged from undertaking a risk assessment in the light of the need for the above data. It is, however, not as difficult as it might at first seem, even for those who have not looked at such clinical data since finishing their degree! However, if a practitioner is unsure it would be wise to consult experts e.g. the local Medicines Information centre or the Breastfeeding Network (BfN) Drugs in Breastmilk Helpline, at least to confirm the understanding of the matter.

The section below is aimed at increasing confidence in making decisions, this follows some worked examples.

In general, data on the relative infant dose, m/p ratio, half-life of the drug and extent of plasma binding can allow a judgement of the extent to which a drug passes into breastmilk. Additionally maternal and infant factors have to be taken into consideration along with the drug safety profile and possible side effects on mother and baby.

Example 1: imipramine

Data taken from Medications and Mothers Milk (Hale 2012 online access).

Relative infant dose quoted as 0.15%. Imipramine is metabolised to desipramine the active metabolite. Since the m/p ratio (0.5–1.5) crosses 1, milk levels might be expected to approximate to those of maternal serum. However, 90% is plasma protein bound and unable to pass into breastmilk, so levels in breastmilk may be assumed to be relatively low. The half-life of the drug is 8–16 hours so there is no opportunity to minimise transfer by feeding immediately before taking the drug even if it has not reached steady state. The low level of transfer is borne out by a published case study of two mothers. Ware (1990) studied two women taking imipramine 50 mg daily for panic attacks. In one baby, levels of imipramine and desipramine, the active metabolite were 91–185 µg per litre, respectively. In the other, only trace levels were detected.

The m/p ratio is high but a small amount of the drug is free to pass into breastmilk so the absolute level of transferring is limited, reflected in the relative infant dose which is well below the 10% level taken as safe.

No paediatric side effects have been reported from this drug being taken by a breastfeeding mother although in theory it could cause the baby to be drowsy and experience a dry mouth. The BNF recommendation is 'caution in breastfeeding, but amounts too small to be harmful'. If the baby exhibited drowsiness or significant weight loss, it should be monitored or a decision could be made for the mother to stop the drug and see if the baby's behavior returned to normal or if deemed essential to formula feed her baby.

Example 2: diclofenac

Data taken from Medications and Mothers Milk (Hale 2012 online access).

Relative Infant Dose quoted as 1%. Because of the very high plasma binding (99.7%), very little drug is available to pass into breastmilk, hence no m/p ratio has been determined. The half-life is very short (1.1 hours) and the mother could be advised to feed just before taking the tablet to minimise transfer further as the medication may be taken in short acute doses or on an as required regime. Non-steroidal drugs, as a class, are often transferred into breastmilk at very low levels hence their widespread use for immediate post-partum pain.

Diclofenac is preferable to naproxen in mothers with babies less than 6 weeks. Naproxen has a half-life of 12–15 hours, an m/p ratio of 0.01 and plasma protein binding of 99.7%, and the relative infant dose is 3.32%. The longer half-life is of marginally more concern in younger babies. One case of a 7-day-old baby with prolonged bleeding, haemorrhage and acute anaemia has been reported by Hale (2010).

Example 3: ranitidine

Data taken from Medications and Mothers Milk (Hale 2012 online access).

Relative Infant Dose quoted as 4.5%. The pharmacological data would suggest that this drug can readily permeate breastmilk and from the m/p ratio (1.9–6.7) would appear to concentrate in breastmilk. Additionally plasma protein binding data (15%) suggest that much of the drug is free to pass into breastmilk. It has, however, only limited bio-availability (50%).

A single case study (Kearns et al. 1985) showed that following a 150 mg dose given to the mother twice a day for 2 days, an infant consuming 1 l of breastmilk per day, would ingest 2.6 mg in 24 hours. This can be compared with an unlicensed paediatric dose of 1 mg per kg three times a day used for gastro-oesophageal reflux in infants from 1 month to 2 years (BNFC).

Although this drug appears to concentrate in breastmilk, using case report data and knowledge of pharmacokinetics we can deduce that it reaches levels which are sub-therapeutic and no paediatric concerns have been reported. Ranitidine has a relative infant dose of 4.5% (Hale 2012 online access).

Key points

- Information on the transfer of drugs into breastmilk is not readily available to healthcare practitioners, but is available in specialised sources.
- It is possible to determine the probable safety of a drug from its pharmacokinetic properties.
- There is a drug within most classes on which we have some data on safety.
- The drug with data on transfer into breastmilk should ideally be chosen.
- The relative infant dose is a simple guide to safety but is only available in specialised texts.
- Recommending that a mother ceases or interrupts breastfeeding in order to take a drug should be undertaken only as a last resort having taken all other factors into consideration.
- Where no data exist the process on which safety decisions were made should be documented and discussed with the mother.

Chapter 7

Professional responsibility and counselling

The dilemma of taking prescription drugs during breastfeeding

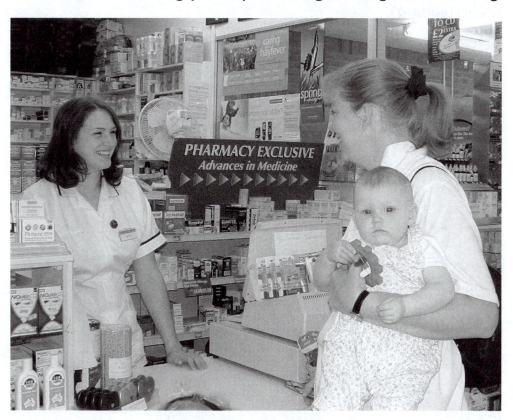

The dilemma of prescribing drugs during lactation lies in the decision in terms of which is more important – the potential risk of the drug in breastmilk or the lack of breastmilk? Before prescribing/recommending a drug we need to consider some questions:

- How essential is the need for this particular drug if a mother is breastfeeding?
- Is it possible to substitute it with a drug of which we have more data in terms of its passage from mother to infant?
- Do we know whether it would be safe for her infant if the mother continues to breastfeed while on this drug?
- Would she choose to continue breastfeeding without any medication? Is this decision sensible taking into account her medical condition?

In other words, can we prescribe/recommend this drug for a breastfeeding mother without jeopardising the safety of her baby or would it be safer to suggest that she stops breastfeeding temporarily or permanently, and that the baby is fed with artificial supplements?

How do mothers perceive the dilemma of drugs during breastfeeding?

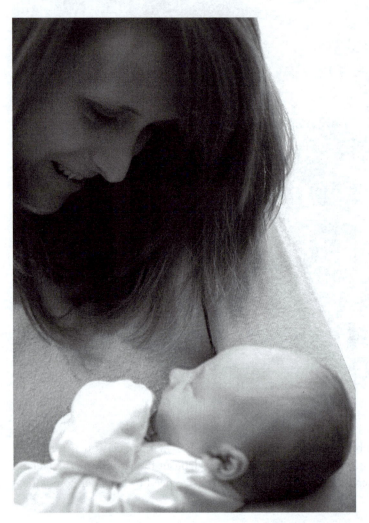

It is interesting to look at how mothers may view this dilemma differently. Research in Canada (Ito 1993) showed that of 203 mothers who phoned a telephone helpline (Motherisk) for information on the safety of antibiotics which they had been prescribed, 125 were followed up by a telephone call within 32 weeks to characterise breastfeeding patterns during antimicrobial therapy. Of those followed up, 15% (19) had chosen not to take the medicine and continue to breastfeed rather than expose their baby to the risk, while 7% (7) of the remaining 106 had stopped breastfeeding during therapy. All mothers had been assured that the risk to their baby was minimal and had been given full information on potential side effects. The authors suggest that doctors need to be aware of the risks of non-compliance with drug regimens and the potential negative impact of breastfeeding even with full information on safety.

A study of 1000 women, 1000 doctors and 1000 pharmacists undertaken as part of a PhD research study (Jones 2000) looked at the experiences and attitudes of the groups to breastfeeding and drugs in breastmilk. Of the women who had been advised to give up breastfeeding, 58.3% reported that they had refused to take the medication. Comments that they made are enlightening of the attitudes which some mothers have on preventing 'pollution' of their breastmilk.

> I was unwilling to take any drugs and endured flu, sinusitis and a tooth infection without any drugs for three and a half years. I don't feel leaflets give enough detail and so little is known about a wide range of drugs on the market I don't think it is worth the risk.

Other mothers are posed with different outcomes as a result of temporarily interrupting breastfeeding.

> I was told to stop breastfeeding by my health visitor; my GP said it was up to me. I wanted to continue and express temporarily but I felt too ill. Other people around me were advising me to continue bottle-feeding as my baby was enjoying it. I stopped totally before my baby was 2 weeks old.

The polarity map

In light of the known disadvantages of not breastfeeding which have been identified, it may be thought that the dilemma 'would it be safer to suggest that she stops breastfeeding temporarily or permanently, and that the baby is given artificial milk supplements' is easily resolved. However, evidence for the benefits does not take into account individual cases, in which the health professional and mother find themselves.

It may be useful to look at the dilemma in terms of a polarity map (Johnson 1996).

The two polarities of the dilemma could be to continue breastfeeding in the presence of the medication or cease breastfeeding and use artificial formula. There is, in fact, an intermediate solution which is to temporarily express breastmilk to maintain the supply while substituting with formula. However, for the purposes of this discussion long-term medication will be assumed so that this is not possible.

First, we need to identify the positive aspects for each polarity:

Continue breastfeeding	Cease breastfeeding
• Mothers wish • Continued advantages of breast-milk for mother and baby • Baby unwilling to feed from a bottle	• No passage of drug to the baby • Professional responsibility not to use a drug outside of licence unless necessary • Safety of baby assured by lack of exposure to the drug

It may be possible to identify further positive in each polarity, but in order to simplify the explanation we will minimise the options.

Then we identify the negative aspects for each polarity:

Continue breastfeeding	Cease breastfeeding
• Passage of drug to baby • Professional accountability in absence of safety data/licences application • Baby's health may be jeopardised	• Mother's wish to continue to breastfeed • Loss of advantages of breastmilk to mother and baby • Difficulties in changing feeding method for mother and baby

Again there may be further arguments for the negative benefits for each decision.

These points are then used to devise the polarity map, which we will return to as we examine the responsibility of the professional, and how it influences decision-making.

Positive for continued breastfeeding	*Positive for formula*
• Mothers wish • Continued advantages of breastmilk for mother and baby • Baby unwilling to feed from a bottle	• No passage of drug to the baby • Professional responsibility not to use a drug outside of licence unless necessary • Safety of baby assured by lack of exposure to the drug • Safety of baby
Breastfeeding with medicine ———————————————————— **Formula**	
• Passage of drug to baby • Professional accountability in absence of safety data/licences application • Baby's health may be jeopardised	• Mother's wish to continue to breastfeed • Loss of advantages of breastmilk to mother and baby • Difficulties in changing feeding method for mother and baby
Negative aspects of continued breastfeeding	*Negative aspects of formula*

The healthcare professional making the recommendation to the mother needs to be confident in their own mind where within the polarity map they feel comfortable in taking responsibility and where the mother feels most comfortable with the decision. An example of the use of this decision aid is given below.

Christine's story

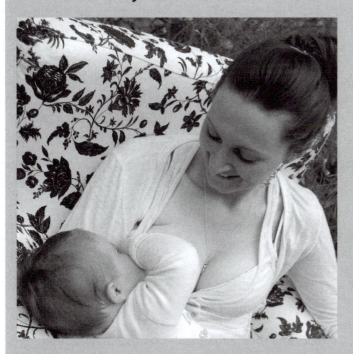

Christine has a daughter Megan who is 4 months old and fully breastfed. Christine has a history of manic depression but has been relatively well since the delivery, maintained on a low dose of haloperidol 0.5 mg three times a day. She recently experienced a psychotic episode and was admitted to a mother and baby unit. It is intended that olanzapine is initiated. There are concerns about the safety of this for Megan as it is unlicensed for use during lactation. Christine's partner Oliver asks to discuss the options with staff as they have both been committed to breastfeeding Megan exclusively for a minimum of 6 months as there is a family history of atopic diseases on both sides of the family.

The medical concerns are around Christine's mental state. Megan has been given breastmilk from a store which Christine had built up and frozen and has as yet not been given any formula. The risk of formula may exacerbate her risk for atopic diseases in the future which Oliver and Christine are keen to minimise.

If we consider the polarity map:

- Christine is keen to breastfeed.
- There are potential risks to Megan if she is formula fed.
- Olanzapine is not licensed in lactation so there is a professional responsibility.

- The doctor does not have information on the risks of the drug on the baby so feels unable to prescribe it unless Christine stops breastfeeding.
- Oliver is very clear that he and Christine are unwilling for Megan to stop breast-feeding at this time.
- Christine urgently needs medication for her condition.

The information we need to fully inform the decision is what the risk is for Megan:

- How much drug will she receive through her mother's breastmilk – theoretical or measured?
- What are the potential side effects?
- Are there any long-term safety studies?
- Are there any studies at all of the effects on babies of the drug passing through breastmilk?

Using information from Hale (2012 online access) and LactMed (2012)

m/p ratio	0.38
Half-life	21–54 hours
Plasma protein binding	93%
Oral bioavailability	>57%
Relative infant dose	1.2%

Croke (2003) studied five mothers and their babies and took nine milk samples. The median relative infant dose was 1.6% and there were no apparent ill effects in the infants.

In a study of seven mothers (Gardiner 2003) taking between 5–20 mg per day, The median infant dose of olanzapine ingested through milk was 1.02% of the maternal dose. Olanzapine was measured in plasma and milk with high-performance liquid chromatography over a dose interval (for six patients) and olanzapine was below the level of detection in the plasma of these babies. All infants were healthy and displayed no adverse effects.

Friedman (2003) studied one baby whose mother took olanzapine 5 mg from the third trimester and during breastfeeding. Her infant was large for gestational age and had Erb's palsy (which resolved), and it remained healthy at six months.

In another study of a single infant breastfed for 2 months during maternal intake of 10 mg per day. No abnormalities were found in growth and development during 11 months of follow up (Kirchheiner 2000). A poster presentation by Goldstein (2002) reported on the exposure of 23 infants – four had adverse events reported – two deemed unrelated to olanzapine. The other two cases were judged to be possibly related: somnolence, diarrhoea and nappy rash in one infant, and lethargy, poor suck-ing and shaking in a post-mature infant.

The relative infant dose of 1.2% is well below the 10% level that is accepted to be safe. There are small studies (n<23), but the results appear to indicate that the amount transferred into breastmilk is low and the babies have remained healthy during the study period of up to 11 months.

So we have information on the amount of drug transferred (low), incidence of side effects (low) and a few limited longitudinal studies.

Balancing this information with the needs of Christine, the wishes of the parents that the baby continues to be breastfed, and the potential risks of formula, we can develop the polarity map.

Positive for continued breastfeeding	*Positive for formula*
• Mother's wish • Continued advantages of breastmilk for mother and baby • Baby unwilling to feed from a bottle • Reduced risk of atopy	• Limited passage of drug to the baby • Professional responsibility (the responsibility is to balance risk and benefit with the knowledge gained from reference sources) • Safety of baby (may be greater risk of atopy with formula)
Breastfeeding with medicine	**Formula**
• Passage of drug to baby appears limited from research • Professional accountability – data to evaluate risk are available • Baby's health may be jeopardised (low risk)	• Mother's wish to continue to breastfeed • Loss of advantages of breastmilk to mother and baby • Difficulties in changing feeding method for mother and baby
Negative aspects of continued breastfeeding	*Negative aspects of formula*

This information may enable us to discuss with the parents what the potential risks are to the baby of exposing it to an unlicensed drug (and what that means), and what the potential risks of substituting formula are. We can then take professional responsibility for that decision, the reasons for which should be clearly documented in the patient's notes for clarification and to inform any other practitioners who become involved subsequently.

Involving the parents in decision-making

Using any drug during pregnancy or breastfeeding has a background risk. The final decision to take the medicine may be said to be the mothers, if she has been provided with sufficient information, given in a form, which she can access and comprehend.

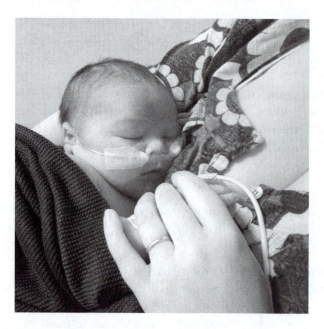

The relative risks of all of the options need to be explored in the mother's own individual circumstances, bearing in mind the severity of her illness and the maturity of her baby.

It should be borne in mind that each mother and baby pair is unique and that no two consultations with regards to a medicine taken during breastfeeding will be the same. Below are other examples taken from real-life queries, of how information might be provided to the mother and how this might affect her decision on whether or not to continue breastfeeding or take a particular drug.

Kelly's story

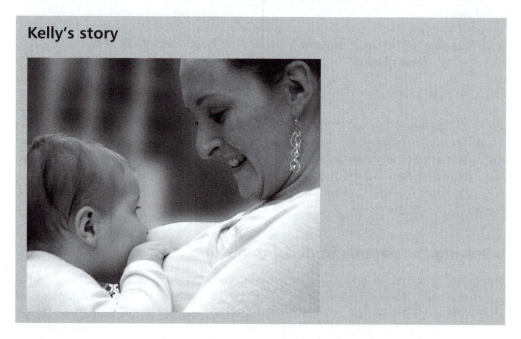

Kelly is 40 years old and the mother of a 15-month-old Jack. She has just been diagnosed with cancer of the bowel and is about to undergo a combination of radiotherapy and chemotherapy with fluorouracil. She understands that she needs to interrupt breastfeeding while actively having intravenous infusions of chemotherapy. She is also aware that she may feel very tired and low afterwards, but would very much like to resume breastfeeding if possible between courses of chemotherapy as she and Jack enjoy the experience.

Fluorouracil is an anti-metabolite and there is no data on the transfer of the drug into breastmilk. There are metabolites with long half-life (Hale 2012 online access), so it would be unwise to jeopardise the safety of Jack by attempting to continue to breastfeed.

However, Kelly needs to be counselled about the benefits and risks in this situation. It is vital that she receives her optimal therapy to increase her survival chances, but to dismiss her wish to continue to breastfeed would be unfair in her vulnerable situation. She would benefit from understanding the risks of the drug to Jack, discussing the benefits of the therapy for her, allowing her to reach her own decision that there is no alternative. Unfortunately, in many such situations mothers are abruptly told that the baby no longer benefits from breastmilk, and is left without discussion and understanding, to stop breastfeeding before the therapy begins.

Louise's story

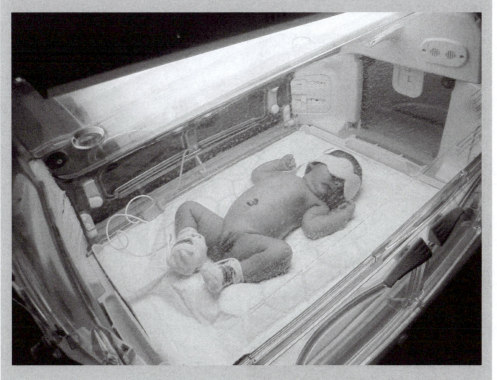

Louise has just given birth to a 28-week gestation baby who is having breathing difficulties and is currently on a respirator in the special care baby unit (SCBU). Long term, she has taken 5 mg three times a day of diazepam initially for panic attacks but is now dependent on it. She wants to breastfeed and the unit are keen for her baby to receive breastmilk because of the risk of necrotising enterocolitis.

Diazepam has a long half-life and an active metabolite desmethyldiazepam (Hale 2012 online access; Lactmed 2012; Martindale 2005), which may accumulate, particularly in a baby who is premature with immature renal and hepatic function. It can also produce lethargy, sedation and poor suckling. In view of the health of the baby already, exposure to diazepam through breastmilk may produce additional risks.

Louise is very keen to breastfeed but realises that she is putting her baby at risk from exposure to the diazepam. After discussion with the staff, it is arranged that she will receive cognitive behaviour therapy to help her deal with her panic attacks while she slowly discontinues the drug. In the meantime, she will be helped to maintain her lactation – pumping and dumping her milk – and her baby will receive donor breastmilk until Louise is able to stop taking diazepam.

The support of Louise and her baby would involve multi-disciplinary teamworking – supporting both Louise and her baby but would have health benefits for both of them, over and above the benefits of breastfeeding.

Information on the use of medication from the mother's viewpoint

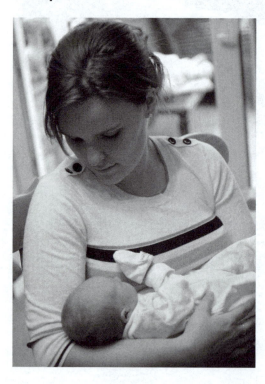

In the 1995 study (Jones 2000), 56.5% of mothers reported receiving some form of medication in the first five days of their baby's life, the majority of these perhaps, not surprisingly, being analgesics. Once discharged from hospital, 54.9% were prescribed medicines by their GP and 53.7% had purchased a drug from a pharmacy while they were breastfeeding.

Comments made by the mothers buying medicines from their local community pharmacy were diverse.

> I returned from Spain with Campylobacter and was ill for 3 weeks; the pharmacist was very thorough and advised just one dose of loperamide. I needed more but could not and did not take it. I had to put up with it and wait for it to get out of my system.

One wonders on what basis the pharmacist made the recommendation for one single dose? The BNF states 'amount probably too small to be harmful'. There was no reason that the mother could not have continued the medication to alleviate her symptoms.

> I had conjunctivitis and I asked the chemist if I could use eye drops and he said no.

The transfer of eye drops into breastmilk is likely to be very low and the only concerns raised have been around beta-blockers e.g. timolol. There is no evidence to support restriction of antibacterial eye drops. The most likely explanation is that the pharmacist looked up chloramphenicol and assumed that the warning of bone marrow toxicity applied to the eye drops as well as oral preparations.

> The pharmacist advised that what I was buying was OK but without checking; the leaflet inside said it was not OK to take whilst breastfeeding.

The impact of patient information leaflets would appear to have added confusion in this case. Where manufacturers have not included safety during breastfeeding in their licence application, a statement advising against use or referral to a doctor must be included. It may be that the pharmacist was correct but the contradiction in the form of written information over-rode his input in the view of the mother who assumed he was incorrect. It is perhaps interesting to note her comment that he did not check adding to her belief in the written information.

Professional decisions and liability

As has already been stated, the literature contains little information on which to base clinical judgements. If a healthcare professional provides information to a parent about the safety of a drug to be used by a breastfeeding mother outside of the drug's licence application, they must be prepared to take professional responsibility for that information. It may be advisable to record the sources consulted and information provided to the parent so that in the event of any later queries full documentation of the event is available. It is now commonplace for professionals to be held accountable for the information or perceived 'advice' given because of the limitations of information available when the licence application is undertaken.

Phrasing of information to parents

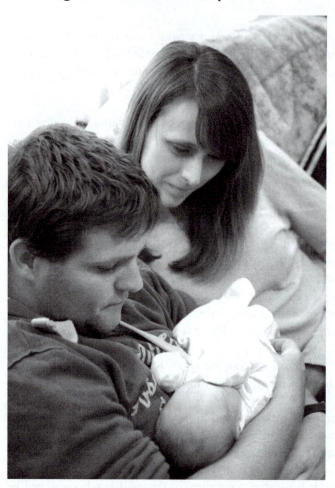

The way in which information is presented has a considerable impact on the way in which it is perceived. For instance, a teratology risk of 3% is reported as being seen as less acceptable than a 97% chance of having an unaffected baby (Jasper 2001). This has a parallel with the food industry stating 'only 3% fat' or '97% fat free'.

It is also important that information is presented to the parents at a level commensurate with their understanding and that medical jargon and abbreviations are avoided. The perception of information can also be altered by facts picked up from other sources such as the media, positive or negative influences of family and friends and in the light of their own personal experiences to date. There are very few instances when an instant answer is essential and a delay to check facts is preferable.

Counselling skills

The dictionary definitions of 'counsel' are: the act of exchanging opinions and ideas/consultation; advice or guidance, especially as solicited from a knowledgeable person; and to recommend.

The British Association for Counselling & Psychotherapy (British Association for Counselling & Psychotherapy 2012) definition of counselling is that:

> Counselling takes place when a counsellor sees a client in a private and confidential setting to explore a difficulty the client is having, distress they may be experiencing or perhaps their dissatisfaction with life, or loss of a sense of direction and purpose. It is always at the request of the client. Counselling is a way of enabling choice or change or of reducing confusion. It does not involve giving advice or directing a client to take a particular course of action.

In this context, counselling skills are those involved with listening to the patient rather than the provision of information or advice, a role with which healthcare professionals are more familiar. It has a common base with many of the principles underlying concordance, ensuring agreement with the patient on the action, which shall be taken.

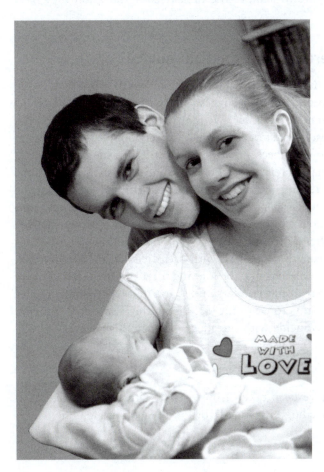

Counselling involves listening to the patient in a non-judgmental and empathetic manner. The skills of reflection and clarification of information heard are important to ensure that the patient, in this case mother, is able to explore the dilemmas of her situation fully. Counselling in its purest form is very difficult in most situations within a healthcare setting. What is possible is empathetic listening and the provision of information on which to base future actions. Being aware of body language may also allow the practitioner to judge the way that the patient has received the information. For example she may avoid eye contact as a means of ignoring the information or may turn away to block the discussion. Alternatively she may visibly relax, smile and make good eye contact if she is receptive to advice.

Mothers receive feeding advice and information from a variety of sources. They generally trust the information and expertise of healthcare professionals but can become concerned if their baby does not appear to fit the 'norms' described by the experts. So having a baby who feeds more frequently than has been suggested, may lead a mother to perceive her breastmilk as deficient in quality or quantity. Breastfeeding exclusively for six months may appear extremely difficult in the face of significant problems. Not only do these mothers need correct information, they need a supportive and empathetic approach which involves listening to their concerns and acknowledging concerns if they are to achieve the breastfeeding duration they have chosen (Shealy *et al.* 2008).

How is counselling different from medical advice?

Healthcare practitioners are used to providing advice, a solution to a problem based on their judgement of the situation. We may suggest alternatives and provide some explanation to enable patients to make a choice. We may explain why we see a particular course of action is in the best interest of the patient. Rarely do we ask patients at any length what they want to do and check how the options feel to them.

When we are considering scenarios relating to breastfeeding and particularly to the use of medication during breastfeeding we need to understand the viewpoint of the mother. It may seem simple to advise her to stop breastfeeding without taking into consideration that milk supply does not cease instantly. We may also forget that the act of feeding from a bottle is different from sucking at the breast and may not be easy for a baby. We may ignore the feelings associated with breastfeeding for that mother. It is as important to acknowledge that she may be looking for a reason to stop but we cannot assume that is true. We may need to understand that a mother feeding an older child may feel strongly that she wants to wean the child from the breast at a mutually convenient time which may not coincide with our ideas of when this time is.

Scenarios

All of the following scenarios have been taken from real-life situations according to phone calls taken on the Breastfeeding Network Drugs in Breastmilk Helpline.

Scenario 1

A doctor decides that Amy with an 8-week-old baby, exclusively breastfed baby needs drug x to treat her current medical condition. He looks in his immediately available reference sources and tells her: 'there is no information on the safety of this drug according to the manufacturers so you need to stop breastfeeding now. After all the baby is 8 weeks old now, you've given him a good start and the goodness of the milk is less now so he would be better on the bottle, wouldn't he? So here's the prescription, everything clear, good, fine. Thank you. Goodbye.'

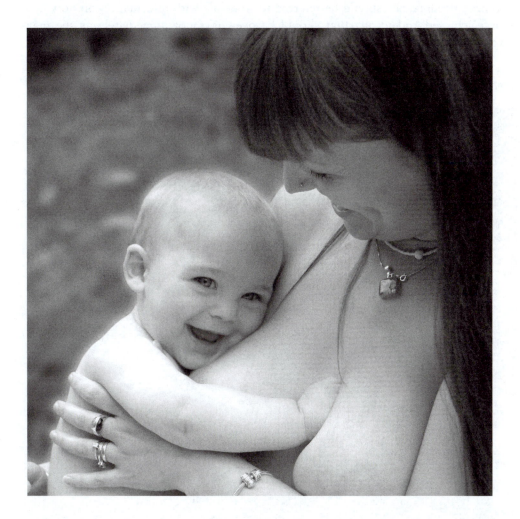

Amy leaves the surgery somewhat confused. Is it true that she has to stop breastfeeding? Are there alternative sources of information other than the drug manufacturer? Is there an alternative drug she could have and carry on breastfeeding? What if she doesn't take the drug? Is it true that her milk has no goodness left after 8 weeks? How does she stop breastfeeding?

The answer to Amy's questions depends on the condition for which she is being treated. The manufacturer is unlikely to have licensed the drug, as clinical trials are not mandatory and would be unethical. We can consult the BNF for Children. If a drug is licensed or used outside of license to treat children, it is likely to be safe in levels passing through breastmilk. We can look at the pharmacokinetic data and assess the risk to the baby. Frequently there are alternative drugs about which we do have more safety data.

The statement that her breastmilk has no residual goodness is factually inaccurate: breastmilk continues to have goodness for 2 years and beyond. If Amy does need to stop breastfeeding, she should be referred to someone with information on how this is best achieved and ideally that should be over days not immediately as she may develop engorgement or mastitis.

Scenario 2

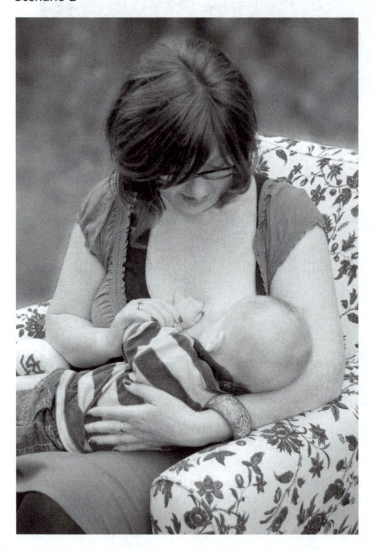

Dr Brown tells Annabel who has a 3-month-old baby: 'I think this is the best drug to treat you, we don't know a lot about how much gets through to the baby though I know some women have taken it. Quite honestly I wouldn't let my wife breastfeed on it but it is up to you. If you want to carry on breastfeeding it's up to you.'

Dr Brown has used specific advice and subtle cues, which as Anderson (2003) comments may shorten the duration of breastfeeding in the face of medication prescribed.

Scenario 3

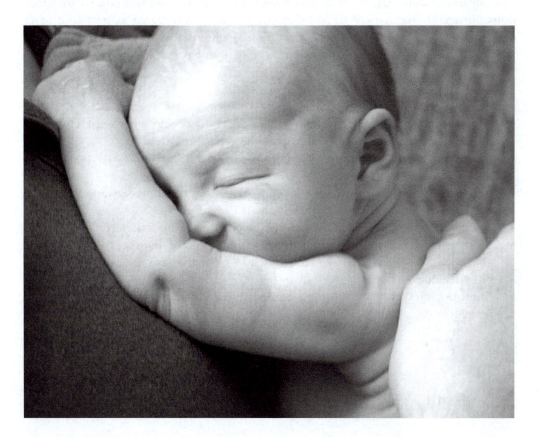

Susan has gone to see Dr Stewart. He has suggested that she needs a drug but admits that he does not know what effect it may have on baby Jack who is only 2 weeks old.

Susan is keen to carry on breastfeeding as Jack is doing well and she has ulcerative colitis herself, which she knows can be linked with formula milk (mothers with ulcerative colitis pass on a genetic predisposition to their children to develop the condition and it is also linked with being formula fed in infancy) (Klement *et al.* 2004). Dr Stewart says that he will check with the local pharmacist and telephone her later. He gives her a prescription but tells her not to get it dispensed until he calls her. He calls the local community pharmacist who in turn consults the local medicines information service. They decide that drug b would be just as effective because it has more safety data. Dr Stewart telephones Susan and advises her to collect a different prescription but to be aware that drug b may cause some loose bowel motions for Jack but that this is not harmful. After discussion Susan opts to wait and see if her condition improves without medication but will collect drug b if she needs to.

In this case Dr Stewart takes time to consider the prescribing decision and consults more widely. The team find a suitable drug but have some concerns for the baby. Loose bowel motions would be inconvenient but not dangerous but given the option Susan chooses to wait. This is a good example of multi-professional working and support for the mother who is allowed to take the final decision on her treatment.

Counselling skills may seem time-consuming in primary and secondary care situations but enable the patient to feel that she has been considered as part of a team deciding on the optimal treatment. Lactation is one of the few situations where a prescribing decision has implications on more than one person.

Key points

- Use of a polarity map may help practitioners to decide whether it is safe to prescribe a specific drug for a mother while she is breastfeeding.
- Mothers may see the decision-making process in a different way to a healthcare professional.
- Active listening skills may be employed to help a mother to understand the risk of prescribing a medication to her while she is breastfeeding.
- The risks of prescribing during lactation depend on information available.
- Mothers may need to feel part of the prescribing decision in order to feel comfortable with any perceived risks to their child from the drug or the need to stop breastfeeding.
- Multi-disciplinary team working has advantages for all professionals and the patient.

Part II
The safety of drugs in breastmilk

Chapter 8

Information on level of drugs into breastmilk

It is not the purpose of this book to produce a definitive reference manual of the transfer of *all* drugs into breastmilk. The aim is to link an understanding of the health implications of lack of breastmilk, the mechanism of breastfeeding and general information on the safety of drugs in breastmilk into one accessible volume for healthcare professionals, volunteers and mothers.

The information for the passage of drugs into breastmilk has been taken from a variety of sources including Medications and Mothers' Milk (Hale 2012 online access), LactMed (2012 online access), Martindale:the Complete Drug Reference 35th edition (2007), the BNF and the Children's BNF (2012 online access), and from the National Electronic Library for Medicines (2012 online access) and PubMed searches (US National Library of Health online access), but analysed in light of the experience of running the Breastfeeding Network Drugs in Breastmilk Helpline over the past 16 years.

There can be no substitute for individual decision-making, taking into account the mother and child to be exposed to medication. This information is intended as a guide with supporting references and pharmacokinetic datawhere available. Limitations of licensing application should not be seen as evidence of risk but as a limitation of the present drug-licensing system requirements.

It is important to remember that the presence of a drug in breastmilk does not usually equate to meaningful risk to the baby. Drugs are also metabolised by the infant and oral bio-availability, first-pass metabolism and prevention of gastric absorption due to the presence of milk all affect the potency of the drug. It is useful to compare the level with what could be given directly to the baby if it is used to treat children. Very few, if any, drugs passing through breastmilk attain a minimum effective concentration to produce a therapeutic effect.

The risk of a drug passing into breastmilk is not the same as the teratogenic risk of a drug given in pregnancy. However, having become accustomed to avoiding any substance which might be detrimental to the health of the developing foetus, it is often difficult for mothers and healthcare professionals to recognise this. Adverse reactions, such as drowsiness following the use of sedating centrally acting drugs, or apparent diarrhoea with antibiotics, resolve when the mother's therapy ceases. Mothers may also perceive that their milk is contaminated by a drug and choose not to breastfeed during the course of treatment as has already been discussed.

The use of drug in lactation would be greatly simplified by the wider availability of information and post-marketing licence application by manufacturers. This probably requires governmental intervention to produce. In 2005, the US Centers for Disease Control and Prevention (CDC) issued a statement calling for comprehensive, co-ordinated dissemination on the information of safety of drugs in breastmilk (Lagoy 2005).

In May 2008, the US Food and Drug Administration proposed major revisions to the labelling of prescription drugs to provide better information about the effects of medicines used during pregnancy and breastfeeding (FDA 2012). This action followed recognition during the 1990s that the shortcomings of pregnancy and breastfeeding information in prescription drug labelling (information supplied to healthcare professionals which might be adapted for use on patient information leaflets). In February 2011, the final rule was under discussion with a proposal that the lactation section of the labelling should contain the following: If a mother is taking multiple drugs the individual and additive effect on the baby should be borne in mind, particularly in a neonate.

Risk summary

- If appropriate, include a statement that the use of the drug is compatible with breastfeeding.
- Effects of the drug on milk production.
- Whether the drug is present in human milk (and if so, how much).
- The effect of the drug on the breastfed child.

Clinical considerations

- Ways to minimize exposure to the breastfed child, such as timing or pumping and discarding milk.
- Potential drug effects in the child and recommendations for monitoring or responding to these effects.
- Dosing adjustment during lactation.

Data

- Overview of data on which risk summary and clinical considerations are based.

If this were adopted in the UK, prescribing during lactation would be become far less of a dilemma for healthcare professionals. Women who are taking medication need to be informed of the known or possible side effects for which they need to monitor the infant e.g. drowsiness, diarrhoea. They need to know when it is important that these are reported to the prescriber, when the drug needs to be stopped and when the effect is expected and therefore of less significance.

The National Institute for Health and Clinical Excellence (NICE) Maternal and Child Nutrition PH Guideline 11 (NICE PH11 2008) recommended that practitioners should discuss the benefits and risks associated with prescribed medication and encourage the mother to continue breastfeeding. Furthermore, it recommended that Appendix 5 of the BNF should be used only as a guide as it does not contain quantitative data on which to base individual decisions (this appendix has now been incorporated into the individual drug monographs).

This text is intended to assist practitioners in understanding the depth of information available from a variety of sources and how this may be used to inform the use of medication outside of its licence application. The information in this section has been organised to reflect the chapters in the BNF but refers to only the most commonly used drugs. Information has been taken from texts including the Children's BNF but where possible a simple recommendation on safety and adverse effects to be aware of has been made.

It is not possible to provide information on every drug in a book of this type. It is hoped that practitioners can use the reference sources cited to make their own professional decisions on the safety of alternative drugs or use ones on which more safety datais currently available.

Sources used to compile this information

In analysing the safety of the drugs referenced in this chapter I have used specialist sources and texts. Some of the books are standard reference texts e.g. BNF and Martindale. Other sites and authors work dedicated to the safety of drugs in lactation that I have found to be invaluable are described in more detail below.

LactMed

LactMed (Drugs and Lactation data base) is a freely available, web-based data base. Its primary author and founder is Philip O Anderson, PharmD, FASHP. Dr Anderson is a Health Sciences Clinical Professor of Pharmacy at the University of California San Diego Skaggs School of Pharmacy and Pharmaceutical Sciences. The data are peer reviewed by a panel of experts. The entries are fully referenced with links to PubMed abstracts in the majority of cases. The information is organised into a summary, maternal and infant drug levels, effects on breastfed infants, effects on lactation and alternative drugs. LactMed is one specialist area of the National Electronic Library of Medicine and Toxnet. It is available as an app for smart phones.

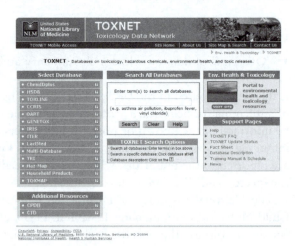

Medications and Mothers' Milk

This book, now in its 15th edition (2012), has been produced by Dr Thomas Hale, who is Professor of Pediatrics, Texas Tech University School of Medicine, is a respected world expert on the safety of drugs in breastmilk. Dr Hale also has founded the InfantRisk Centre, a call centre that provides evidence-based information on the safety of drugs in pregnancy and breastfeeding. It also acts as a training centre for medical and pharmacy students as well as conducting clinical research. It operates a helpline on nausea and vomiting in pregnancy, alcohol and substance misuse and depression, in addition to answering calls on drugs in pregnancy and lactation. As executive director, Dr Hale is supported by several other specialists. The textbook is updated approximately every two years, but also has an online data base accessible via subscription. The InfantRisk (www.infantrisk.com/) centre also operates a searchable discussion forum for parents and healthcare professionals.

Motherisk

Motherisk is based at The Hospital for Sick Children in Toronto and is affiliated to the Organization of Teratology Information Specialists (www.otispregnancy.org/) having been founded initially to provide information on drugs in pregnancy. It has provided training for others to set up similar services worldwide under the mentorship of Assistant Director Adrienne Einarson. It provides helplines on alcohol and substance misuse, morning sickness, HIV as well as the safety of drugs in pregnancy and lactation. It has an interactive website which provides links to many of its published papers. It educates many healthcare professionals each year as well as conducting and publishing research.

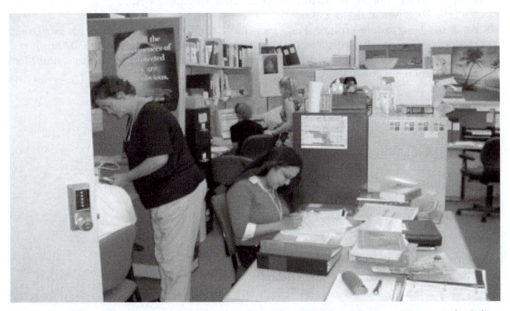

Motherisk Office, photograph taken in 2005 by author showing Adrienne Einerson (far left)

BNF

The recommendation on use of drugs during breastfeeding (accessed March 2012) is included within the text of each drug for reference purposes only. Frequently the information contains a comment on the manufacturer's recommendation that the drug is not used during breastfeeding, as is often repeated in the patient information leaflet. Information within the text provides an evidence base where possible for use during lactation or pharmacokinetic factors which influence the transfer into breastmilk.

The British National Formulary for Children (BNFC)

Any drug which is licensed for use in children is likely to be safe for use by a breast-feeding mother. Levels reached in breastfed infants following maternal consumption are unlikely to reach therapeutic levels (see Figure 6.7, p. 80). It may be possible to compare the theoretical infant dose with the recommended infant dose.

References

British National Formulary, British Medical Association, Royal Pharmaceutical Society, London.

British National Formulary, Children, British Medical Association, Royal Pharmaceutical Society, London.

Hale T, Medications and Mothers' Milk, 2012.

LactMed (http:toxnet.nlm.nih.gov/cgi-bin/sis/htmlgen?LACT).

Lagoy CT, Joshi N, Cragan JD, Rasmussen SA, Report from the CDC: medication use during pregnancy and lactation: an urgent call for public health action, *J Women's Health*, 2005;14:104–9.

Martindale: the Complete Drug Reference 35th edition, London: Pharmaceutical Press, 2007.

National Electronic Library for Medicines NHS (www.nelm.nhs.uk/en).

NICE PH11 2008 (www.nice.org.uk).

US Food and Drug Administration Pregnancy and Lactation Labelling (www.fda.gov/Drugs/DevelopmentApprovalProcess/DevelopmentResourcesperlitreabeling/ucm093307.htm)

US National Library of Medicine, National Institutes of Health (PubMed) (www.ncbi.nlm.nih.gov/pubmed).

Key:

Compatible with breastfeeding   ☺

Avoid during breastfeeding   ☹

Use with care during breastfeeding –
may be associated with some side effects   (?)

Gastro-intestinal system

Antacids

Brand names: *Maalox®*, *Mucogel®*, *Milk of Magnesia®*, *Rennie Rap-Eze®*, *Settlers®*

> **Antacid of choice for mother during breastfeeding based on evidence of benefit and safety for the baby:**
>
> **All antacids are safe during breastfeeding**
> **Choose according to personal preference**

Many women take antacids in the latter stages of pregnancy to overcome the reflux of acid caused by the pressure of the baby in the abdomen. Antacids are also used to treat occasional symptoms of acidity, to reduce heartburn or symptoms associated with gastro-oesophageal reflux (GORD). Dyspepsia often resolves with lifestyle changes.

Aluminium, magnesium and calcium antacids

Simple antacids are composed of a combination of aluminium, magnesium and calcium salts all of which reduce gastric acidity. There is little evidence of effectiveness compared with alginates. Antacids may have peppermint or spearmint flavour added, both of which have historically been used as carminatives. Antacids do not alter the volume of hydrochloric acid produced and rebound secretion may occur in response to an increase in gastric pH.

Aluminium-containing antacids may produce a constipating action if consumed in excess e.g. aluminium hydroxide.

Magnesium-containing products may produce a laxative action if consumed in excess e.g. magnesium trisilicate, magnesium hydroxide (*Milk of Magnesia*).

Calcium-containing antacids generally rely on the neutralising properties of calcium carbonate (*Rennie Rap-Eze®*, *Settlers®*). Many products contain a mixture of ingredients.

> Compatible with breastfeeding – None of the ingredients in antacids are likely to pass into breastmilk as they only act locally to neutralise gastric hydrochloric acid. All antacids can be used during breastfeeding.

Simeticone (activated dimeticone)

Brand names: *Altacite Plus®*, *Asilone®*, *Windcheaters® Maalox Plus®*, *Rennie Deflatine®*, *Remegel Wind Relief®*
US Brands: *Advanced Formula Di-Gel®*, *Alamag Plus®*
Australian brands: *Alucone®*, *De-Gas Extra®*

Simeticone is used to relieve flatulence and abdominal discomfort due to wind. It causes bubbles of gas in the gastro-intestinal (GI) tract to coalesce, aiding dispersion of wind. It is often combined with antacids. It is used alone in paediatric products to relive colic pains in babies e.g. Infacol® (see section on colic).

> Compatible with breastfeeding – Simeticone can be taken during lactation. No effects are likely to be seen in the breastfed infant as it is not absorbed from the gut. It is also used directly in infants to relieve colic.

Alginates

Brand names: *Gaviscon Advance®, Peptac®, Rennie Duo®*

> **Alginate of choice for mother during breastfeeding based on evidence of benefit and safety for the baby:**
>
> **All alginates are safe during breastfeeding**
> **Choose according to personal preference and cost**

Alginates form a pH neutral raft on top of the food contents of the stomach in order to prevent regurgitation and heartburn resulting from irritation of the oesophagus. They are poorly absorbed from the GI tract (15 to 30%) and can be taken during lactation without risk to the baby.

> Compatible with use during breastfeeding – Infant Gaviscon® is also given directly to infants to relieve symptoms of reflux.

Anti-spasmodics

> **Anti-spasmodic of choice for mother during breastfeeding based on evidence of benefit and safety for the baby:**
>
> **Mebeverine or peppermint oil – or if these are ineffective, hyoscine hydrombromide**

Anti-spasmodics are used to relieve the spasmodic pain of irritable bowel syndrome (IBS). IBS can present as abdominal pain with constipation or diarrhoea. Taking anti-muscarinic drugs e.g. dicloverine before food as required may relieve abdominal pain in IBS by reducing intestinal mobility. Smooth muscle relaxants e.g. alverine directly relax intestinal smooth muscle. This drug group may also be useful in relieving symptoms of diverticular disease.

Alverine

Brand name: *Relaxyl®, Spasmonal®*
US brand:
Australian brand: *Alvercol®*

Alverine is widely used to treat symptoms of IBS, but one study shows that it was no better than placebo in providing relief of symptoms (Mitchell 2002). It is licensed for use in patients over the age of 12 years. There is no information on its passage into breastmilk.

The BNF states that limited information is available and that the manufacturer advises it is avoided during breastfeeding.

> Avoid if possible as no information on passage into breastmilk.
> Peppermint Oil or mebeverine are preferable, based on limited research on other drugs.

References

Mitchell SA, Mee AS, Smith GD, Palmer KR, Chapman RW, Alverine citrate fails to relieve the symptoms of irritable bowel syndrome: results of a double-blind, randomized, placebo-controlled trial, *Aliment Pharmacol Ther*, 2002;16:1187–95.

Dicycloverine (dicyclomine) ☹

Brand names: *Merbentyl®, Kolanticon®*
US brand: *Antispas®, Dibent®*
Australian brand: *Merbentyl®*

Dicycloverine (dicyclomine) is an anti-muscarinic drug. In the past it was used to treat infantile colic but following reports of apnoea, its licence for use in infants under 6 months was withdrawn. The adverse reactions occurred in babies under the age of 6 weeks and involved sudden reactions following administration of the drug via a spoon. All children recovered normally (Williams 1994; Edwards 1984; Spoudeas and Shribman 1984). There is also a single case report of a similar reaction in a 12-day-old breastfed baby whose mother took this drug (personal communication reported in Briggs 2005), so it is a drug best avoided in lactation since there are alternative preparations available.

Relative infant dose is quoted as 7% (Hale 2012 online access). Dose for children aged 6 months to 2 years is 5 to 10 mg three or four times daily before feeds (BNFC). The BNF states that it is present in milk, that it should be avoided as apnoea has been reported in an infant.

> Avoid if possible during breastfeeding as has been linked to apnoea in a young baby in one case report. Mebeverine or peppermint oil are preferable, based on limited research on other drugs.

References

Edwards PDL, Dicyclomine in babies, *BMJ*, 1984;288:1230.
Reported as personal communication in Briggs GG, Freeman RK, Yaffe SJ, *Drugs in pregnancy and lactation, 7th ed.*, Baltimore: Williams & Wilkins, 2005

Spoudeas H, Shribman S, Dicyclomine in babies, *BMJ*, 1984;288:1230.
Williams J, Watkin-Jones R, Dicyclomine: worrying symptoms associated with its use in some small babies, *BMJ*, 1984;288:901.

Hyoscine butylbromide

Brand name *Buscopan®*
US brands: *Pamine®*
Australian brands: *Buscopan®*

Hyoscine butylbromide is used to relieve spasms of the gut and colic. It has anti-muscarinic activity so may produce constipation, blurred vision, urinary retention as well as a dry mouth in the mother. It is poorly absorbed from the gut. No levels in breastmilk have been reported from studies. It is licensed at half the adult dose for children over 6 years (10 mg three times daily). Alternative preparations are available so it should be a third-line choice unless merbeverine and peppermint oil are ineffective.

The BNF and BNFC state that the amount secreted into breastmilk is too small to be harmful.

> Probably compatible with breastfeeding as it is licensed in children but there are no reports of levels in breastmilk from studies. BNF says amount is too small to be harmful.
> Peppermint oil or mebeverine are preferable based on limited research on other drugs.

Mebeverine

Brand name: *Colofac®*
US brands:
Australian brands: *Colese®, Colofac®*

Mebeverine is an anti-spasmodic with a direct action on the smooth muscle of the GI tract. It should be taken 20 minutes before meals. It is licensed for use in children above the age of three at a dose of 25 mg three times daily as an adjunct in GI disorders characterised by smooth muscle spasm (BNFC). It is 75% plasma protein bound.

> Compatible with breastfeeding. Licensed for use in children >3 years.

Peppermint oil

Brand name: *Colpermin®, Mintec®*
US brands:
Australian brands:

Peppermint oil is used to relieve abdominal colic and distension due to flatulence. It is an aromatic carminative. There is some evidence that peppermint oil can inhibit cytochrome P450 and may affect the clearance of drugs whose metabolism is mediated by this enzyme (Dresser 2002) so interactions should be borne in mind. Enteric-coated capsules are used to relieve spasms associated with irritable bowel disease but should be swallowed whole, half to one hour before food to avoid irritation of the oesophagus. There is some evidence to support the value of this product in therapy (Pittler and Ernst 1998; Grigoleit and Grigoleit 2005).

Peppermint oil is believed to undergo rapid first-pass metabolism. It is licensed for children over the age of 15 years. There have been anecdotal reports in internet discussions by lactation specialists in the US that it can reduce milk supply but there are currently no studies to prove or disprove these.

The BNF reports that significant levels of menthol in breastmilk are unlikely.

> Compatible with breastfeeding as undergoes rapid first-pass metabolism. Anecdotal reports of implication in low milk supply.

References

Dresser GK, Wacher V, Wong S, Wong HT, Bailey DG, Evaluation of peppermint oil and ascorbyl palmitate as inhibitors of cytochrome P4503A4 activity in vitro and in vivo, *Clin Pharmacol Ther*, 2002;72:247–55.

Grigoleit H-G, Grigoleit P, Peppermint oil in irritable bowel syndrome, *Phytomedicine*, 2005;12:601–6.

Pittler MH, Ernst E, Peppermint oil for irritable bowel syndrome: a critical review and meta-analysis, *Am J Gastroenterol*, 1998;93:1131–5.

H₂ antagonists

Histamine H$_2$-receptor antagonists reduce gastric acid secretion by blocking histamine H$_2$ receptors. They are used to relieve symptoms of GORD and may be used to relieve chronic indigestion. They are known to stimulate prolactin secretion and there have been some reports of gynaecomastasia with cimetidine (Delle Fave *et al.* 1977).

> H$_2$ antagonist of choice for mother during breastfeeding based on evidence of benefit and safety for the baby:
>
> **Ranitidine**

Reference

Delle Fave GF, Tamburrano G, De Magistris L, Natoli C, Santoro ML, Carratu R, Torsoli A, Gynaecomastia with cimetidine, *Lancet*, 1977;309:1319.

Cimetidine

Brand name: *Tagamet*®
Tagamet dual action® (with sodium alginate)

US brands: *Tagamet®*
Australian brands: *Hexal®, Magicul®, Tagamet®*

Cimetidine appears to be actively transported into breastmilk shown by high milk:plasma (m/p) ratios reportedly as high as 5.5 times higher than expected by passive diffusion (Ziemniak *et al.* 1984). Cimetidine binds to cytochrome 450 and potential interactions should be borne in mind.

In a detailed single patient study, Somogyi and Gugler (1979) estimated that even if every feed took place at the maximum milk concentration, the baby would receive only 6 mg per litre per day and no adverse events have been reported. Treatment of term neonates at 20 mg per kg has been suggested. Relative infant dose is quoted as 9.8 to 32.6% (Hale 2012 online access).

The BNF reports that there are significant amount present in milk but that it is not known to be harmful although the manufacturer advises it is avoided.

> Probably compatible with breastfeeding despite high m/p ratio; however, use of ranitidine is preferable.

References

Somogyi A, Gugler R, Cimetidine excretion into breastmilk, *Br J Clin Pharmacol*, 1979;7:627–9.
Ziemniak JA, Wynn RJ, Aranda JV, Zarowitz BJ, Schentag JJ, The pharmacokinetics and metabolism of cimetidine in neonates, *Dev Pharmacol Ther*, 1984;7:30–38.

Ranitidine

Brand name: *Zantac®, Gavalast®*
US brands: *Zantac®*
Australian brands: *Ausran®, Ranitic®, Ranoxyl®*

Although apparently concentrated in breastmilk (Kearns *et al.* 1985), ranitidine is only 50% orally bio-available so the overall level transferred into breastmilk is low. It does not affect cytochrome P450 and so produces fewer interactions (Smith and Kendall 1988). Ranitidine is given directly to babies to relieve reflux at a dose of 2 to 4 mg per kg per day (BNFC). Relative infant dose quoted as 1.3 to 4.6% (Hale 2012 online access). No adverse events in infants have been reported.

The BNF reports that significant amounts are present in milk, but are not known to be harmful.

> Compatible with breastfeeding because poorly bio-available. It is given directly to babies for severe reflux at up to ten times the level transferred via breastmilk.

References

Kearns GL, McConnell RF Jr, Trang JM, Kluza RB, Appearance of ranitidine in breastmilk following multiple dosing, *Clin Pharm*, 1985;4:322–4.

Smith SR, Kendall MJ, Ranitidine versus cimetidine: a comparison of their potential to cause clinically important drug interactions, *Clin Pharmacokinet*, 1988;15:44–56

Famotidine (?)

Brand name: *Pepcid*®, *Pepcid 2*® (with antacid)
US brands: *Pepcid*®
Australian brands: *Amfamox*®, *Ausfam*®, *Famohexal*®, *Pepcid*®, *Pepcidine*®, *Pepzan*®

Famotidine is an alternative H_2 antagonist with lower levels reaching breastmilk. Its oral bio-availability is 40 to 45% and it is weakly bound to plasma proteins. Reduced clearance has been shown in infants below 3 months given it directly (Wenning *et al.* 2005). It is not used in paediatric therapy in the UK (BNFC). Courtney *et al.*'s study of eight women (1988) showed a peak level of drug at 6 hours and an infant dose of 0.01 mg per kg per day following a maternal dose of 40 mg.

The BNF reports that it is present in milk but that it is not known to be harmful although the manufacturer advises it is avoided.

> Use ranitidine as preferred drug in this class since there is reduced clearance of famotidine in infants less than 3 months of age.

References

Courtney TP, Shaw RW, Cedar E, *et al.* Excretion of famotidine in breastmilk, *Br J Clin Pharmacol*, 1988;26:639P.

Wenning LA, Murphy MG, James LP, Blumer JL, Marshall JD, Baier J, Scheimann AO, Panebianco DL, Zhong L, Eisenhandler R, Yeh KC, Kearns GL, Pharmacokinetics of famotidine in infants, *Clin Pharmacokinet*, 2005;44:395–406.

Proton pump inhibitors (PPIs)

> **PPI of choice for mother during breastfeeding based on evidence of benefit and safety for the baby:**
>
> Omeprazole

Proton-pump inhibitors (PPIs) are more effective than H_2 antagonists in healing and relieving the symptoms of oesophagitis. They inhibit the secretion of gastric acid by irreversibly blocking the enzyme system of the gastric parietal cell. They can be used to reduce symptoms of dyspepsia, and GORD, in gastro protection with non-steroidal anti-inflammatory drugs (NSAIDs) and in *Helicobacter pylori* eradication.

Omeprazole

Brand name *Losec*®
US brands: *Prilosec*®, *Zegerid*®
Australian brands: *Losec*®, *Meprazol*®, *Probitor*®

Omeprazole is rapidly destroyed in acid conditions of the stomach below pH 4. It is also given to infants to treat severe gastric reflux.

It is 95% bound to plasma proteins. It is not licensed for use in children below one year but is used outside of its license application at a dose of 700 µg per kg per day for reflux compared with an estimated dose through breastmilk of 3 µg per kg per day passing through breastmilk in the study of one mother (Marshall *et al.* 1998). It is metabolised by the cytochrome P450 system so potential interactions are possible. The BNF reports that it is present in milk but that it is not known to be harmful.

> Compatible with breastfeeding as destroyed at pH <4. Used directly in children with severe reflux.

References

Marshall JK, Thompson AB, Armstrong D, Omeprazole for refractory gastroesophageal reflux disease during pregnancy and lactation, *Can J Gastroenterol*, 1998;12:225–7.

Lansoprazole

Brand name: *Zoton*®
US brands: *Prevacid*®
Australian brands: *Zoton*®

Presumed safe to use during breastfeeding due to instability in gastric acid although there are no studies on levels in breastmilk. Omeprazole is preferred drug in this class.

Lansoprazole is unstable in stomach acid and will be destroyed in the infant's stomach. It is not licensed for use in children but doses of 0.5 to 1 mg per kg daily are used outside of licence application (BNFC). There are no studies of the passage into breastmilk but theoretical absorption from breastmilk is likely to be minimal. Its structural similarity to omeprazole makes it unlikely to cause adverse effects in breastfed babies. The BNF states that it is present in milk in animal studies and that the manufacturer advises it should be avoided.

Rabeprazole

Brand name: *Pariet*®
US brands: *Aciphex*®
Australian brands: *Pariet*®

There is no data on the transfer of rabeprazole into breastmilk although animal studies suggest a high m/p ratio. The relevance to humans is unclear. It is 97% plasma protein bound and it is extensively metabolised in the liver by cytochrome P450 and undergoes degradation by stomach acid if not enteric coated. It also undergoes first-pass metabolism. These factors suggest it should be compatible with breastfeeding although other safer options with more safety data on use in lactation exist. The BNF states that the manufacturer advises it should be avoided as there is no information available on the amount secreted into breastmilk.

> Probably compatible with breastfeeding although there are no studies on levels in breastmilk. Omeprazole is preferred drug in this class.

Esomeprazole

Brand name: *Nexium*®
US brands: *Nexium*®
Australian brands: *Nexium*®

Esomeprazole is the *S*-isomer of omeprazole and although there are no studies on the passage into breastmilk, it seems reasonable to assume transfer is likely to be insignificant. The BNF states that the manufacturer advises it should be avoided as there is no information available on the amount secreted into breastmilk.

> Probably compatible with breastfeeding as it is an isomer of omeprazole, although there are no studies on levels in breastmilk. Omeprazole is preferred drug in this class.

Anti-diarrhoea medication

> **Drug of choice to treat diarhoea in a mother during breastfeeding based on evidence of benefit and safety for the baby:**
>
> **Loperamide and/or rehydration therapy**

Diarrhoea can lead to dehydration, excess water and electrolyte loss. Optimal treatment is oral rehydration. Acute diarrhoea is generally self-limiting and may be seen as the body's attempt to rid itself of the infection. However, many people are unwilling to put up with the inconvenience of frequent, watery stools for more than a short period. Breastfeeding mothers may be concerned that their milk will dry up if their own symptoms of diarrhoea are not treated quickly. Mothers should be encouraged to drink according to thirst and to take rehydrating solutions in addition to anti-motility agents if there is excess fluid loss. Careful hygiene is important but there is no reason to stop breastfeeding if the mother has diarrhoea as she will pass on antibodies to the infection to her baby via the entero-mammary pathway.

  Rehydration products are suitable for artificially fed infants in addition to formula milk during episodes of diarrhoea. Breastfeeding should be continued freely and should not be replaced by rehydration fluids. Exclusively breastfed babies have a very low risk of diarrhoea.

Rehydration therapy

Brand name: *Dioralyte®, Electrolade®*

Rehydration solution sachets contain balanced levels of sugar and salts to correct the electrolyte and fluid balance. They would not affect breastfed babies as no significant levels would be passed into breastmilk. They may prevent dehydration of the mother with severe diarrhoea.

> Compatible with use during breastfeeding as they only restore normal electrolyte balance.

Loperamide

Brand name: *Imodium®, Imodium Plus®* (with simeticone)
US brands: *Neo-Diaral®, Pepto diarrhoea control®*
Australian brands: *Gastro-Stop®, Harmonise®*

Loperamide provides symptomatic relief of diarrhoea by inhibiting gut motility. Only small amounts are found in breastmilk as it is poorly absorbed (Nikodem and Hofmeyr 1992) making this a suitable drug to be taken by a breastfeeding mother. It is licensed to be given to children over the age of 4 years in syrup formulation at a dose of 1 mg three or four times daily for a maximum of 3 days.

For babies and children continued breastfeeding if applicable, and rehydration is generally recommended unless symptoms continue, as loperamide has been associated with toxicity and paralytic ileus.

Relative infant dose is quoted as 0.03% (Hale 2012 online access). The BNF states that the amount secreted into breastmilk is probably too small to be harmful.

> Compatible with breastfeeding as poorly absorbed from the gut.

References

Nikodem VC, Hofmeyr GJ, Secretion of the antidiarrhoeal agent loperamide oxide in breast-milk, *Eur J Clin Pharmacol*, 1992;42:695–6.

Codeine phosphate

The BNF states that the amount secreted into breastmilk is usually too small to be harmful; however, mothers vary considerably in their capacity to metabolise codeine and there is a risk of morphine overdose in infants (Koren *et al.* 2006). One death of an infant has been reported where the mother was an ultra-rapid metabolizer.

A study of two mothers found very low levels of free codeine and its metabolite morphine, in the plasma of breastfed infants whose mothers had taken a 60 mg dose of codeine. It was considered that such levels were sub-therapeutic and unlikely to cause respiratory depression (Naumburg *et al.* 1987). However, concerns raised by Koren are important to take into consideration.

Relative infant dose quoted as 8.1% (Hale 2012 online access). Other preparations such as loperamide may be considered more suitable for a breastfeeding mother (see concern over codeine use under analgesics).

> Use loperamide as alternative if possible to control diarrhoea during breastfeeding as codeine may accumulate in baby and cause respiratory depression.

References

Koren G, Cairns J, Chitayat D, Gaedigk A, Leeder SJ, Pharmacogenetics of morphine poisoning in a breastfed neonate of a codeine-prescribed mother, *Lancet*, 2006;368(9536):704.

Naumburg EG, Meny RG, Findlay J *et al.* Codeine and morphine levels in breastmilk and neonatal plasma, Pediatr Res, 1987;21(4, pt 2):240A. Abstract.

Co-phenotrope (diphenoxylate plus atropine)

Brand name: *Lomotil®*
US brands: *Logen®, Lonox®, Lomotil®*
Australian brands: *Lofenoxal®, Lomotil®*

Co-phenotrope is a synthetic derivative of pethidine but has no analgesic effects. It reduces intestinal motility and is particularly useful in the control of faecal consistency after colostomy or ileostomy. It is rarely used purely as an anti-diarrhoeal drug any more. There is little information on its transfer into breastmilk and its use in lactation is not recommended. Unless there are compelling reasons to use co-phenotrope, loperamide is a safer option.

The BNF states that it may be present in milk.

> Use loperamide as alternative if possible to control diarrhoea during breastfeeding as limited information on amount passing into breastmilk.

Inflammatory bowel disease (IBD)

> Drug of choice to treat inflammatory bowel disease in a mother during breastfeeding based on evidence of benefit and safety for the baby:
>
> Prednisolone and/or mesalazine as necessary to health of mother

Inflammatory bowel disease (IBD) covers two main conditions ulcerative colitis (UC) and Crohn's disease (CD).

In a retrospective study published in 1995 (Kane and Lemieux 2005) of 122 women with IBD, only 44% of patients breastfed their infants and many stopped their drugs before doing so, causing a flare in their bowel condition. The authors of the study suggested that most drugs are considered compatible with breastfeeding but that patients should avoid breastfeeding for four hours after taking corticosteroids. Milk levels are low so this seems an unnecessary recommendation.

A paper on the management of mothers with IBD during pregnancy and lactation was published in July 2008 (Ferguson et al. 2008). The authors quoted earlier data (Caprilli et al. 2006) on the safety of medication to treat IBD during lactation. The table states that loperamide and metronidazole are contra-indicated in breastfeeding while thiopurines (azathioprine), anti-tumour necrosis factor (infliximab) and fluoro-quinolones (e.g. ciprofloaxacin) are probably compatible but provides no further data. This paper would be unlikely to support anyone prescribing for a mother with IBD without access to further supporting data, despite its position in a prodigious peer-reviewed journal.

In a paper published in 2008, Mikhailov and Furner looked at the impact of genetic factors and breastfeeding on the development of IBD. The preponderance of evidence suggests that breastfeeding is a protective factor for IBD, with a greater effect for CD than UC. The relationship between breastfeeding in infancy and subsequent development of IBD was first evaluated in the early 1960s. A meta-analysis (Klement and Reif 2005) has shown that there was a protective effect of breastfeeding on the development of UC and CD. However, the authors suggested that further studies are required to examine the genetic predisposition to IBD. In face of the risks of not being breast-fed and a potential predisposition to babies of mothers with IBD developing the condition themselves, it would seem reasonable to avoid the use of formula milk in these children.

References

Caprilli R, Gassull MA, Escher JC, Moser G, Munkholm P, Forbes A, Hommes DW, Lochs H, Angelucci E, Cocco A, Vucelic B, Hildebrand H, Kolacek S, Riis L, Lukas M, de Franchis R, Hamilton M, Jantschek G, Michetti P, O'Morain C, Anwar MM, Freitas JL, Mouzas IA, Baert F, Mitchell R, Hawkey CJ; European Crohn's and Colitis Organisation, European evidence based consensus on the diagnosis and management of Crohn's disease: special situations, *Gut*, 2006;55:i36–58

Ferguson CB, Mahsud-Dornan S, Patterson RN, Inflammatory bowel disease in pregnancy, *BMJ*, 2008;337:a427

Kane S, Lemieux N, The role of breastfeeding in post-partum disease activity in women with inflammatory bowel disease, *Am J Gastroenterol*, 2005;100:102–105.

Klement E, Reif S, Breastfeeding and risk of inflammatory bowel disease, *Am J Clin Nutr*, 2005;82:486.

Mikhailov TA, Furner SE, Breastfeeding and genetic factors in the etiology of inflammatory bowel disease in children, *World J Gastroenterol*, 2008;15(3):270–279.

Prednisolone

Corticosteroids are often used in active disease with high doses to induce remission, followed by reduced dose as the inflammatory response is dampened.

Prednisolone is extensively bound to plasma proteins and passes into breastmilk in small quantities. In patients with disease confined to the distal colon or rectum, local topical therapy with suppositories or enemas of corticosteroids may be appropriate. Rectal formulations are poorly absorbed. In a study of three women receiving intravenous prednisolone of 50 mg over 6 hours only 0.025% of the dose appeared in breastmilk (Greenberger 1993).

Maternal doses of prednisolone up to 40 mg produce low levels in milk and would not be expected to cause any adverse effects in breastfed infants (Greenberger *et al.* 1993; McKenzie *et al.* 1975; Ost *et al.* 1985). High-dose steroids (>40 mg) are rarely necessary long term and so can be used in breastfeeding.

The BNF recommends waiting 4 hours after administration if possible to minimise exposure – this may not be practical advice for most breastfeeding mothers.

The maximum level in breastmilk occurs one hour after dosage. Even at a maternal dose of 80 mg the maximum level of drug in breastmilk was recorded by Ost was 317 µg per litre. Prednisolone is licensed for UC or CD at a dose of 2 mg per kg to a maximum of 60 mg in children over the age of 2 years.

With prolonged high doses over 40 mg monitoring of the infant for growth may be advisable but no reports of problems have been reported in the literature and this may be only a theoretical problem (Committee on Safety of Medicines, Medicines Control Agency 1998). This recommendation refers to direct levels administered to the child and not to the level being taken by a breastfeeding mother.

The benefit of treatment with corticosteroids during pregnancy and breastfeeding outweighs the risk to the baby. The BNF states that prednisolone appears in small amounts in breastmilk but maternal doses of up to 40 mg daily are unlikely to cause systemic effects in the infant; infants should be monitored for adrenal suppression if the mothers are taking a higher dose.

> Compatible with breastfeeding in doses ≤40 mg daily as extensively plasma protein bound. In higher, prolonged doses monitor baby for limited growth, in theory.

References

Committee on Safety of Medicines, Medicines Control Agency. Systemic corticosteroids in pregnancy and lactation, *Current Problems* 1998;24

Greenberger PA, Odeh YK, Frederiksen MC, Atkinson AJ Jr, Pharmacokinetics of prednisolone transfer to breastmilk, *Clin Pharmacol Ther*, 1993;53:324–8.

McKenzie SA, Selley JA, Agnew JE, Secretion of prednisolone into breastmilk, *Arch Dis Child*, 1975;50:894–6.

Ost L, Wettrell G, Bjorkhem I, Rane A, Prednisolone excretion in human milk, *J Pediatr*, 1985;106:1008–11.

Azathioprine

Brand name: *Imuran*®
US brands: Azasan®, Imuran®
Australian brands: Azahexal®, Azamun®, Azapin®, Imuran®, Thioprine®

Azathioprine is an immunosuppressive anti-metabolite. It is converted to mercaptopurine in the body. It has a corticosteroid-sparing effect and is widely used to produce and maintain remission in IBD, as well as conditions such as lupus and rheumatoid arthritis.

Traditionally, breastfeeding by mothers taking azathioprine has been discouraged because of theoretical risks of infant bone marrow suppression, susceptibility to infection, growth retardation and pancreatitis. According to recent research (Gardiner *et al.* 2007) breastfeeding need not be withheld in infants whose mothers are taking azathioprine. Gardiner *et al.* studied four mothers taking azathioprine. The metabolites 6-MP and 6-TGN were undetectable in neonatal blood and no clinical signs of immunosuppression were observed in the infants. Similarly Moretti *et al.* (2006) studied four babies and measured levels of 6-MP in breastmilk and neonatal blood for drug levels, white cell and platelet counts. Levels of metabolites were below the level of detection in the neonates and no clinical signs of immunosuppression were observed. Sau *et al.* (2007) studied ten women and similarly found no immunosuppression. Women taking azathioprine should therefore not be discouraged from breastfeeding.

It is licensed to be given to children over the age of 2 years at a dose of 2 mg per day initially for severe UC and CD. Relative infant dose is quoted as 0.07% to 0.3% (Hale 2012 online access).

The BNF states that it is present in milk in low concentrations, that there is no evidence of harm in small studies and the drug may be considered if the potential benefit outweighs the risk.

> Compatible with breastfeeding according to more recent studies; metabolites undetectable in infant's blood and no signs of immunosupression in small studies.

References

Gardiner SK, Gearry RB, Roberts RL, Zhang M, Barclay ML, Begg EJ, Exposure to thiopurine drugs through breastmilk is low based on metabolite concentrations in mother-infant pairs, *Br J Obstet Gynecol*, 2007;114:498–501.

Moretti ME, Verjee Z, Ito S, Koren G, Breastfeeding during maternal use of azathioprine, *Ann Pharmacother*, 2006;40:2269–72.

Sau A, Clarke S, Bass J, Kaiser A, Marinaki A, Nelson-Piercy C, Azathioprine and breastfeeding – is it safe?, *BJOG*, 2007;114:498–501.

Sulphasalazine

Brand name: *Salazopyrin®*
US Brands: *Azulfidine®*
Australian brands: *Pyralin®, Salazopyrin®*

Sulphasalazine is metabolised to sulphapyridine and 5-aminosalicylic acid (mesalazine). Small amounts of sulphasalazine and its sulphapyridine metabolites are excreted in breastmilk. Bloody diarrhoea in one breastfed infant, whose mother was taking sulphasalazine 3 g daily, has been reported. The mother was a slow acetylator with a relatively high blood concentration of sulphapyridine, which contributed to the appearance of the drug in the infant's blood and this reaction may be concluded as rare (Branski *et al.* 1986). A small study initially involving 17 mother–child pairs (Esbjörner *et al.* 1987) concluded sulphasalazine treatment could continue throughout pregnancy and lactation. The study found negligible amounts of sulphasalazine, and its main metabolite sulphapyridine, were transferred to the child via breastfeeding. The authors did, however, warn that this conclusion could not be applied to a prematurely born child or a child with haemolytic disease. Jarnerot and Into-Malberg (1979) studied 12 patients with IBD. Of 31 milk samples obtained, only five had detectable levels of sulphasalazine. Azad Khan *et al.* (1979) have reported no cases of adverse drug reactions to sulphasalazine in ten years of working in clinics, treating UC throughout pregnancy and the puerperum.

It is licensed to be given directly to children with IBD from the age of 2 years at 10 to 15 mg per kg four to six times daily to treat an acute attack. Relative infant dose quoted as 0.3 to 1.1 % (Hale 2012 online access).

The BNF states that babies should be monitored for diarrhoea.

Probably compatible with breastfeeding, be alert for bloody diarrhoea in baby.

References

Azad Khan AK, Truelove SC, Placental and mammary transfer of sulphasalazine, *Br Med J*, 1979;2:1553.
Branski D, *et al.* Bloody diarrhea—a possible complication of sulfasalazine transferred through human breastmilk, *J Pediatr Gastroenterol Nutr*, 1986;5:316–17.
Esbjörner E, Järnerot G, Wranne L, Sulphasalazine and sulphapyridine serum levels in children to mothers treated with sulphasalazine during pregnancy and lactation, *Acta Paediatr Scand*, 1987;76:137–42.
Jarnerot G, Into-Malberg MB, Sulphasalazine treatment during breast feeding, *Scand J Gastroenterol*, 1979;14:869–71.
Jenss H, Weber P, Hartmann F, Aminosalicylic acid and its metabolite in breastmilk during lactation, *Am J Gastroenterol*, 1990;85:331.
Klotz U, Harings-Kaim A, Negligible excretion of 5-aminosalicylic acid in breastmilk, *Lancet*, 1993;342:618–19.
Nelis GF, Diarrhoea due to 5-aminosalicylic acid in breastmilk, *Lancet*, 1989;i:383.

Mesalazine

Brand name: *Asacol®, Pentasa®, Mesren®, Ipocol®, Salofalk®, Mezavant®*
US brands: *Asacol®, Canasa®, Pentasa®, Rowasa®*
Australian brands: Mesasal®, Pentasa®, Salofalk®

Mesalazine may cause headache and GI disturbances, such as nausea, diarrhoea and abdominal pain in mothers. However, 80% of patients who are unable to tolerate sulphasalazine are able to tolerate mesalazine. Tablets are enteric coated to delay absorption until after they have passed through the stomach. The drug is poorly absorbed from the GI tract. The concentrations of mesalazine in maternal plasma and breastmilk in a woman taking 500 mg three times daily, were 410 and 110 ng per ml respectively. The authors concluded that the amount of mesalazine distributed into breastmilk was small and that it was compatible with breastfeeding. Maternal use of mesalazine 500 mg suppositories twice daily has been associated with watery diarrhoea in one breastfed infant. It seems likely to have been an idiosyncratic response (Jenss *et al.* 1990; Klotz and Harings-Kaim 1993; Nelis 1989).

Most products are not licensed for children below the age of 12 years. Relative infant dose quoted as 0.1 to 8.8% (Hale 2012 online access). The BNF states that diarrhoea in a breastfed infant has been reported but that negligible amounts can be detected in breastmilk; monitor infant for diarrhoea.

> Compatible with breastfeeding, measured levels low. Be alert for watery diarrhoea.

References

Jenss H, Weber P, Hartmann F, Aminosalicylic acid and its metabolite in breastmilk during lactation, *Am J Gastroenterol*, 1990;85:331.
Klotz U, Harings-Kaim A, Negligible excretion of 5-aminosalicylic acid in breastmilk, *Lancet*, 1993;342:618–19.
Nelis GF, Diarrhoea due to 5-aminosalicylic acid in breastmilk, *Lancet*, 1989;i:383.

Balsalazide

Brand name: *Colazide®*
US brands: *Colazide®*
Australian brands: *Colazide®*

Very little of the oral dose of balsalazide is absorbed from the upper GI tract, and almost the entire dose reaches its site of action in the colon. It is broken down by the colonic bacterial into 5-aminosalicylic acid (mesalazine), which is active, and 4-aminobenzoylalanine, an inert carrier. It is used to treat mild to moderate UC and to maintain remission. As it is metabolised to mesalazine, safety in breastfeeding may be assumed to be similar although there are no studies. It is used in children over 12 years although only licensed in adults (>18 years).

The BNF states that breastfed babies should be monitored for diarrhoea.

> Probably compatible with breastfeeding as metabolised to mesalazine, although there are no studies of levels in breastmilk. As with mesalazine, be alert for watery diarrhoea.

Olsalazine

Brand name: *Dipentum®*
US brands: *Dipentum®*
Australian brands: *Dipentum®*

Olsalazine may be associated with watery diarrhoea as an adverse effect. This may be reduced if the medication is taken on a full stomach. A study involving one woman with CD found that olsalazine was undetectable in the breastmilk for 48 hours after a single 500 mg dose, and although small amounts of the metabolite acetylated 5-aminosalicylic acid were detected in breastmilk the infant showed no adverse effects during the study period (Miller *et al.* 1993).

It is not licensed in children less than 12 years of age. Relative infant dose quoted as 0.9% (Hale 2012 online access). The BNF states babies should be monitored for diarrhoea.

> Probably compatible with breastfeeding although only one study has measured levels of drug in breastmilk. Be alert for watery diarrhoea.

Reference

Miller LG, Hopkinson JM, Motil KJ, Corboy JE, Andersson S, Disposition of olsalazine and metabolites in breastmilk, *J Clin Pharmacol*, 1993;33:703.

Infliximab

Brand name: *Remicade®*
US brands: *Remicade®*
Australian brands: *Remicade®*

In 2002, NICE (NICE 2002) recommended that this drug be only used for the treatment of severe, active CD when treatment with immunosuppressant drugs and corticosteroids is not tolerated or has failed. It should only be initiated by consultant gastroenterologists. Infections are common in patients treated with infliximab or other drugs that inhibit tumour necrosis factor (TNF). The incidence of tuberculosis is particularly marked. Blood dyscrasias, including leucopenia, thrombocytopenia, pancytopenia and aplastic anaemia, have been reported rarely with TNF inhibitors; in some cases the outcome was fatal. Infliximab is a large molecular weight antibody and preliminary results suggest it is too large to pass into breastmilk and it is not orally bio-available. It is distributed primarily in the vascular compartment and has a terminal elimination half-life of 8 to 9.5 days. After recommended doses, infliximab has been detected in serum for at least 8 weeks. It is suggested that use by a mother should not preclude breastfeeding based on this data (Peltier *et al.* 2001; Forger *et al.* 2004; Mahadevan *et al.* 2005; Vasiliauskas *et al.* 2006).

The BNF states that the amount in breastmilk is too small to be harmful which has superceded the recommendation that the manufacturer advised that breastfeeding should be avoided for at least 6 months after last dose.

> Compatible with breastfeeding due to poor bio-availability and hence low-level absorption by the infant.

References

Forger F, Matthias T, Oppermann M *et al.* Infliximab in breastmilk, *Lupus*, 2004;13:753. Abstract.

NICE Crohns Disease – infliximab 2002 (www.nice.org.ukguidanceindex.jsp?action= byID&o=11454).

Mahadevan U, Kane S, Intentional infliximab use during pregnancy for induction or maintenance of remission in Crohn's disease, *Aliment Pharmacol Ther*, 2005;21:733–8.

Peltier M, James D, Ford J, Wagner C, David H, Hanauer S, Infliximab levels in breastmilk of a nursing Crohn's patient, *Am J Gastroenterol*, 2001;96(9 Suppl. 1):S312. Abstract.

Vasiliauskas EA, Church JA, Silverman N, Barry M, Targan SR, Dubinsky MC, Case report: evidence for transplacental transfer of maternally administered infliximab to the newborn, *Clin Gastroenterol Hepatol*, 2006;4:1255–8.

Laxatives

> **Drug of choice to treat constipation in a mother during breastfeeding based on evidence of benefit and safety for the baby:**
>
> **Bulk and osmotic laxatives are safe in normal doses; stimulant laxatives should be reserved for use if these have proved ineffective**
> **Choose on clinical symptoms, cost and personal preference**

The definition of constipation is very individual but is generally held to be a disruption of normal faecal frequency and consistency. Many new mothers may report difficulties following delivery due to perineal sutures and opiate analgesics, which make the passage of firm stools uncomfortable. Initial management consisting of lifestyle advice is good practice e.g. increased natural fibre in the diet, increased fluid intake (particularly water rather than tea and coffee or carbonated drinks) and increased exercise. If this has failed to improve symptoms, a bulk or osmotic laxative may be recommended, neither of which involve passage of a drug into breastmilk so can safely be recommended in breastfeeding.

Bulk-forming laxatives

Brand names: ispaghula husk – *Fybogel®, Regulan®*; sterculia – *Normacol®*; methylcellulose – *Celevac®*

Bulk-forming laxatives take up to 72 hours to produce a full effect but are particularly useful for relief of small, hard stools as they increase faecal mass, which stimulates peristalsis. These preparations require adequate fluid intake and should not be taken before bedtime in case they cause obstruction. These products are not absorbed from the gut and are not contra-indicated in breastfeeding.

Compatible with breastfeeding as not absorbed from the gut.

Osmotic laxatives

Osmotic laxatives increase the amount of water in the large bowel by drawing it back or retaining it. There may be a delay of up to 48 hours in achieving full effect. There is no contra-indication in breastfeeding.

Lactulose may also be given directly to children but is rarely, if ever, necessary in breastfed babies.

Compatible with breastfeeding as not absorbed into breastmilk.

Macrogols – manufacturers advise avoidance during breastfeeding but these products are used in children aged over two years. Macrogol 3350 is not absorbed from the GI tract and cannot therefore pass into breastmilk e.g. *Movicol®*, *Idrolax®*. These products may also be used in bowel preparations prior to colonoscopy – *Klean-Prep®*.

Compatible with breastfeeding as not absorbed into breastmilk.

Magnesium hydroxide is poorly absorbed from the gut. Low doses are used as antacids (*Milk of Magnesia®*), higher doses (25 to 50 ml) as laxatives. It may be mixed with liquid paraffin to form an emulsion (*Milpar®*).

Compatible with breastfeeding as not absorbed into breastmilk.

Stimulant laxatives

Stimulant laxatives stimulate nerve endings in the mucosa of the colon to produce a laxative effect. They are more prone to misuse by patients who wish to produce frequent bowel motions in an attempt to lose weight. They should not be used regularly as this may produce loss of water and electrolytes in particular potassium. It may also lead to loss of tone in the colon. They frequently produce abdominal cramping.

In normal doses there is no contra-indication in breastfeeding (BNF).

Bisacodyl – *Dulcolax®*
US brands: *Bisa-Lax®, Gentlax®*
Australian brands: *Bisalax®, Duralax®*

Senna – *Senokot®, Manevac®* – may colour mother's urine yellow-brown or red depending on pH
US brands: *Senokot®, Dosaflex®*
Australian brands: *Senokot®*, Dantron – *Co-danthramer®*, Normax® – may colour the mother's urine and has been reported to increase bowel activity of breastfed baby; generally, only used in terminally ill patients as has been shown to be carcinogenic in animal studies.
Sodium picosulphate – *Ducolax perles®* – stimulates the bowel following metabolism by colonic bacteria. It is usually effective in 6 to 12 hours although bowel preparation may occur more rapidly. It is not known to be present in breastmilk.
Australian brand: *Durolax SP®*

> Compatible with breastfeeding in normal doses.

Stool softener

Docusate – *Dioctyl®* – an anion surfactant which probably acts as faecal softener as well as stimulant laxative. It does pass into breastmilk according to the BNF although the amount is unknown. As this drug is minimally absorbed from the GI tract the amount in breastmilk is likely to be extremely small. It is licensed for use in children over the age of 2 years.

US brands: *Colace®, Dioctyn®, Docusoft®*
Australian brands: *Coloxyl®, Rectalad®*

> Compatible with breastfeeding in normal doses.

Laxative enemas or suppositories

Laxative enemas or suppositories may be given in extreme cases of constipation – these would not be absorbed systemically. They act within an hour of use but are generally only used as an acute measure and rarely in younger patients. There is no contra-indication in breastfeeding.

Phosphate enema – *Fletchers®, Fleet®*
Sodium citrate enema – *Microlax®, Microlette®*
Glycerine suppositories

> Compatible with breastfeeding as not absorbed systemically.

Bowel-cleansing solutions

Bowel-cleansing solutions are used to clear the bowel prior to colonoscopy or radio-logical examinations of the bowel. During dosage solid foods are discontinued but adequate fluid consumption of clear fluids should be continued. There is no contra-indication in breastfeeding. The BNF says that the manufacturers advise use only if essential as no information is available.

Macrogol 3350 – *Klean Prep*® – is not absorbed from the GI tract
Sodium picosulphate – *Picolax*® (a mixture with magnesium citrate) – not present in breastmilk
Phosphate enema – *Fleet*® – is not absorbed from the GI tract

Compatible with breastfeeding as not excreted in breastmilk.

Reference

Friedrich C, Richter E, Trommeshauser D, de Kruif S, van Iersel T, Mandel K, Gessner U, Lack of excretion of the active moiety of bisacodyl and sodium picosulphate into human breast-milk: an open-label, parallel group, multiple dose study in healthy lactating women, *Drug Metab Pharmacokinet*, 2011;26(5):458–64.

Haemorrhoidal preparations

Drug of choice to treat haemorroids in a mother during breastfeeding based on evidence of benefit and safety for the baby:

All products are compatible with breastfeeding, use depends on clinical symptoms, cost and personal preference

Haemorrhoids and anal fissures are often an unfortunate result of pregnancy or a prolonged second stage of labour resulting in extreme discomfort for the mother trying to sit to feed her baby. Preparations often combine corticosteroids, local anaes-thetics and soothing agents. Sufficient absorption from topical application to haemorrhoids is very unlikely. Any associated constipation should be dealt with to produce softer bowel motions and the mother encouraged to consume more fibre and ensure an adequate fluid intake.

Ingredients vary with brands, some are available to purchase over the counter and others only available on prescription. Examples: *Anugesic HC*®, *Anusol*®, *Anusol HC*®, *Proctosedyl*®, *Scheriproct*®, *Ultraproct*®, *Xyloproct*®, *Proctafoam HC*®, *Perianal*®, *Germaloids*®

Compatible with breastfeeding as not absorbed into breastmilk.

Glyceryl trintrate ointment

Brand name: *Rectogesic*®

An anal fissure is a superficial tear in the mucosa of the distal anal canal characterised by pain on defecation, rectal bleeding, and spasm of the anal sphincter. Healing, which is usually achieved within 2 weeks, may be helped by management with bran and bulk laxatives and topical local anaesthetics for pain relief. In women, about one in ten cases occur during childbirth. However, some patients continue to experience pain for longer. Glyceryl trinitrate (GTN) ointment can be used for the treatment of chronic anal fissures. It helps to relax the anal muscle, reduce pain, relieve the spasm of the muscles and improve the blood supply to the fissure. Studies (Gorfine 1995; Lund 1996; Scholefield 2003; Lund and Scholefield 1998; Nelson 2004) have reported benefit from topical application of GTN, although a high rate of spontaneous resolution with placebo has been reported in some studies (Bailey *et al.* 2002; UKMI 2006). A study carried out at Mothersafe, Royal Women's Hospital, Sydney showed no adverse effects in a group of babies whose mothers used GTN ointment. The 43 mothers reported a high rate of side effects 28 experienced headache (three with headache and dizziness) and seven with dizziness or lightheadedness without headache in the mothers. None of them reported any side effects in their babies, despite very close scrutiny (Taylor and Kennedy 2008; UKMI 2011).

The BNF says that there is no information available and that the manufacturers advise use only if potential benefit outweighs risk.

Compatible with breastfeeding from studies.

References

Bailey HR, Beck DE, Billingham RP, Binderow SR, Gottesman L, Hull TL, Larach SW, Margolin DA, Milsom JW, Potenti FM, Rafferty JF, Riff DS, Sands LR, Senagore A, Stamos MJ, Yee LF, Young-Fadok TM, Gibbons RD; Fissure Study Group, A study to determine the nitroglycerin ointment dose and dosing interval that best promote the healing of chronic anal fissures, *Dis Colon Rectum*, 2002;45:1192–9.

Gorfine SR, Topical nitroglycerin therapy for anal fissures and ulcers, *N Engl J Med*, 1995;333:1156–7.

Lund JN, Armitage NC, Scholefield JH, Use of glyceryl trinitrate ointment in the treatment of anal fissure, *Br J Surg*, 1996;83:776–7.

Lund JN, Scholefield JH, Follow-up of patients with chronic anal fissure treated with topical glyceryl trinitrate, *Lancet*, 1998;352:1681.

Nelson R, A systematic review of medical therapy for anal fissure, *Dis Colon Rectum*, 2004;47:422–31.

Scholefield JH, Bock JU, Marla B, Richter HJ, Athanasiadis S, Pröls M, Herold A., A dose finding study with 0.1%, 0.2%, and 0.4% glyceryl trinitrate ointment in patients with chronic anal fissures, *Gut*, 2003;52:264–9.

Taylor T, Kennedy D, Safety of topical glyceryl trinitrate in the treatment of anal fissure in breastfeeding women, *Birth Defects Research Part a – Clinical and Molecular Teratology*, 2008;82:411. Abstract.

UKMI Medicines Q and A, Is topical glyceryl trinitrate for anal fissure compatible with breast-feeding? 2011.
UKMI New Drug Information, Glyceryl trinitrate 0.4%, 2006.

Cardiovascular system

Diuretics

> **Diuretic of choice to treat a mother during breastfeeding based on evidence of benefit and safety for the baby:**
>
> **All diuretics should be avoided unless essential for health of the mother**

Diuresis is not generally advised in breastfeeding due to the inherent risk of reducing the volume of breastmilk. Great care should be taken if diuretic use is considered essential.

Bendroflumethiazide

Brand name: *Aprinox®*
US brands: *Naturetin®*
Australian brands:

Bendroflumethiazide, a thiazide diuretic, has been used to suppress lactation at a dose of 5 mg twice daily (Stout 1962). The risk of reducing milk established supply at a dose of 2.5 mg is unknown (Healy 1961).

BNF data recommends that the amount in breastmilk is too small to be harmful but that large doses may suppress lactation.

> Avoid if possible as may suppress lactation. Use ACE inhibitor, beta blocker or calcium channel blockers as alternative antihypertensive unless diuresis is essential.

References

Healy M, Suppressing lactation with oral diuretics, *Lancet*, 1961;1:1353–4.
Stout G, Suppression of lactation, *Br Med J*, 1962;1:1150. Letter.

Indapamide

Brand name: Natrilix®
US brand: *Lozol®*
Australian brands: *Dapa-Tabs®; Indahexal®, Insig®, Napamide®, Natrilix®*

Indapamide is a diuretic with similar effects to thiazides but fewer reported effects on blood glucose concentrations. It is assumed to have the same potential to reduce breastmilk production. There is no data on transfer into breastmilk. The BNF says that it is present in milk and that the manufacturer advises it should be avoided.

Avoid if possible due to lack of safety data and risk of lactation suppression. Use ACE inhibitor, beta blocker or calcium channel blockers as alternative anti-hypertensive unless essential.

Furosemide

Brand name: *Lasix*®
US brand: *Lasix*®
Australian brands: *Frusehexal*®, *Frusid*®, *Lasix*®, *Uremide*®, *Urex*®

Furosemide is a loop diuretic with a short duration of action. It is used to treat cardiac and respiratory problems in neonates. There are no reports of levels in breastmilk and the risk of intense diuresis reducing breastmilk, make it a drug which should only be used if the maternal need is great. Cominos *et al.* (1976) studied the use of furosemide with reduced fluid intake and breast binding on breastmilk suppression. It is unknown how much the drug contributed to the breastmilk suppression but this occurred within 3 days.

BNF data recommend that the amount in breastmilk is too small to be harmful but that it may inhibit lactation.

Avoid if possible as may suppress lactation. Use ACE inhibitor, beta blocker or calcium channel blockers as alternative antihypertensive unless essential.

Reference

Cominos DC, van der Walt A, van Rooyen AJ, Suppression of post-partum lactation with furosemide, *S Afr Med J*, 1976;50:251–2.

Bumetanide

Brand name: *Burinex*®
US brands: *Bumex*®
Australian brands: *Burinex*®

Bumetanide is a potent loop diuretic similar in action to furosemide. There is no data on transfer into breastmilk.

BNF data report that the manufacturer advises avoid if possible as there is no information available and that it may inhibit lactation.

Avoid if possible due to lack of safety data and risk of lactation suppression. Use ACE inhibitor, beta blocker or calcium channel blockers as alternative antihypertensive unless essential.

ACE inhibitors

> ### ACE inhibitor of choice in a mother during breastfeeding based on evidence of benefit and safety for the baby:
>
> ### Enalapril

In the absence of data on the transfer of many ACE inhibitors into breastmilk it may be prudent to use enalapril or captopril on which there is more information. However, a class effect may be expected and if another ACE inhibitor is essential there seems little reason to discontinue breastfeeding. Small levels of the drugs on which we do have data are transferred into breastmilk. ACE inhibitors are contra-indicated in pregnancy. The most commonly reported adverse effect in patients taking ACE inhibitors is a cough due to raised levels of bradykinin.

Enalapril

Brand name: *Innovace®*
US brands: *Vasotec®*
Australian brands: *Alphapril®, Amprace®, Auspril®, Enahexal®, Enalabell®, Renitec®*

Redman *et al.* (1990) studied five women taking 20 mg enalapril, it was not detectable after 4 hours in four of the five women while the average peak level of enalaprilat (the metabolite of enalapril) was 1.7 µg per litre. No adverse events were reported in four babies exposed to maternal levels of 5 to 10 mg. Huttenen *et al.* (1989) studied three women after single doses of enalapril up to 10 mg. Enalaprilat levels were not detected and the concentration of ACE activity in milk was unchanged. Rush *et al.* (1989) deduced that the total amount of enalapril and its metabolite to which a baby would be exposed was 2 µg of enalaprat while unlicensed use of enalapril from 1 month (BNFC) is 100 µg per kg per day. Relative infant dose quoted as 0.2% (Hale 2012 online access).

BNF data recommend that the drug is avoided in the first few weeks after delivery due to the risk of profound neonatal hypotension; it can be used in older infants if essential, but recommends that the infant's blood pressure is monitored.

> Compatible with breastfeeding. Amount transferred into breastmilk is significantly less than can be given directly to a baby more than 1 month of age.

References

Huttunen K, Gronhagen-Riska C, Fyhrquist F, Enalapril treatment of a nursing mother with slightly impaired renal function, *Clin Nephrol*, 1989;31:278. Letter.

Redman CWG, Kelly JG, Cooper WD, The excretion of enalapril and enalaprilat in human breastmilk, *Eur J Clin Pharmacol*, 1990;38:99.

Rush JE, Snyder DL, Barrish A, Hichens M, Comment on Huttunen K, Gronhagen-Riska C, Fyrquist F, Enalapril treatment of a nursing mother with slightly impaired renal function, *Clin Nephrol*, 1989;31:278, *Clin Nephrol*, 1991;35:234. Letter.

Captopril

Brand name: *Capoten*®
US brands: *Capoten*®
Australian brands: *Acenorm*®, *Capoten*®, *Captohexal*®, *Topace*®

Devlin and Fleiss' study (1981) of 12 women showed that the concentration of captopril in breastmilk was about 1% of maternal plasma, equivalent to 4.7 µg per litre in breastmilk of mothers taking 300 mg daily and no adverse effects were noted in the babies. Captopril is widely used to treat paediatric patients at a neonatal dose of 10 to 50 µg per kg two or three times daily, although outside of licence application. It can be used to treat breastfeeding women if an ACE is required, although its clinical use has largely declined to be superseded by newer drugs in this class.

BNF data recommend that the drug is avoided in the first few weeks after delivery due to the risk of profound neonatal hypotension; it can be used in older infant if essential but recommends that the infant's blood pressure is monitored.

> Compatible with breastfeeding. Amount transferred into breastmilk is significantly less than can be given directly to a baby more than 1 month of age.

Reference

Devlin RG, Fleiss PM, Captopril in human blood and breastmilk, *J Clin Pharmacol*, 1981;21:110–113.

Ramipril

Brand name: *Tritace*®
US brands: *Tritace*®
Australian brands: *Ramace*®, *Tritace*®

There is no data available on transfer into breastmilk. Ramipril has an active metabolite ramiprilat, which is approximately 56% plasma protein bound. Although there is no evidence that safety is not a class effect, the use of enalapril with its available safety data may be prudent.

> Probably compatible with breastfeeding if class effect assumed but no studies to substantiate this. Use enalapril if possible.

Lisinopril

Brand name: *Zestril*®, *Carace*®
US brands: *Prinivil*®, *Zestril*®
Australian brands: *Fibsol*®, *Liprace*®, *Lisinobell*®, *Lisodur*®, *Prinivil*®, *Zestril*®

There is no information on the transfer of lisinopril into breastmilk, although the oral bio-availability is only 29%. It is not significantly bound to plasma proteins. Although there is no evidence that safety is not a class effect, the use of enalapril with its available safety data may be prudent. The BNF recommends that it is avoided as no information is available.

> Probably compatible with breastfeeding if class effect assumed but no studies to substantiate this. Use enalapril if possible.

Perindopril

Brand name: *Coversyl*®
US brands:
Australian brands: *Coversyl*®

There is no data available on the transfer of perindopril into breastmilk. It is metabolised to perindoprilat which is the active drug. Plasma protein binding is reported to be 10 to 20% and oral bio-availability is 65 to 75%. Although there is no evidence that compatability is not a class effect, the use of enalapril with its available safety data may be prudent.

> Probably compatible with breastfeeding if class effect assumed but no studies to substantiate this. Use enalapril if possible.

Beta blockers

> **Beta blocker of choice in a mother during breastfeeding based on evidence of benefit and safety for the baby:**
>
> **Metoprolol, propranolol or labetalol**

Beta blockers are used in pregnancy to treat pre-eclampsia or eclampsia but may increase the risk of neonatal hypoglycaemia, particularly if the baby is born prematurely.

Reference

Baby Friendly Initiative, Hypoglycaemia policy guidelines.

Atenolol

Brand name: *Tenormin*®, *Tenormin LS*®, *Tenoret*®
US brands: *Tenormin*®
Australian brands: Anselol®, Atehexal®, Noten®, Tenormin®, Tensig®

Atenolol diffuses into breastmilk in concentrations similar to or higher than those in maternal blood demonstrated by m/p ratios of 1.5 to 6.8. Despite this, the authors calculated the infant would only be exposed to 0.13 mg per day following a maternal dose of 50 mg per day (Liedholm 1983). Cyanosis and bradycardia in a 5-day-old term infant associated with maternal intake of 50 mg atenolol twice daily in breast-milk has been reported. The infant recovered when breastfeeding was interrupted (Schimmel *et al.* 1989). Other authors have reported no adverse effects in 15 infants aged 3 days to 2 weeks exposed to 50 to 100 mg atenolol (Bhamra *et al.* 1983; White *et al.* 1984; Kulas *et al.* 1984). It is not licensed for use in children under the age of 12 years. Relative infant dose quoted as 6.6% (Hale 2012 online access).

Atenolol has low plasma protein binding and therefore passes more freely into breastmilk. Caution is particularly advised in neonates because of the renal excretion of this drug. Babies whose mothers are on beta blockers with low plasma protein binding should be observed for symptoms of hypoglycaemia.

The BNF recommends that it is present in milk in greater amounts than some other beta blockers; toxicity due to beta blockade is possible and the infant should be monitored and atenolol used with caution (Baby Friendly Initiative 2012).

> Use labetalol, metoprolol or propranolol as alternative if possible particularly in neonates.

References

Baby Friendly Initiative, Hypoglycaemia policy guidelines.

Bhamra RK, Thorley KJ, Vale JA, Thorley KJ, Vale JA, Holt DW, High-performance liquid chromatographic measurement of atenolol: methodology and clinical applications, *Ther Drug Monit*, 1983;5:313–18.

Kulas J, Lunell N-O, Rosing U, Lunell NO, Rosing U, Stéen B, Rane A, Atenolol and metoprolol. A comparison of their excretion into human breastmilk, *Acta Obstet Gynecol (Scand Suppl.)*, 1984;Suppl. 118:65–9.

Liedholm H, Transplacental passage and breastmilk accumulation of atenolol in humans, *Drugs*, 1983;25(Suppl. 2):217–18.

Schimmel MS, Eidelman AI, Wilschanski MA, Shaw D Jr, Ogilvie RJ, Koren G, Toxic effects of atenolol consumed during breastfeeding, *J Pediatr*, 1989;114:476–8.

Thorley KJ, McAinsh J, Levels of the beta-blockers atenolol and propranolol in the breastmilk of women treated for hypertension in pregnancy, *Biopharm Drug Dispos*, 1983;4:299–301.

White WB, Andreoli JW, Wong SH, Cohn RD, Atenolol in human plasma and breastmilk, *Obstet Gynecol*, 1984;63:42S–44S.

Labetalol

Brand name: *Lopressor®, Trandate®*
US brands: *Normodyne®, Trandate®*
Australian brands: *Presolol®, Trandate®*

Michael's study of 25 patients (1979) taking between 330 and 800 mg labetalol daily showed a m/p ratio less than 1, although one patient taking 1200 mg daily produced milk samples where the concentration in milk exceeded that in maternal plasma. Lunell *et al.*'s study (1985) produced similar results. However, no baby in these studies exhibited any adverse drug reactions. Mirpuri *et al.* (2008) reported that a 26-week premature baby exhibited bradycardia and premature beats when tube fed expressed breastmilk from its mother who was receiving 300 mg labetalol twice daily. Its condition returned to normal when formula milk was substituted.

Labetalol is more extensively plasma protein bound (50%) than atenolol. It is not licensed for use in children. Relative infant dose quoted as 0.2 and 0.6% (Hale 2012 online access).

The BNF recommends that it is present in milk but that the amount is probably too small to be harmful although it is advisable to monitor the infant for possible symptoms of alpha- and beta blockade.

Compatible with breastfeeding because of low levels transferred into breastmilk.

References

Lunell NO, Kulas J, Rane A, Transfer of labetalol into amniotic fluid and breastmilk in lactating women, *Eur J Clin Pharmacol*, 1985;28:597–9.

Michael CA, Use of labetalol in the treatment of severe hypertension during pregnancy, *Br J Clin Pharmacol*, 1979;8(Suppl. 2):211S–215S.

Mirpuri J, Patel H, Rhee D, Crowley K, What's mom on? A case of bradycardia in a premature infant on breastmilk, *J Invest Med*, 2008;56:409

Metoprolol

Brand name: *Lopressor®*
US brands: *Lopresor®, Toprol®*
Australian brands: *Betaloc®, Lopresor®, Metohexal®, Metrol®, Minax®, Toprol®*

Studies have shown that metoprolol also produces m/p ratios in excess of 1 (Sandström and Regårdh 1980; Liedholm *et al.* 1981). However, the absolute level of drug transferring to the baby is small and studies have failed to detect metoprolol at significant levels in infant plasma (Kuklas *et al.* 1984). Although the drug is well-absorbed, it undergoes extensive first-pass metabolism. It is 12% bound to plasma proteins. No adverse events have been reported in babies exposed to metoprolol via breastmilk (Ho *et al.* 1999; Lindeberg *et al.* 1984). It is not licensed for use in children. Relative infant dose quoted as 1.4% (Hale 2012 online access).

The BNF recommends that it is present in milk but that the amount is probably too small to be harmful although it is advisable to monitor the infant for possible symptoms of beta blockade.

Compatible with breastfeeding because of low levels transferred into breastmilk.

References

Ho TK, Moretti ME, Schaeffer JK, Ito S, Koren G, Maternal beta-blocker usage and breast-feeding in the neonate, *Pediatr Res*, 1999;45:67A. Abstract 385.

Kulas J, Lunell NO, Rosing U, Stéen B, Rane A, Atenolol and metoprolol: a comparison of their excretion into human breastmilk, *Acta Obstet Gynecol (Scand Suppl.)*, 1984;118:65–9.

Liedholm H, Melander A, Bitzén PO, Helm G, Lönnerholm G, Mattiasson I, Nilsson B, Wåhlin-Boll E, Accumulation of atenolol and metoprolol in human breastmilk, *Eur J Clin Pharmacol*, 1981;20:229–31.

Lindeberg S, Sandstrom B, Lundborg P, Regårdh CG, Disposition of the adrenergic blocker metoprolol in the late-pregnant woman, the amniotic fluid, the cord blood and the neonate. Acta Obstet Gy

Sandström B, Regårdh C-G, Metoprolol excretion into breastmilk, *Br J Clin Pharmacol*, 1980;9: 518necol Scand Suppl. 1984;suppl 118:61-4.

Bisoprolol

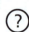

Brand name: *Cardicor®, Emcor®*
US brands: *Zebeta®*
Australian brands: *Bicor®*

Bisoprolol is almost completely absorbed from the GI tract and undergoes only minimal first-pass metabolism resulting in an oral bio-availability of approximately 90%. It is 30% plasma protein bound. It is a cardio-selective beta-blocker. Its pharmacokinetic properties suggest that it may accumulate particularly in neonates and its use should be avoided unless essential. Other beta blockers demonstrate better safety data in lactation.

The BNF recommends that the amount of most beta blockers in breastmilk is probably too small to be harmful although it is avisable to monitor the infant for possible symptoms of beta blockade.

> Use labetalol, metoprolol or propranolol as alternative if possible especially in neonates.

Propranolol

☺

Brand name: *Inderal®, Inderal LA®, Half Inderal®*
US brands: *Inderal®, InnoPran®*
Australian brands: *Deralin®, Inderal®*

Propranolol is almost completely absorbed from the GI tract but undergoes first-pass metabolism. It is highly lipid soluble and is approximately 90% plasma protein bound. It has at least one active metabolite but the impact of this is unclear. The half-life of propranolol is 3 to 6 hours. It is used to treat children with hypertension initially at a dose of 1 mg per kilogram but can be increased to 2 to 4 mg per kg per day in divided doses. It is also used to prevent migraines in children under the age of 12 at dose of 20 mg two or three times daily. It crosses the blood–brain barrier and the placenta. It is present in breastmilk.

In adults it may be used to lower blood pressure, to relieve symptoms of hyperthyroidism, to prevent migraines or to prevent panic attacks.

In a study of three women (Smith 1983) it was calculated that the maximum dose likely to be ingested by a breastfed infant would be less than 0.1% of the maternal dose. A m/p ratio range of 0.33 to 1.65 was reported. Bauer estimated that the maximal dose of cumulative propranolol to which a breastfed infant would be exposed at a maternal dose of 40 mg four times daily would be 21 µg per 24 hours. This dose is considerably less than the therapeutic dose of propranolol for infants. No adverse effects have been reported in breastfed infants whose mothers were receiving propranolol. The relative infant dose is quoted as 0.3 and 0.5% (Hale 2012 online access)

The BNF recommnds that the amount of most beta blockers in breastmilk is probably too small to be harmful although it is advisable to monitor the infant for possible symptoms of beta-blockade.

> Compatible with breastfeeding because of low levels transferred into breastmilk determined in studies.

References

Bauer JH, Pape B, Zajicek J, Groshong T, Propranolol in human plasma and breastmilk, Am J Cardiol, 1979;43(4):860–2.

Smith MT, Livingstone I, Hooper WD, Eadie MJ, Triggs EJ, Propranolol, propranolol glucuronide, and naphthoxylactic acid in breastmilk and plasma, *Ther Drug Monit*, 1983;5(1):87–93.

Angiotensin II receptor antagonists

> **Sartan (ARB) of choice in a mother during breastfeeding based on evidence of benefit and safety for the baby:**
>
> **Avoid if possible and use ACE inhibitor due to lack of data**
> **Candesartan might be assumed to produce lowest levels**

This group of drugs is given to patients who are unable to tolerate ACE inhibitors to treat hypertension and heart failure. As with ACE inhibitors, this group of drugs is contra-indicated in pregnancy. There is no data on transfer into breastmilk and the use of ACE inhibitors is recommended. This class of drug might be expected to produce low levels in breastmilk because of the high protein binding and low bio-availability but no data exists to support this assumption.

Candesartan

Brand name: *Amias®*
US brands: *Atacand®*
Australian brands: *Atacand®*

Candesartan has a bio-availability of around 14% when taken orally. It is more than 99% plasma protein bound. There appears to be no studies on passage into breastmilk. It should only be used if essential to the health of the mother.

> Avoid if possible and use ACE inhibitor due to lack of data. If use of a sartan (ARB) is essential likely to be the most compatible due to high level of plasma. protein binding

Irbesartan

Brand name: *Aprovel®*
US brands: *Avalide®*
Australian brands: *Avapro®*

The oral bio-availability of this drug is higher than the other class drugs (60 to 80%) and is 96% bound to plasma proteins. Based on pharmacokinetic assumptions it may be a less beneficial choice. There is no data on transfer into breastmilk.

The BNF states that information on the use of angiotensin-II receptor antagonists in breastfeeding is limited. They are not recommended in breastfeeding and alternative treatment options, with better established safety information during breastfeeding, are available.

> Avoid if possible and use ACE inhibitor due to lack of data. If use of a sartan (ARB) is essential likely to be the most compatible due to high level of plasma protein binding.

Losartan ?

Brand name: *Cozaar®*
US brands: *Cozaar®*
Australian brands: *Cozaar®*

This drug undergoes extensive first-pass metabolism and has bio-availability of only 33%. It has an active metabolite but both prodrug and metabolite are more than 98% plasma protein bound. There is no data on transfer into breastmilk and only limited data on use in children.

The BNF states that information on the use of angiotensin-II receptor antagonists in breastfeeding is limited. They are not recommended in breastfeeding and alternative treatment options, with better established safety information during breastfeeding, are available.

> Avoid if possible and use ACE inhibitor due to lack of data. If use of a sartan is essential likely to be the most compatible due to high level of plasma protein binding.

Valsartan

(?)

Brand name: *Diovan*®
US brands: *Diovan*®
Australian brands:

Valsartan has a bio-availability of 23% and is 94 to 97% plasma protein bound. There is no data on transfer into breastmilk.

The BNF states that information on the use of angiotensin-II receptor antagonists in breastfeeding is limited. They are not recommended in breastfeeding and alternative treatment options, with better established safety information during breastfeeding, are available.

> Avoid if possible and use ACE inhibitor due to lack of data. If use of a sartan is essential likely to be the most compatible due to high level of plasma protein binding.

Calcium channel blockers

> **Calcium channel blocker of choice in a mother during breastfeeding based on evidence of benefit and safety for the baby:**
>
> **Nifedipine**

Calcium channel blockers interfere with the movement of calcium into cells. The drugs act in different ways according to their site of action.

Nifedipine

Brand name: *Adalat*®
US brands: *Afeditab*®, *Nifediac*®, *Nifedical*®, *Procardia*®
Australian brands: *Adefin*®, *Nifecard*®, *Nifehexal*®, *Nypine*®

Nifedipine relaxes vascular smooth muscle and dilates coronary and peripheral arteries. It has activity in reducing blood pressure and in the treatment of Reynaud's phenomenon.

Nifedipine is almost completely absorbed from the GI tract but undergoes extensive first-pass metabolism. It is up to 98% bound to plasma proteins. It is used to treat hypertension (Penny and Lewis 1989; Ehrenkranz *et al.* 1989) and also to improve circulation in Reynaud's phenomenon (cold extremities and nipple vasospasm) in doses up to 30 mg daily (Lawlor-Smith and Lawlor-Smith 1996; Garrison 2002; Anderson *et al.* 2004). Side effects for the mother include flushing and headache, which may limit its usefulness. It is present in breastmilk but in levels too small to be harmful and there have been no reports of adverse effects in babies (see section on Reynaud's phenomenon, p. 51).

In Taddio et al's study (1996) of 21 women taking 40 mg Nifedipine daily the babies were estimated to be exposed to 0.1% of the maternal weight adjusted dose via breastmilk. Nifedipine is widely used to treat pre-eclampsia and eclampsia in the mother together with methyldopa or a beta blocker. Ehrenkranz *et al.* (1989) studied one woman who took 10, 20 or 30 mg three times daily on different days. Using the maximum dose transferred by the 30 mg regimen, the authors estimated that the baby would be exposed to the authors estimated that an exclusively breastfed infant would receive an estimated maximum of 7.5 µg per kg of nifedipine daily. Its relative infant dose is quoted as 2.3–3.4% (Hale 2012 online access).

The BNF reports that the amount secreted into breastmilk is too small to be harmful but that manufacturer advises it should be avoided.

> Compatible with breastfeeding.

References

Anderson JE, Held N, Wright K, Raynaud's phenomenon of the nipple: a treatable cause of painful breastfeeding, *Pediatrics*, 2004;113(4):e360–4.

Ehrenkranz RA, Ackerman BA, Hulse JD, Nifedipine transfer into human milk, *J Pediatr*, 1989;114:478–80.

Garrison CP, Nipple vasospasm, Raynaud's syndrome, and nifedipine, *J Hum Lact*, 2002;18(4):382–5.

Lawlor-Smith LS, Lawlor-Smith CL, Raynaud's phenomenon of the nipple: a preventable cause of breastfeeding failure?, *Med J Aust*, 1996;166:448. Letter.

Penny WJ, Lewis MJ, Nifedipine is excreted in human milk, *Eur J Clin Pharmacol*, 1989;36:427–8.

Taddio A, Oskamp M, Ito S, *et al.* Is nifedipine use during labour and breastfeeding safe for the neonate?, *Clin Invest Med*, 1996;19(4 Suppl.):S11. Abstract.

Amlodipine

Brand name: *Istin*®
US brands: *Norvasc*®, *Amvaz*®
Australian brands: *Norvasc*®

Amlodipine has an oral bio-availability of 60 to 65% and is 97.5% bound to plasma proteins. It has been used to treat hypertension in children. It has a prolonged terminal half-life of 30 to 50 hours. No data exist on transfer into breastmilk. Other agents may be preferred to reduce blood pressure during lactation.

The BNF reports that there is no information available on the transfer into breastmilk and that the manufacturer advises it should be avoided.

> Use alternatives if possible due to long terminal half-life.

Diltiazem

Brand names: Adizem®, *Dilzem®, Tildiem®, Calcicard®*
US brands: *Cardizem®, Cartia®, Dilacor®, Dilt-XR®, Diltia®, Taztia®, Tiazac®*
Australian brands: *Cardizem®, Coras®, Diltahexal®, Dilzem®, Vasocardol®*

Diltiazem is used for its antiarrhythmic, anti-anginal and antihypertensive properties but rarely in women of childbearing age unless there are very specific indications from the medical history. It is rarely used simply to treat hypertension.

Okada *et al.* (1985) studied one mother who took diltiazem 60 mg four times daily and found that concentrations in breastmilk were similar to those in serum. Lubbe (1987) studied a mother and her twins. She breastfed while taking diltiazem for 6 months and no adverse effects were noted in the children. It is an option to treat breastfeeding mothers if they are unable to tolerate other anti-hypertensives. Relative infant dose quoted as 0.9% (Hale 2012 online access).

The BNF states that a significant amount is found in breastmilk and although there is no evidence of harm it should be avoided unless there is no safer alternative.

> Use alternatives if possible due to limited safety data.

References

Lubbe WF, Use of diltiazem during pregnancy, *NZ Med J*, 1987;100(818):121.
Okada M, Okada M, Inoue H, Nakamura Y, Kishimoto M, Suzuki T, Excretion of diltiazem in human milk, *N Engl J Med*, 1985;312:992–3.

Alpha blockers

> **Alpha blocker of choice in a mother during breastfeeding based on evidence of benefit and safety for the baby:**
>
> **Avoid unless essential to mother's health**

This class of drugs are generally only used in addition to other drugs with poorly controlled blood pressure. They are not normally used as first line or monotherapy

Doxazosin

Brand name: *Cardura®*
US brands: *Cardura®*
Australian brands:

In animal studies doxazosin appears to accumulate in breastmilk according to the manufacturers. Whether this is applicable to humans is unknown as there are no reported studies on passage into human milk. An active transport mechanism leading to concentration is hypothesised. This drug should only be used in extreme circumstances and with close monitoring of the infant, if at all.

The manufacturer advises avoid during breastfeeding as it accumulates in milk.

Avoid if possible due to lack of data and possible accumulation in breastmilk.

Terazosin

Brand name: *Hytrin®*
US brands: *Hytrin®*
Australian brands: *Hytrin®*

Terazosin has bio-availability of 90% and is up to 94% protein bound. The antihypertensive activity is attributed to a metabolite. There is no data on transfer into breastmilk (BNF).

Avoid as no information on passage into breastmilk.

Anti-coagulants

Anti-coagulant of choice in a mother during breastfeeding based on evidence of benefit and safety for the baby:

Warfarin, heparin, low molecular weight heparinoids as necessary are all safe to use

A thrombus is a stationary blood clot composed of fibrin and platelets and other cellular elements. Thrombosis is the occlusion of a vein or artery by a thrombus. An embolus is a fragment of a thrombus, which may occlude a blood vessel resulting in an embolism. Venous thrombosis usually results from poor blood circulation and can be precipitated by obesity, immobility or heart failure but may also be associated with clotting disorders resulting from pregnancy.

Thrombolytic medication may be used in an emergency situation. Thromboprophylaxis may also be necessary for women with a history of recurrent miscarriage or with a history of thrombosis or obesity. Such prophylaxis is generally continued for several weeks after delivery and may therefore have implications for breastfeeding.

Warfarin

Brand name: *Marevan®*
US brands: *Coumadin®, Jantovan®*
Australian brands: *Coumadin®, Marevan®*

Warfarin is contra-indicated in pregnancy as it crosses the placenta and may harm the foetus. However, heparin and the heparinoids are too large to cross the placenta and are therefore generally prescribed until delivery although warfarin may then be substituted for the post-natal period.

Orme *et al.* (1977) measured drug concentrations in the plasma and milk of 13 lactating women receiving 2 to 12 mg of warfarin daily. Plasma concentrations in the mothers varied from 1.6 to 8.5 µmol per litre (equivalent to 0.5 and 2.6 µg per ml) but none was detectable in the breastmilk or in the plasma of the seven infants who were breastfed (limit of detection 0.08 µmol per litre or 25 ng/ml). No anti-coagulant effect was found in the three breastfed infants tested. McKenna *et al.* (1983) studied two mothers but found no evidence of the drug or any anti-coagulant effect in the babies.

Warfarin interacts with many drugs so care should be taken in co-prescribing and international normalised ratio (INR) measurements should be repeated as necessary. Premature infants who are being breastfed may benefit from vitamin K supplements to prevent any possibility of haemorrhage of which they are at greater risk. It is not licensed for use in children.

The BNF states that it is not excreted in breastmilk and that there is no evidence of harm.

Compatible with breastfeeding as limited transfer.

References

McKenna R, McKenna R, Cole ER, Vasan U, Is warfarin sodium contraindicated in the lactating mother?, *J Pediatr*, 1983;103:325–7.

Orme ML, Lewis PJ, de Swiet M, Serlin MJ, Sibeon R, Baty JD, Breckenridge AM, May mothers given warfarin breastfeed their infants?, *BMJ*, 1977;1:1564–5.

Heparin

Heparin is not absorbed from the GI tract and does not cross the placenta, or pass into breastmilk. It has to be given by injection, generally sub-cutaneously, due to its lack of oral bio-availability. Its high molecular weight prevents it being transferred into breastmilk and any that could pass, would not be absorbed by the infant from its own GI tract. It can safely be used during breastfeeding.

The BNF states that it is not excreted in milk due to its high molecular weight.

Compatible with breastfeeding due to limited bio-availability.

Low molecular weight heparinoids

Low molecular weight heparinoids have a molecular weight less than 8000. They generally have a greater bio-availability and a longer half-life than heparin after subcutaneous injection but remain poorly absorbed from the gut so can be used during breastfeeding.

The BNF states that due to the relatively high molecular weight of these drugs and inactivation in the GI tract, passage into breastmilk and absorption by the nursing infant are likely to be negligible; however, manufacturers advise avoid.

Compatible with breastfeeding due to limited bio-availability.

Enoxaparin

Brand name: *Clexane®*
US brands: *Lovenox®*
Australian brands: *Lovenox®*

Enoxaparin was studied by Guillonneau *et al.* (1996) in 12 women receiving 10 to 20 mg: after 5 to 7 days of exclusive breastfeeding their infants showed no change in anti-coagulant activity or evidence of bleeding. The relative molecular size (though smaller than heparin) is still too large to be expected to pass into breastmilk. It is not licensed for use in children but used outside of licence for neonates at 1.5 to 2 mg twice daily. The BNF states that the manufacturer advises it is avoided as no information is available.

Compatible with breastfeeding, due to large molecular weight and poor transfer into breastmilk.

Reference

Guillonneau M, de Crepy A, Aufrant C, Hurtaud-Roux MF, Jacqz-Aigrain E, L'allaitement est possible en cas de traitement maternel par l'enoxaprine, *Arch Pediatr (Paris)*, 1996;4:513–14.

Tinzaparin

Brand name: *Innophep®*
US brands: *Innophep®*

Tinzaparin is similarly large. Although there are no studies on transfer into breastmilk, there is no reason to suggest that it will pass though to the baby due to its lack of oral bio-availability.

It is not licensed for use in children but is used outside of licence for babies 1 to 2 months old. The BNF states that the manufacturer advises it should be avoided as no information is available.

Probably compatible with breastfeeding, due to large molecular weight although no studies on transfer into breastmilk.

Dalteparin ☺

Brand name: *Fragmin*®
US brands: *Fragmin*®
Australian brands: *Fragmin*®

Dalteparin is a low molecular weight heparin with anti-coagulant properties. It is a large molecule with no oral bio-availability and may be expected not to penetrate breastmilk. This was confirmed by a study of two women receiving 5,000 and 10,000 units, respectively. No drug was detected in their breastmilk (Harenberg *et al.* 1987). In another study (Richter *et al.* 2001) of 15 patients who had undergone caesarian section, breastmilk levels measured were less than 0.037 IU per ml and no adverse events were reported. As the drug is not orally bio-available the levels in milk are irrelevant as the baby will not be able to absorb any present.

It is not licensed for use in children but is used outside of licence for neonates. The BNF states that there is no information on passage into breastmilk.

> Probabably compatible with breastfeeding, due to large molecular weight and limited information from studies.

References

Harenberg J, Leber G, Zimmermann R, Schmidt W, [Prevention of thromboembolism with low-molecular weight heparin in pregnancy], *Geburtshilfe Frauenheilkd*, 1987;47:15–18.
Richter C, Sitzmann J, Lang P, Weitzel H, Huch A, Huch R, Excretion of low molecular weight heparin in human milk, *Br J Clin Pharmacol*, 2001;52:708–10.

Anti-platelet agents

> **Anti-platelet of choice in a mother during breastfeeding based on evidence of benefit and safety for the baby:**
>
> **Aspirin dispersible 75 mg**

Anti-platelets decrease platelet aggregation and may inhibit thrombus formation. Clopidogrel is largely used where there is an allergic reaction to aspirin because of the increased cost. Both drugs are equally gastro-irritant so may need to be used with a PPI or H_2 antagonist for protection. There is some concern over a potential interaction between clopidogrel and omeprazole and esomeprazole, with the anti-platelet effect of clopidogrel being diminished.

References

Kwok CS, Loke YK, Effects of proton pump inhibitors on platelet function in patients receiving clopidogrel: a systematic review, *Drug Saf*, 2012;35(2):127–39.

Kwok CS, Loke YK, Inconsistencies surrounding the risk of adverse outcomes with concomitant use of clopidogrel and proton pump inhibitors, Expert Opin Drug Saf, 2012;11(2):275–84.

Clopidogrel and proton pump inhibitors: interaction—updated advice Drug Safety Update April 2010 (www.mhra.gov.uk/Safetyinformation/DrugSafetyUpdate/CON087711).

Aspirin dispersible 75 mg

Aspirin 75 mg acts by decreasing platelet adhesiveness irreversibly inhibiting aggregation. It is not used during treatment of thrombosis but may be used in cases of recurrent miscarriage and post myocardial infarction (MI) and stroke or to decrease cardiovascular risk. There is little evidence that enteric-coated tablets are less likely to increase the risk of GI bleeds and may be less effective in their anti-platelet activity as well as more expensive.

Although aspirin is not recommended during breastfeeding at analgesic doses of 600 mg four times a day, due to its association with Reye's syndrome, use of the small dose as an anti-platelet may be considered to be acceptable. In the absence of the risk of association of Reye's syndrome, aspirin would be a drug compatible with lactation due to its pharmacokinetic properties. Before the link with Reye's syndrome was identified, the children's dose of aspirin was 75 mg four times a day. Relative infant dose is quoted as 2.5 to 10.8% (Hale 2012 online access).

The BNF states that it should be avoided due to possible risk of Reye's syndrome. Regular use of high doses could impair platelet function and produce hypoprothrombinaemia in infant if neonatal vitamin K stores are low.

Compatible with breastfeeding if necessary at 75 mg daily, avoid as an analgesic.

Clopidogrel

Brand name: *Plavix*®
US brands: *Iscover*®, *Plavix*®
Australian brands: *Plavix*®

Clopidogrel is considerably more expensive than aspirin 75 mg and is generally only used in the UK where there is intolerance to aspirin, following insertion of stents into blocked cardiac blood vessels or for stroke prophylaxis. Little is known about the levels of clopidogrel secreted into breastmilk. Clopidogrel irreversibly modifies the platelet adenosine diphosphate (ADP) receptor so any reaching the baby would have a long-term affect. There are no human studies but rat studies have shown passage into milk. This significance in human treatment is unknown.

The BNF reports that the manufacturer advises it is avoided.

Avoid if possible die to lack of safety data. Use aspirin dispersible 75 mg if possible.

Lipid-regulating drugs

> **Statin of choice in a mother during breastfeeding based on evidence of benefit and safety for the baby:**
>
> **Avoid if possible, no long-term outcome studies of impact on baby of lowered cholesterol**

Raised cholesterol levels may have a genetic basis but are also associated with a high-fat diet. A diet rich in saturated fat and cholesterol and poor in fibre can produce hyper-cholesterolaemia. Obesity is often linked with raised cholesterol as is lack of exercise, and smoking. Drug-treatment centres around the use of statins (HMGCoA reductase inhibitors) which reduce the production of cholesterol in the liver. However, their place during lactation is unclear as cholesterol is an essential part of development of cells and disruption may have unknown long-term effects for the child. Given that raised cholesterol levels can frequently be reduced by modified diet and increased exercise, cessation of statin therapy during pregnancy and lactation is unlikely to be critical. However, very raised levels from familial hyper-cholsterolaemia may need individual consideration.

Simvastatin

Brand name: *Zocor*®
US brands: *Zocor*®
Australian brands: *Lipex*®, *Simvabell*®, *Simvahexal*®, *Simvar*®, *Zimstat*®, *Zocor*®

There is no data on the transfer of simvastatin into breastmilk but it is 95% plasma bound, has a long half-life and undergoes extensive hepatic first-pass metabolism so levels might be assumed to be low. However, we do not have data on the effect of breastmilk with lowered fat levels. It is not licensed for use in children.

The BNF reports that the manufacturer advises avoidance due to lack of information.

> Avoid as no information on passage into breastmilk. Follow a low-fat diet and increased exercise to lower cholesterol.

Atorvastatin

Brand name: *Lipitor*®
US brands: *Lipitor*®
Australian brands: *Lipitor*®

There are no human studies on the transfer of atorvastatin into breastmilk but it is 98% plasma bound and has a half-life of 14 hours. However, the half-life of inhibitory activity for CoA reductase is approximately 20 to 30 hours due to the contribution of active metabolites. It undergoes first-pass metabolism and breastmilk levels may be assumed to be low. It is not licensed for use in children.

According to the BNF manufacturer advises it should be avoided in breastfeeding as there is no information available.

> Avoid as no information on passage into breastmilk. Follow a low-fat diet and increased exercise to lower cholesterol.

Respiratory system

> **Respiratory drug choice in a mother during breastfeeding based on evidence of benefit and safety for the baby:**
>
> **According to needs of the mother**
> **Inhaled drugs, theophylline and prednisolone can be taken as normal during pregnancy and breastfeeding**

SIGN guidelines (2011) refer to the fact that asthma may worsen during pregnancy. In a study of 366 pregnancies, symptoms worsened in 36% of women (Schatz 1988). Studies by Schatz and Wendel (1995, 1996) in the United States suggest that 11 to 18% of pregnant women with asthma will have at least one emergency department visit for acute asthma and of these 62% will require hospitalisation.

Asthmatic women should be encouraged to breastfeed and reassured that medication is not contra-indicated during lactation. (Turner *et al.* 1980). However, a recent study (Kramer *et al.* 2007) failed to find an association between breastfeeding and a reduction in asthma or allergic symptoms. The report represents further data collected from the Promotion of Breastfeeding Intervention Trial (PROBIT) study. The authors comment that the incidence of allergy in the study population is particularly low while representative of other studies in Eastern Europe. Results cannot therefore be extrapolated to western societies with a higher background incidence.

References

Kramer MS, Matush L, Vanilovich I, Platt R, Bogdanovich N, Sevkovskaya Z, Dzikovich I, Shishko G, Mazer B; Promotion of Breastfeeding Intervention Trial (PROBIT) Study Group, Effect of prolonged and exclusive breastfeeding on risk of allergy and asthma: cluster randomised trial, *BMJ*, 2007;335(7624):815.

Schatz M, Harden K, Forsythe A, Chilingar L, Hoffman C, Sperling W, Zeiger RS, The course of asthma during pregnancy, post partum, and with successive pregnancies: a prospective analysis, *J Allergy Clin Immunol*, 1988;81:50917.

Schatz M, Zeiger RS, Hoffman CP, Harden K, Forsythe A, Chilingar L, Saunders B, Porreco R, Sperling W, Kagnoff M, Perinatal outcomes in the pregnancies of asthmatic women: a prospective controlled analysis, *Am J Respir Crit Care Med*, 1995;151:11704.

SIGN British guidelines on the management of asthma (www.sign.ac.uk).

Turner ES, Greenberger PA, Patterson R, Management of the pregnant asthmatic patient, *Ann Intern Med*, 1980;93:90518.

Wendel PJ, Ramin SM, Barnett-Hamm C, Rowe TF, Cunningham FG, Asthma treatment in pregnancy: a randomized controlled study, *Am J Obstet Gynecol*, 1996;175:1504.

Bronchodilators

> **Bronchodilator of choice in a mother during breastfeeding based on evidence of benefit and safety for the baby:**
>
> **Inhaled bronchodilators can be used as normal during breastfeeding**

Short acting beta$_2$ agonists are used to produce immediate relief of bronchospasm and used when required by asthmatic and chronic obstructive pulmonary disease (COPD) patients. Inhalation produces negligible blood levels (less than 10%) and can be used safely during breastfeeding. Oral medication, though rarely used, now can produce tremors, palpitations, tachycardia and headache in the mother and infant. Short-acting beta$_2$ agonists are widely used to treat children using spacer devices to deliver the inhaled drug.

Salbutamol

Brand names: *Salamol®, Ventolin®, Airomi®, Asmasal®*
US brands: *Accuneb®, ProAir®, Proventil®, Ventolin®, VoSpire®*
Australian brands: *Airomir®, Asmol®, Butamol®, Epaq®, Respax®, Ventolin®*

Salbutamol is readily absorbed from the GI tract but is subject to first-pass metabolism in the liver. Inhaled salbutamol acts directly on the tissues within the lung. Any absorption via the oral route is as a result of inhaler technique and swallowing of the dose. Spacer devices may reduce this. Salbutamol inhalers can be used as normal during breastfeeding (BNF). Licensed for use in children by inhalation.

> Compatible with breastfeeding due to first-pass metabolism of any drug absorbed from the GI tract.

Terbutaline

Brand name: *Bricanyl®*
US brands: *Bricanyl®*
Australian brands: *Bricanyl®, Brethine®*

Terbutaline is variably absorbed from the GI tract and about 60% of the absorbed dose undergoes first-pass metabolism and trace amounts are secreted into breastmilk. Inhaled terbutaline produces minimal blood levels and can be used as normal during lactation (BNF). It is licensed for use in children by inhalation.

> Compatible with breastfeeding due to first-pass metabolism of any drug absorbed from the GI tract.

Long-acting beta₂ agonists

Long-acting beta$_2$ agonists are used in addition to corticosteroid inhalers. They do not relieve acute asthma attacks but are a part of prevention therapy if regular use of inhaled corticosteroids has failed to control symptoms.

Salmeterol

Brand name: *Serevent®*
US brands: *Serevent®*
Australian brand: *Serevent®*

Salmeterol produces negligible plasma concentrations after inhalation (80 to 90 µg per litre in patients treated regularly over several months (Cazzola *et al.* 2002). There are no reports of levels measured in breastmilk but as maternal plasma levels are virtually undetectable, such measurements are unlikely to be possible. It is licensed for use in children by inhalation from 5 years. Inhaled drugs can be taken as normal during breastfeeding (BNF).

> Compatible with breastfeeding as minimal levels in maternal plasma.

References

Cazzola M, Testi R, Matera MG, Clinical pharmacokinetics of salmeterol, *Clin Pharmacokinet*, 2002;41:19–30.

Formoterol

Brand name: Atimos®, Oxis®
US brands: Foradile®
Australian brands: Foradil®, Oxis®

Formoterol is believed to achieve such minuscule plasma levels that breastmilk concentrations are not likely to be measurable. It is licensed for use in children by inhalation from 6 years. Inhaled drugs can be taken as normal during breastfeeding (BNF).

> Compatible with breastfeeding as minimal levels in maternal plasma following inhalation.

Corticosteroids

> **Corticosteroid of choice in a mother during breastfeeding based on evidence of benefit and safety for the baby:**
>
> **Inhaled corticosteroids can be used as normal during breastfeeding**
> **Oral prednisolone can be used to treat exacerbations**

Corticosteroid inhalers are widely used in the management of asthma, and benefit some patients with COPD. An inhaled corticosteroid such as beclometasone dipropionate, budesonide or fluticasone is added to therapy if symptomatic relief with a bronchodilator is needed regularly. Corticosteroid inhalers are unlikely to produce clinically significant levels in breastmilk and should be used regularly at normal doses to protect the health of the mother. A short 'rescue' course of oral corticosteroid (prednisolone) may be needed at for an acute exacerbation.

Prednisolone

Brand name: *Deltacortil®*
US brands: *Prednisol®, Prelone®, Predcor®*
Australian brands: *Predsol®, Predsolone®, Solone®, Redipred®*

Prednisolone is secreted in breastmilk. For maternal doses of 40 mg daily the nursing infant is exposed to minimal amounts of steroid with no clinically significant risk (see section on corticosteroids in IBD). The BNF recommends that prednisolone appears in small amounts in breastmilk but maternal doses of up to 40 mg daily are unlikely to cause systemic effects in the infant, who should be monitored for adrenal suppression if the mothers are taking a higher dose.

> Compatible with breastfeeding at dose ≤40 mg daily.

Beclometasone

Brand names: *Clenil®, Qvar®* (Some brands are licensed for children, others are not because of alcohol contact, licensed age depends on brand).
US brands: *Beclovent®, Qvar®*
Australian brands: *Becloforte®, Becotide®, Qvar®*

Beclometasone reaches clinically insignificant levels in maternal plasma after inhalation so passage into breastmilk poses no threat. The BNF recommends that inhaled drugs, can be taken as normal during breastfeeding.

> Compatible with breastfeeding due to low systemic absorption following inhalation.

Budesonide

Brand names: *Pulmicor®, Symbicort® (with formoterol)*
US brands: *Pulmicor®*
Australian brands: *Pulmicor®, Symbicort® (with formoterol).*

Budsonide reaches clinically insignificant levels in maternal plasma after inhalation so passage into breastmilk poses no threat. It is licensed for use in children by inhalation, via a spacer device. The BNF recommends that inhaled drugs can be taken as normal during breastfeeding.

> Compatible with breastfeeding due to low systemic absorption following inhalation.

Fluticasone

Brand names: *Flixotide®, Seretide® (with salmeterol)*
US brands: *Flovent®, Flixotide®, Advair® (with salmeterol)*
Australian brands: *Flixotide®, Seretide® (with salmeterol)*

Fluticasone reaches clinically insignificant levels in maternal plasma after inhalation so passage into breastmilk poses no threat. It is licensed for use in children by inhalation from 4 years. The BNF recommends that inhaled drugs can be taken as normal during breastfeeding.

> Compatible with breastfeeding due to low systemic absorption following inhalation.

Theophylline

Brand names: *Nuelin S®, Slo-Phyllin®, Uniphyllin Continus®* (prescription should be by brand due to variations in rate of absorption)
US brands: *Accurbon®, Aerolate®, Asmalix®, Elixomin®, Elixophyllin®, Slo-Phyllin®*
Australian brands: *Nuelin S®*

Theophylline is an oral bronchodilator used to treat asthma. It has a narrow therapeutic index and needs regular blood level monitoring. It also interacts with other medications and care should be taken in co-prescribing. In a study of three mothers, less than 1% of the maternal dose of theophylline was found to be excreted into breastmilk. (Stec *et al.* 1980; Reinhardt 1983). In a further study of five mothers, Yurchak and Jusko (1976) estimated the level at less than 10%. One baby in the study exhibited irritability on the days on which its mother took the drug. Relative infant dose is quoted as 5.9% (Hale 2012 online access).

The BNF states that it is present in breastmilk and that irritability in babies exposed through breastmilk has been reported but that theophylline can be taken as normal during breastfeeding. It is licensed for use in children from 2 years.

> Compatible with breastfeeding but observe for irritability following one single case report.

References

Reinhardt D, Richter O, Brandenburg G, Pharmacokinetics of drugs from the breast-feeding mother passing into the body of the infant, using theophylline as an example, Monatsschr Kinderheilkd, 1983;131:66–70.

Stec GP, Greenberger P, Ruo TI, Henthorn T, Morita Y, Atkinson AJ Jr, Patterson R, Kinetics of theophylline transfer to breastmilk, *Clin Pharmacol Ther*, 1980;28:404–8.

Yurchak AM, Jusko WJ, Theophylline secretion into breastmilk, *Pediatrics*, 1976;57:518–20.

Leukotriene receptor antagonists

Leukotriene receptor antagonists are of benefit in exercise-induced asthma and in patients with associated rhinitis. There is little information on levels secreted into breastmilk but they are licensed for use in children. Due to the high level of plasma protein binding, levels in breastmilk are likely to be low. Levels of zafirlukast are reduced when the drug is administered with food.

Montelukast (?)

Brand name: *Singulair®*
US brands: *Singulair®*
Australian brands: *Singulair®*

Montelukast is licensed for use in children from 6 months. Hale (online access 2012) suggests that levels passing into breastmilk are probably quite low, while the BNF reports that manufacturers advise avoiding its use during breastfeeding unless use is essential.

> Probably compatible with breastfeeding but there is no data on levels transferring into breastmilk.

Zafirlukast

Brand name: *Accolate®, same in US and Australia*

The manufacturers state that Zafirlukast is secreted into breastmilk. Relative infant dose is quoted as 0.7% (Hale 2012 online access). It is licensed for use in children from 12 years.

The BNF reports that it is present in breastmilk and that the manufacturer advises it should be avoided during breastfeeding.

Probably compatible with breastfeeding but there is no data on levels transferring into breastmilk.

Anti-histamines

Antihistamine of choice in a mother during breastfeeding based on evidence of benefit and safety for the baby:

Loratadine

Allergies may be seasonal (hayfever or seasonal rhinitis) or an acute reaction e.g. urticarial rash. There are two types of anti-histamines: those that cause drowsiness and second-generation products that do not produce drowsiness and are generally only taken once a day.

Hayfever can commence in March or later depending on the allergen to which the mother is sensitive. Other people may be sensitive to dust mite or animal fur that persists all year round. The symptoms are debilitating and untreated may make life unpleasant for the sufferer with runny nose and streaming eyes.

Sedating anti-histamines are valuable in preventing and treating urticaria. Sedating anti-histamines used over a prolonged period have the potential to reduce weight gain in the baby by producing excessive somnolence. Used for a short period e.g. to counteract the effects of hives, their use is not unreasonable.

The BNF states that significant amounts of some anti-histamines are present in breastmilk although not known to be harmful manufacturers advise avoiding use in mothers who are breastfeeding.

Cetirizine

Brand names: *Zirtek®, Piriteze®, Benadryl One a Day®*
US brands: *Zyrtek®*
Australian brands: *Zyrtek®*

Cetirizine is readily absorbed from the GI tract and reaches its peak concentration within half an hour. It is highly bound to plasma proteins and has an elimination half-life of about 10 hours. It has been detected in breastmilk. It does not appear to cross the blood–brain barrier to a significant extent and therefore has low levels of sedation in normal doses. It is licensed for children over the age of 6 months in the US and 2 years in the UK for symptoms of allergic rhinitis. The BNF states that significant amounts of some anti-histamines are present in breastmilk – although not known to be harmful, manufacturers advise avoiding use in mothers who are breastfeeding.

Compatible with breastfeeding due to high plasma protein binding limiting transfer into breastmilk.

Levocetirizine

Brand name: *Xyzal®*
US brands:
Australian brands:

Levocetirizine is the R-enantiomer of cetirizine and has similar action. There is no data on its transfer into breastmilk, but there is no reason to suggest it should be any less compatible with breastfeeding than the parent compound. The dose should be reduced in renal patients so it is probably best avoided where the baby has reduced renal function e.g. prematurity; neonatal period. It is licensed for use in children over the age of 2 years in syrup form. The BNF states that significant amounts of some anti-histamines are present in breastmilk – although not known to be harmful, manufacturers advise avoiding use in mothers who are breastfeeding.

> Probably compatible with breastfeeding as it is the R-enantiomer of cetirizine but no data on levels transferred are available.
> Use cetirizine or loratadine unless use is essential.

Loratadine

Brand name: *Clarityn®*
US brands: *Alavert®, Claritin®, Clear-Atadine®, Tavist-ND®*
Australian brands: *Claratyne®, Lorastyne®*

Loratadine is a long-acting, non-sedating anti-histamine and is used to children from age 2 years. No adverse effects have been seen in breastfeeding infants whose mothers were receiving loratadine. After a single oral dose of loratadine, Hilbert *et al.* (1988) measured a maximum dose in the breastmilk of six mothers of 29.2 µg per litre, 2 hours after the mother took 40 mg and a total excretion of 11.7 µg of loratadine and its metabolite desloratadine via breastmilk. In the normal UK dose of 10 mg daily this would represent approximately 3 µg passing to the baby. Relative infant dose quoted as 0.3% (Hale 2012 online access). It is licensed for use in children over 2 years at a dose of 5 mg daily. The BNF states that significant amounts of some anti-histamines are present in breastmilk – although not known to be harmful, manufacturers advise avoiding use in mothers who are breastfeeding.

> Compatible with breastfeeding. Preferred antihistamine for regular use during breastfeeding.

References

Hilbert J, Radwanski E, Affrime MB, Perentesis G, Symchowicz S, Zampaglione N, Excretion of loratadine in human breastmilk, *J Clin Pharmacol*, 1988;28:234–9.

Desloratadine

Brand name: *Neoclarityn*®
US brands: *Clarinex*®
Australian brands: *Clarinex*®

Desloratadine is the active metabolite of loratadine. There is no data on the transfer into breastmilk. The prodrug loratadine is generally well tolerated and is a better choice in breastfeeding mothers at this time, although data from the Hilbert *et al.* (1988) study may be extrapolated. It is licensed for use in children over 1 year at a dose of 1.25 mg daily. The BNF states that significant amounts of some anti-histamines are present in breastmilk. Although not known to be harmful, manufacturers advise avoiding use in mothers who are breastfeeding.

> Probably compatible with breastfeeding as it is the active metabolite of loratadine but no data on levels transferred are available.
> Use loratadine unless choice is essential.

Reference

Hilbert J, Radwanski E, Affrime MB, Perentesis G, Symchowicz S, Zampaglione N, Excretion of loratadine in human breastmilk, *J Clin Pharmacol*, 1988;28:234–9.

Fexofenadine

Brand name: *Telfast*®
US brands: *Allegra*®
Australian brands: *Fexotabs*®, *Telfast*®, *Xergic*®

Fexofenadine is a non-sedating anti-histamine. No adverse reports have been made on its use in lactation. Milk levels of fexofenadine have not been measured but data has been collected on the parent compound terfenadine (Lucas *et al.* 1995). In a telephone follow-up study of 25 infants exposed to terfendine, three mothers reported irritability in their infants but no medical attention was sought (Ito *et al.* 1993). Terfenadine itself was withdrawn from use following association with ventricular arrhythmias including torsade de pointes in some patients at high doses or in patients with liver disease. This effect has not been noted with the metabolite. It is licensed for use in children over 6 years.

The BNF states that significant amounts of some anti-histamines are present in breastmilk. Although not known to be harmful manufacturers advise avoiding use in mothers who are breastfeeding.

> Probably compatible with breastfeeding but no data on levels fexofenadine transferring into breastmilk although there are studies on terfenadine. Observe infant for irritability. Use loratadine unless choice is essential.

References

Ito S, Blajchman A, Stephenson M, Eliopoulos C, Koren G, Prospective follow-up of adverse reactions in breastfed infants exposed to maternal medication, *Am J Obstet Gynecol*, 1993;168:1393–9.

Lucas BD Jr, Purdy CY, Scarim SK, Benjamin S, Abel SR, Hilleman DE, Terfenadine pharmacokinetics in breastmilk in lactating women, *Clin Pharmacol Ther*, 1995;57:398–402.

Mizolastine

Brand name: *Mizollen®*
US brands:
Australian brands:

Mizolastine has a weak potential to prolong QT intervals and should not be used in patients with significant cardiac or hepatic disease, with hypokalaemia or other electrolyte imbalance, or with known or suspected QT prolongation. It is a non-sedating anti-histamine with a long duration of action. It is licensed for use over the age of 12 years but there is no data on transfer into breastmilk. The BNF states that significant amounts of some anti-histamines are present in breastmilk – although not known to be harmful, manufacturers advise avoiding use in mothers who are breastfeeding.

> Avoid if possible especially if the baby has concurrent cardiac problems. No data on levels transferring so use of other non-sedating antihistamines preferable. Use loratadine unless choice is essential.

Chlorpheniramine

Brand name: *Piriton®*
US brands: *Aller-Chlor®, Allergy Relief®, Allergy® Chlo-Amine®, Chlor-Pro® Chlor-Trimeton®*
Australian brands:

In the Ito *et al.* study (1993) no parents reported no adverse reactions were reported in the infants exposed through breastmilk. It is not licensed to be given to children under one year but is used outside of its licence where necessary at a dose of 1 mg twice daily (BNFC). It undergoes considerable first-pass metabolism and has a duration of action of 4 to 6 hours. There is no data on transfer into breastmilk but the pharmacokinetic information and use in children provides a reasonable level of information to support use in lactation in short courses or for the relief of night-time maternal itching when babies are unlikely to wake for feeds. It is licensed for use in children over 1 year. The BNF states that significant amounts of some anti-histamines are present in breastmilk – although not known to be harmful, manufacturers advise avoiding use in mothers who are breastfeeding.

> Use alternatives if possible for regular use. Suitable for short-term use. Observe baby for sedation and slow weight gain. Use loratadine unless choice is essential.

Reference

Ito S, Blajchman A, Stephenson M, Eliopoulos C, Koren G, Prospective follow-up of adverse reactions in breastfed infants exposed to maternal medication, *Am J Obstet Gynecol*, 1993;168:1393–9.

Promethazine

Brand name: *Phenergan®, Avomine®, Sominex®*
US brands: *Phenergan®, Phenadox®*
Australian brands: *Avomine®, Insonn-eze®*

Promethazine has been associated with sudden infant death when administered directly to infants (Kahn and Blum 1979, 1982; Kahn *et al.* 1985, Stanton 1983, Pollard and Rylance 1994, Starke *et al.* 2005). Kahn prospectively studied 52 victims of sudden infant death syndrome (SIDS), 32 near miss and 175 controls. He found 23% of SIDS infants, 22% of the near-miss infants but only 2% of controls were taking a phenothiazine medication. They suggested that these drugs can cause central and obstructive apnoea as well as reduced arousal. The European Commission reported that it was likely that the risk of apnoea is associated with all sedative drugs.

Promethazine is widely used to reduce nausea particularly associated with travel sickness as well as symptomatic relief of urticaria and as an over-the-counter (OTC) hypnotic for short-term use. There is no data available on transfer into breastmilk but it is believed that it does pass into breastmilk. It is licensed for use in children over 2 years. Chlorpheniramine is probably a safer option as a sedating anti-histamine for a breastfeeding mother unless there are compelling reasons to use promethazine. The BNF states that significant amounts of some anti-histamines are present in breastmilk – although not known to be harmful, manufacturers advise avoiding use in mothers who are breastfeeding.

> Use alternatives if possible, ideally non-sedative anti-histamine or chlorpheniramine if sedative anti-histamine is necessary.

References

Kahn A, Blum D, Possible role of phenothiazines in sudden infant death, *Lancet*, 1979;ii:364–5.
Kahn A, Blum D, Phenothiazines and sudden infant death syndrome, *Pediatrics*, 1982;70:75–8.
Kahn A, Hasaerts D, Blum D, Phenothiazine-induced sleep apneas in normal infants, *Pediatrics*, 1985;75:844–7.
Pollard AJ, Rylance G, Inappropriate prescribing of promethazine in infants, *Arch Dis Child*, 1994;70:357.
Stanton AN, Sudden infant death syndrome and phenothiazines, *Pediatrics*, 1983;71:986–7
Starke PR, Weaver J, Chowdhury BA, Boxed warning added to promethazine labeling for pediatric use, *N Engl J Med*, 2005;352:2653

Mucolytics

Mucolytics may affect sputum viscosity and structure and patients have reported alleviation of their symptoms, but no consistent improvement has been demonstrated in lung function.

Carbocisteine ⓘ

Brand name: *Mucodyne®*
US brands:
Australian brands:

Carbocisteine is used for its mucolytic activity in respiratory disorders associated with productive cough. Mucolytics may be useful in some patients with COPD but such use is unlikely in the age group generally considered to be breastfeeding mothers.

There is no information on the passage into breastmilk (BNF) but it is licensed for use in children from 2 years of age at a stating dose of 62.5 mg four times daily.

> No information on passage into breastmilk although safety likely as used in children.

Cough preparations

> **Cough mixture of choice in a mother during breastfeeding based on evidence of benefit and safety for the baby:**
>
> **There is little evidence of benefit for cough mixtures**
> **Simple linctus and mixtures containing guaifenesin are safe as used in children's medicines**
> **Remedies that cause drowsiness or contain decongestants are best avoided.**

A cough is a physiological protective mechanism. Symptoms can be divided into a productive and non-productive cough.

Expectorants have long been used on the grounds that increasing the volume of secretions in the respiratory tract facilitates removal by ciliary action and coughing. However, clinical evidence of efficacy is lacking, and many authorities consider expectorants to be of no value other than as a placebo. Commonly used expectorants include ammonium salts, guaifenesin, ipecacuanha and sodium citrate. Products containing these ingredients remain popular with patients who spend many millions of pounds annually on their purchase. There is no evidence that products containing guaifenesin, ipecacuanha and sodium citrate are harmful for breastfeeding mothers and may help to alleviate symptoms. Guaifenesin is found in many children's cough remedies.

Of the commonly used cough suppressants, pholcodine and dextromethorphan are considered to have fewer adverse effects than codeine. However, there is little evidence that these drugs are effective in severe cough at licensed doses. These ingredients are also used in preparations for children and have not been shown to exhibit respiratory depression at normal doses. Levels secreted in breastmilk are unlikely to reach clinical significance.

Demulcents provide a protective coating in the pharynx and reduce coughing in consequence. Examples include glycerol, honey, liquorice and syrup based on sucrose. These can all be used safely by breastfeeding mothers.

Combinations of cough and cold remedies have little clinical evidence of effectiveness but their use is a matter of habit and personal preference. Combinations including oral decongestants should be avoided as they can reduce breastmilk supply.

Medicines and Healthcare products Regulatory Agency (MHRA) per Commission on Human Medicines (CHM) advice (March 2008 and February 2009)

Children under 6 years should not be given OTC cough and cold medicines containing the following ingredients:

- brompheniramine, chlorpheniramine, diphenhydramine, doxylamine, promethazine or triprolidine (anti-histamines);
- dextromethorphan or pholcodine (cough suppressants);
- guaifenesin or ipecacuanha (expectorants); and
- phenyleprind, pseudoephedrine, ephedrine, oxymetazoline or xylometazoline (decongestants).

OTC cough and cold medicines can be considered for children aged 6 to 12 years after basic principles of best care have been tried. Children should not be given more than one cough and cold preparation at a time because different brands may contain the same active ingredient, care should be taken to give the correct dose.

Nasal decongestants

Nasal decongestant of choice in a mother during breastfeeding based on evidence of benefit and safety for the baby:

There is little evidence of benefit for oral decongestants in preference to topical forms. Simple saline drops are cheap and effective
If necessary, use steam inhalation, nasal drops or spray of decongestant

Nasal congestion may be a symptom of the common cold or of allergic rhinitis. The common cold is usually self-limiting and lasts for 4 to 10 days. Symptoms include nasal discharge and stuffiness, sneezing, sore throat and cough. Sympathomimetic agents are widely used for symptomatic relief produced by vasoconstriction.

Products containing ephedrine sodium chloride 0.9%, phenylephrine, naphazoline, oxymetazoline and xylometazoline can be used topically as nasal drops or sprays. Use should be restricted to less than 7 days or rebound congestion may be produced.

Pseudoephedrine

Brand names: *Sudafed®, Contac non Drowsy® and in combination with other ingredients Day and Night Nurse®, Lemsip Flu®, Medinite®, Benylin 4 Flu®* and many other products
US brands: A*frin®, Allermed®, Cenafed®, Congestaid®, Decofed®, Seudotabs®, Sudafed®* and others
Australian brands: *Demazin Sinus®, Dimetapp Sinus®, Logican Sinus®, Sudafed®* and others

In a study of 8 lactating women exposed to a single tablet of 60 mg pseudoephedrine, a reduction in milk production of 24% was measured (Aljazaf *et al.* 2003). The authors suggest that mothers exposed to the drug in late-stage lactation are more sensitive to the drug and experience a greater loss in milk production. This response should be borne in mind in recommending the drug during lactation. Nasal congestion is generally self-limiting and moist steam inhalation has been shown to be beneficial in treating cold symptoms without risk to lactation or the breastfed baby. There is no reason to suppose that the action of phenylephrine is any different to pseudoephedrine in the reduction of breastmilk supply and its use should be considered in the same way.

Small amounts of pseudoephedrine are known to transfer into breastmilk. Its use is discouraged in children under the age of 6 (see MHRA advice above). Findlay *et al.* (1984) studied 3 mothers and found levels of pseudoephedrine higher in breastmilk than plasma but that the level over 12 hours was 250 to 330 µg following a 60 mg dose, a level not high enough to warrant cessation of breastfeeding. In the study by Ito *et al.* (1993) 20% of mothers reported irritability in babies following exposure through breastmilk. Relative infant dose quoted as 4.7% (Hale 2012 online access).

The BNF states that the amount present in breastmilk is too small to be harmful.

> Avoid as possible as reports of lowered milk supply. Use topical nose sprays or drops as alternative to oral preparations if possible.

References

Aljazaf K, HaleTW, Ilett KF, Hartmann PE, Mitoulas LR, Kristensen JH, Hackett LP. Pseudoephedrine: effects on milk production in women and estimation of infant exposure via breastmilk, *Br J Clin Pharmacol*, 2003;56(1):18–24. Findlay JW, Butz RF, Sailstad JM, Warren JT, Welch RM, Pseudoephedrine and triprolidine in plasma and breastmilk of nursing mothers, *Br J Clin Pharmacol*, 1984;18:901–6.

Ito S, Blajchman A, Stephenson M, Eliopoulos C, Koren G, Prospective follow-up of adverse reactions in breastfed infants exposed to maternal medication, *Am J Obstet Gynecol*, 1993;168:1393–9.

Phenylephrine

Brand names: *Sudafed Non drowsy® and* in combination with other ingredients *Beechams all in one®*, *Lemsip cold and flu®* and many other products
US brand names: *AH-chewD®*, *Lusonal®*, *Sinex®*, *Sudafed PE®* *and others*
Australian brand Names: *Albalon Relief®*, *Nyal decongestant®*, *Prefrin®*, *Sudafed PE®*

The transfer of phenylephrine into breastmilk is unlikely to be great due to poor bio-availability but no measurements are available. It's use is discouraged in children under 6 years (see MHRA advice above). As with pseudoephedrine possible reduction in breastmilk supply is possible.

> Avoid as possible as reports of lowered milk supply. Use topical nose sprays or drops or saline drops as alternatives if possible.

Centrally acting drugs

Hypnotics

> **Hypnotic of choice in a mother during breastfeeding based on evidence of benefit and safety for the baby:**
>
> **If essential, hypnotics can be taken: be aware of risks of co-sleeping**
> **Sleep disturbances may indicate post-natal depression which may require a more effective treatment**

Insomnia is defined as the inability to achieve or maintain sleep. It may occur short term or become chronic. Insomnia may be a manifestation of an underlying condition such as depression. The use of hypnotics is generally recommended at the lowest effective dose for as short a period as possible with an emphasis on sleep hygiene and non-pharmacological measures. Tolerance develops within a very short space of time (3 to 14 days). Benzodiazepines are generally regarded as the drugs of first choice. Temazepam is indicated if falling asleep is a problem while a longer-acting drug such as nitrazepam is better for early wakening. Dependence can become a problem with regular or frequent use and withdrawal leads to rebound insomnia. Use during lactation should be discouraged, as the mother may be unresponsive to the needs of the baby. Co-sleeping after taking sedatives produces an increased risk of SIDS (see Caring for your baby at night, Baby Friendly UK 2011).

Committee on Safety of Medicines advice

1 Benzodiazepines are indicated for the short-term relief (two to four weeks only) of anxiety that is severe, disabling or subjects the individual to unacceptable distress, occurring alone or in association with insomnia or short-term psychosomatic, organic or psychotic illness.
2 The use of benzodiazepines to treat short-term 'mild' anxiety is inappropriate and unsuitable.
3 Benzodiazepines should be used to treat insomnia only when it is severe, disabling, or the individual is caused extreme distress.

References

Caring for your baby at night, Baby Friendly UK, 2011 www.unicef.org.uk/BabyFriendly/Resources/Resources-for-parents/Caring-for-your-baby-at-night/

Nitrazepam   (?)

Brand names: *Mogadon®*
US brands:
Australian brands: Mogadon®, *Alodorm®*

Matheson *et al.* (1990) studied nine women who received 5 mg nitrazepam nightly for 5 nights. No adverse effects were noted in the infants. The average amount of nitrazepam received by the breastfed baby in the morning was calculated to increase from 1 to 1.5 µg per 100 ml over the 5 days. The authors concluded that nitrazepam was compatible with breastfeeding in the immediate post-natal period but that further studies were necessary to confirm safety in the longer term. Relative infant dose is quoted as 2.9% (Hale 2012 online access). It is not licensed for use in children.

The BNF recommends that benzodiazepines are present in milk, and should be avoided if possible during breastfeeding.

> Avoid if possible. Use for a short a time as possible. Observe baby for drowsiness. Avoid falling asleep with the baby in bed, on a chair or sofa.

References

Matheson I, Lunde PK, Bredesen JE, Midazolam and nitrazepam in the maternity ward: milk concentrations and clinical effects, *Br J Clin Pharmacol*, 1990;30:787–93.

Temazepam

Brand names:
US brands: *Restoril*®
Australian brands: *Euhypnos*®, *Normison*®

Temazepam is 96% plasma protein bound. It is a short-acting bendodiazepine with a half-life reportedly between 8 and 15 hours. It is used in short-term management of insomnia but should not be used for more than 14 to 28 days. Lebedevs *et al.* (1992) studied 10 women all with babies less than 15 days old. The mothers were given 10 to 20 mg for 2 nights before milk levels were studied. No adverse effects were noted in any of the babies. Temazepam levels were detected in breastmilk in only one of 10 mothers. The authors considered that breastfed neonates would ingest negligible amounts of temazepam. It is not licensed for use in children.

The BNF recommends that benzodiazepines are present in milk, and should be avoided if possible during breastfeeding.

> Avoid if possible. Use for a short a time as possible. Observe baby for drowsiness. Avoid falling asleep with the baby in bed, on a settee or chair.

Reference

Lebedevs TH, Wojnar-Horton RE, Yapp P, Roberts MJ, Dusci LJ, Hackett LP, Ilett KF, Excretion of temazepam in breastmilk, *Br J Clin Pharmacol*, 1992;33:204–6.

Zolpidem

Brand name: *Stilnoct*®
US brands: *Amblen*®
Australian brands: *Stilnox*®

Zolpidem is an imidazopyridine with similar sedative properties to the benzodi-azepines but minimal anxiolytic properties. It has a rapid onset and a short duration of action, and is used as a hypnotic in the short-term management of insomnia. It undergoes first-pass metabolism and has an oral bio-availability of 70%. It is 92% bound to plasma proteins. Hale reports a personal communication case report of a baby who became excessively somnolent when its mother took 100 mg sertraline and 10 mg zolpidem which resolved when the hypnotic was discontinued (Hale 2012 online access). In five women given a 20 mg dose of zolpidem (normal dose 10 mg), after 3 hours the amount of drug detected in breastmilk ranged between 0.76 and 3.88 µg. This is taken to indicate the peak level to which the baby would be exposed. (Pons *et al.* 1989). No detectable zolpidem was found in subsequent milk samples.

The BNF reports that there is only a small amount secreted into breastmilk but that it should be avoided.

> Avoid if possible. Use for a short a time as possible. Observe baby for drowsiness. Avoid falling asleep with the baby in bed, on a settee or chair.

References

Reported in HaleT, Medications and Mothers' Milk (2010) as a personal communication
Pons G, Francoual C, Guillet P, Moran C, Hermann P, Bianchetti G, Thiercelin JF, Thenot JP, Olive G, Zolpidem excretion in breastmilk, *Eur J Clin Pharmacol*, 1989;37:245–8.

Zopiclone ⓘ

Brand name: *Zimovane*®
US brands:
Australian brands: *Imovane*®

Zopiclone has similar sedative and anxiolytic activity to those of the benzodiazepines. It is claimed to initiate sleep rapidly, without reduction of total rapid-eye-movement (REM) sleep. Matheson *et al.* (294) studied 12 women who took a single dose of zopiclone 7.5 mg in the early post-natal period. They found low levels of transfer via breastmilk equivalent to 1.4% of the weight-adjusted maternal dose. The babies were not allowed to breastfeed for up to ten hours but displayed no adverse effects when they resumed breastfeeding.

The BNF reports that it is secreted into breastmilk and that it should be avoided.

> Avoid if possible. Use for a short a time as possible. Observe baby for drowsiness. Avoid falling asleep with the baby in bed, on a settee or chair.

Reference

Matheson I, Sande HA, Gaillot J, The excretion of zopiclone into breastmilk, *Br J Clin Pharmacol*, 1990;30:267–71.

Anxiolytics

> **Anxiolytic of choice in a mother during breastfeeding based on evidence of benefit and safety for the baby:**
>
> **Excessive anxiety may indicate post-natal depression**
> **Behavioural therapy should be the first option if available**

Anxiolytics are used to relive anxiety disorders. Management of anxiety is best achieved by non-pharmacological methods such as counselling and cognitive behavioural therapy. Unfortunately these are often not available immediately and drugs may be prescribed in the interim. Short-term bendodiazepine use is the most common pharmacological method. Long-term use should be minimised because on dependence –

normally occurs with 4 weeks. Anti-depressants may be used for generalised anxiety disorders, particularly selective serotonin re-uptake inhibitors (SSRIs). Use of anxiolytics in lactating women is generally discouraged due to the possibility of sedation of the infant and consequential reduction in feeding efficacy and limited weight gain. However, levels entering breastmilk are relatively low and short term use with careful supervision is possible (McElhatton 1994; Birnbaum *et al.* 1999).

References

Birnbaum CS, Cohen LS, Bailey JW, Grush LR, Robertson LM, Stowe ZN, Serum concentrations of anti-depressants and benzodiazepines in nursing infants: a case series, *Pediatrics*, 1999;104:104.

McElhatton PR, The effects of benzodiazepine use during pregnancy and lactation, *Reprod Toxicol*, 1994;8:461–75.

Diazepam   ⑦

Brand names: *Valium*®
US brands: *Diastat*®
Australian brands: *Antenex*®, *Ducene*®, *Valium*®, *Valpam*®

Diazepam is also a drug which may be abused in large doses. Close observation of the baby should be undertaken and the mother encouraged to reduce the dosage as far as possible under supervision of a detoxification service if necessary. Diazepam has a long half-life (with terminal metabolite being present for 2 to 5 days) and accumulation is possible. The plasma elimination is further extended in neonates due to poor hepatic function. It is 98% plasma protein bound. A shorter-acting anxiolytic is preferable for use for more than a few days particularly in neonates.

Brandt (1976) conducted a study of four post-natal women who were given 10 mg diazepam at bedtime for six nights. He concluded that even with a neonate, a maternal dose of 10 mg produced breastmilk levels too small to cause any untoward effects in the baby. Erkkola and Kanto (1972) studied three infants whose mothers were taking 10 mg diazepam three times daily from delivery. The babies were observed for 6 days during which period no symptoms of sedation were noticed. However, Patrick *et al.* (1972) reported on a single mother taking the same dose. At 8 days of age (three days after the mother commenced diazepam) symptoms of lethargy, EEG changes and weight loss were apparent in the infant and attributed to the diazepam exposure. Relative infant dose quoted as 7.1% (Hale 2012 online access). It is licensed for use in children only to control convulsions.

The BNF suggests that benzodiazepines are present in milk, and should be avoided if possible during breastfeeding.

Diazepam is used to relieve muscular spasm following back injuries and use for a short period of time should not preclude it from use by lactating mothers in these circumstances. However, babies should be observed for sedation.

> Avoid if possible. Use for a short a time as possible. Observe baby for drowsiness. Avoid falling asleep with the baby in bed on a settee or chair.

References

Brandt R, Passage of diazepam and desmethyldiazepam into breastmilk, *Arzneimittelforschung*, 1976;26:454–7.

Erkkola R, Kanto J, Diazepam and breastfeeding, *Lancet*, 1972;299:1235–6. Letter.

Patrick MJ, Tilstone WJ, Reavey P, Diazepam and breastfeeding, *Lancet*, 1972;299:542–3. Letter.

Lorazepam

Brand names: *Ativan®*
US brands: *Ativan®*
Australian brands: *Ativan®*

Lorazepam is 85% bound to plasma proteins and is 90% bio-available. Half-life is reported as 10 to 20 hours. A post-partum study (Summerfield and Nielsen 1985) found clinically insignificant amounts of lorazepam in breastmilk even at a dose of 2.5 mg twice daily for the first 5 days post-natally. Whitelaw *et al.* (1981) estimated that an exclusively breastfed infant would be exposed to 7 µg per kg per day with a maternal dose of 2.5 mg twice daily The single infant studied showed no signs of sedation. The dose used is in this study is more than the usual maximum of 2 mg daily. Relative infant is dose quoted as 2.5% (Hale 2012 online access). It is licensed for use in children only to control convulsions.

The BNF suggests that benzodiazepines are present in milk, and should be avoided if possible during breastfeeding.

> Avoid if possible. Use for a short a time as possible. Observe baby for drowsiness. Avoid falling asleep with the baby in bed on a settee or chair. May be preferable to diazepam as it has a shorter half-life and no active metabolites.

References

Summerfield RJ, Nielsen MS, Excretion of lorazepam into breastmilk, *Br J Anaesth*, 1985;57:1042–3.

Whitelaw AG, Cummings AJ, McFadyen IR, Effect of maternal lorazepam on the neonate, *BMJ (Clin Res Ed)*, 1981;282(6270):1106–1108.

Anti-psychotics

Psychosis involves disordered thinking and loss of contact with reality due to delusions and or hallucinations. There may be accompanying mood or behavioural disturbances. Management of such patients may be complex but with the newer atypical agents they may lead normal lives including having and raising children. Symptoms of schizophrenia may be divided into positive and negative accompanied by hallucinations or apathy.

Typical anti-psychotics

The BNF states that although the amount present in breastmilk is probably too small to be harmful, animal studies indicate possible adverse effects of these drugs on developing nervous system and therefore it is advisable to discontinue breastfeeding during treatment.

> **Antipsychotic of choice in a mother during breastfeeding based on evidence of benefit and safety for the baby:**
>
> **The drug which best controls symptoms in the mother, is the most important consideration**

Chlorpromazine (?)

Brand name: *Largactil*®
US brands: *Thorazine*®
Australian brands: *Largactil*®

Chlorpromazine has a long half-life (30 hours with additional metabolites with further long half-lives) and is particularly sedating. Chlorpromazine is about 95 to 98% bound to plasma proteins and undergoes considerable first-pass metabolism to some active metabolites. Reports of drowsiness in breastfed infants appear to be restricted to high maternal doses. It is a member of the phenothiazines which have been linked with apnoea and increased risk of SIDS although no reports of infant deaths have been published It is given directly to children for a variety of reasons. It is associated with extra-pyramidal side effects in the mother and galactorrhoea. It has in the past been recommended to increase breastmilk supply but is rarely used for this purpose because of the side-effect profile (Zuppa *et al.* 2010).

Ayd (1964) studied six mothers and babies and identified no discernible effects in the babies who were breastfed from birth and studied for up to 3 months. Wiles *et al.* (1978) studied four babies, two of whom were breastfed. One of the breastfed babies showed signs of lethargy and measurable serum levels of 92 ng per ml chlorpromazine while the other had lower levels of drug (7 ng per ml) in the serum and suffered no adverse effects. Relative infant dose quoted as 0.3% (Hale 2012 online access).

The BNF reports that there is limited information available on the short- and long-term effects of anti-psychotics drugs on the breastfed infant. Animal studies indicate possible adverse effects of anti-psychotics medicines on the developing nervous system.

Observe baby for drowsiness. Avoid falling asleep with the baby in bed, on a settee or chair. Mother may have excessive milk supply due to antidopaminergic effect.

References

Ayd FJ, Children born of mothers treated with chloropromazine during pregnancy, *Clin Med*, 1964;71:1758–63.

Wiles DH, Orr MW, Kolakowska T, Chlorpromazine levels in plasma and milk of nursing mothers, *Br J Clin Pharmacol*, 1978;5:272–3.

Zuppa AA, Sindico P, Orchi C, Carducci C, Cardiello V, Romagnoli C, Safety and efficacy of galactogogues: substances that induce, maintain and increase breastmilk production, *J Pharm Pharm Sci*, 2010;13(2):162–74.

Haloperidol

Brand name: *Serenace*®, *Haldol*®
US brands: *Haldol*®
Australian brands: *Haldol*®, *Serenace*®

Haloperidol has been reported to have a plasma elimination half-life ranging from about 12 to 38 hours after oral doses. It is 92% bound to plasma proteins. It undergoes first-pass metabolism. Like chlorpromazine it is also said to increase prolactin levels. There are concerns of decline in developmental scores and extra-pyramidal effects in babies exposed through their mother's milk. Haloperidol is associated with less sedation than chlorpromazine in patients. A study of one woman, taking 5 mg twice daily, was undertaken by Whalley *et al.* (1981). After 4 weeks the infant was feeding well and showing no signs of sedation and on day 21 of therapy, the mother's milk level was 4 µg per litre. The baby was breastfed for 6 weeks and monitoring up to 12 months of age showed all developmental milestones had been reached.

Stewart *et al.* (1980) studied one woman given a mean dose of slightly less than 30 mg haloperidol for 6 days. The milk levels were reported to be 5 ng per ml. At a dose of 12 mg, a sample taken 9 hours after the medication was taken was 2 ng per ml. Licensed product information (company information) reports that there have been isolated cases of extra-pyramidal effects in breastfed infants. Yoshida *et al.* (1997) prospectively studied 12 women who breastfed. He reported some concerns on babies exposed to combinations of anti-psychotics or high doses of single agents failing to reach developmental milestones. Relative infant dose quoted as 2.1 to 12% (Hale 2012 online access).

The BNF reports that there is limited information available on the short- and long-term effects of anti-psychotic drugs on the breastfed infant. Animal studies indicate possible adverse effects of anti-psychotics medicines on the developing nervous system.

Observe baby for drowsiness. Avoid falling asleep with the baby in bed, on a settee or chair.

References

ABPI Medicines Compendium, Haldol® (http: emc.medicines.org.uk).

Stewart RB, Karas B, Springer PK, Haloperidol excretion in human milk, *Am J Psychiatry*, 1980;137:849–50.

Whalley LJ, Blain PG, Prime JK, Haloperidol secreted in breastmilk, *Br Med J (Clin Res Ed)*, 1981;282(6278):1746–1747.

Yoshida K, Smith B, Craggs M, Kumar RC, Investigation of pharmacokinetics and possible adverse effects in infants exposed to tricyclic anti-depressants in breastmilk, *J Affective Disord*, 1997;43:225–37.

Sulpiride   (?)

Brand names: *Dolmatil®, Sulpitil®*
US brands:
Australian brands:

Sulpiride is 40% bound to plasma proteins and is poorly bio-available. It is a selective dopamine antagonist and is said to elevate mood. It has been used to increase breast-milk production (Aono *et al.* 1982; Zuppa *et al.* 2010) but most studies have been poorly designed with supplements and drop-out rates making it difficult to interpret the results (Ylikorkala *et al.* 1982; Ylikorkala *et al.* 1984; Polatti 1982; Badroui *et al.* 1978; Barguno *et al.* 1988).

It has been suggested that sulpiride is less likely to cause tardive dyskinesia than chlorpromazine but extra-pyramidal side effects are reported. It can produce agitation. Adverse effects in breastfed babies have not been reported (Polatti 1984). Theoretical infant dose through breastmilk is quoted as 0.29 mg per kg per day with a relative infant dose quoted as 2.7 to 20.7% (Hale 2012 online access). Although the relative infant dose is higher than the 10% level normally agreed as considered compatible with breastfeeding, the poor bio-availability limits the absolute amount absorbed by the baby and hence the low theoretical infant dose.

The BNF reports that there is limited information available on the short- and long-term effects of anti-psychotics drugs on the breastfed infant. Animal studies indicate possible adverse effects of anti-psychotics medicines on the developing nervous system..

Although it has been used as a galactagogue in developing countries, its use cannot be recommended when there are safer alternatives.

Observe baby for drowsiness. Avoid falling asleep with the baby in bed, on settee or chair. Mother may have excessive milk supply.

References

Aono T, Aki T, Koike K, Kurachi K, Effect of sulpiride on poor puerperal lactation, *Am J Obstet Gynecol*, 1982;143:927–32.

Badroui MHH, Hefnawi F, Hegab M *et al.* The effect of a nonhormonal drug used as a contraceptive method and lactation stimulant after delivery, *Fertil Steril*, 1978;30:742. Abstract.

Barguno JM, del Pozo E, Cruz M, Figueras J, Failure of maintained hyper prolactinemia to improve lactational performance in late puerperium, *J Clin Endocrinol Metab*, 1988;66:876–9.

Polatti F, Brambilla A, Mandelli, Forgione A, Can pharmacologic hyper prolactinemia and breastsuction induce lactation in women with normal menstrual cycles?, *Clin Exp Obstet Gynecol*, 1984;11:123–5.

Polatti F, Sulpiride isomers and milk secretion in puerperium, *Clin Exp Obstet Gynecol*, 1982;9:144–7.

Ylikorkala O, Kauppila A, Kivinen S, Viinikka L, Sulpiride improves inadequate lactation, *Br Med J (Clin Res Ed)*, 1982;285(6337):249–251.

Ylikorkala O, Kauppila A, Kivinen S, Viinikka L, Treatment of inadequate lactation with oral sulpiride and buccal oxytocin, *Obstet Gynecol*, 1984;63(1):57–60.

Zuppa AA, Sindico P, Orchi C, Carducci C, Cardiello V, Romagnoli C, Safety and efficacy of galactogogues: substances that induce, maintain and increase breastmilk production, *J Pharm Pharm Sci*, 2010;13(2):162–74.

Atypical anti-psychotics

Atypical anti-psychotics may be better tolerated with fewer extra-pyramidal side effects. However, they do produce weight gain and a risk of hyperglycaemia which may need to be monitored regularly.

> **Antipsychotic of choice in a mother during breastfeeding based on evidence of benefit and safety for the baby:**
>
> **The drug which best controls symptoms in the mother, is the most important consideration**

Amisulpiride

Brand names: *Solian*®
US brands:
Australian brands: *Solian*®

Amisulpiride has fewer side effects than the typical anti-psychotics but agitation and insomnia are reported. It is 16% plasma protein bound and 48% orally bio-available. It also increases prolactin and may lead to galactorrhoea (Teoh *et al.* 2010).

There is limited information on transfer into breastmilk. Ilett *et al.* (2010) studied one mother who was keen to undertake partial breastfeeding on 250 mg desvenlafaxine daily and 100 mg amilsulpiride twice daily. Measurements on levels in milk and the plasma of mother and baby over a 24-hour period, gave a relative infant dose of 6.1% for amisulpride. No abnormalities in development were noted in a paediatric assessment and the mother planned to continue partial breastfeeding.

The same team studied one mother prescribed 400 mg amisulpiride while breast-feeding her 13-month-old child. Nine days after commencing the medication milk and maternal blood samples were taken over a 24-hour period. A relative infant dose of 10.7% was calculated based on an assumed intake of 0.15 litres per kg per day. The child showed no acute drug related adverse effects but the authors recommended cessation.

The BNF recommends that it should be avoided as there is no information available.

Little information on passage into breastmilk.

References

Ilett KF, Watt F, Hackett LP, Kohan R, Teoh S, Assessment of infant dose through milk in a lactating woman taking amisulpride and desvenlafaxine for treatment-resistant depression, *Ther Drug Monit*, 2010;32(6):704–7.

Teoh S, Ilett KF, Hackett LP, Koha R, Estimation of rac-amisulpride transfer into milk and of infant dose via milk during its use in a lactating woman with bipolar disorder and schizophrenia, *Breastfeed Med*, 2011;6(2):85–8.

Aripiprazole (?)

Brand names: *Ablify®*
US brands: *Ablify®*
Australian brands: *Ablify®*

Aripiprazole is 87% orally bio-available and 99% plasma protein bound. The mean elimination half-life of the drug and metabolites is up to 95 hours and may be extended. The incidence of extra-pyramidal effects is low and tardive dyskinesia has been reported infrequently.

In a case study of one mother 6 months post-partum taking aripiprazole 15 mg daily, milk levels after 11 and 12 days of therapy were found to be 13 and 14 µg per litre by Schlotterbeck (Schlotterbeck *et al.* 2007). Two cases of galactorrhea apparently caused by aripiprazole have been reported (Mendhekar and Andrade 2005; Ruffatti *et al.* 2005) while Mendhekar *et al.* (2006) reported one woman who took it in pregnancy was unable to establish lactation.

It is present in milk in animal studies and should be avoided (BNF).

Little information on passage into breastmilk.

References

Mendhekar DN, Sunder KR, Andrade C, Aripiprazole use in a pregnant schizoaffective woman, *Bipolar Disord*, 2006;8:299–300.

Mendhekar DN, Andrade C, Galactorrhea with aripiprazole, *Can J Psychiatry*, 2005;50:243. Letter.

Ruffatti A, Minervini L, Romano M, Sonino N, Galactorrhea with aripiprazole, *Psychother*

Psychosom, 2005;74:391–2.
Schlotterbeck P, Leube D, Kircher T, Hiemke C, Grunder G, Aripiprazole in human milk, *Int J Neuropsychopharmacol*, 2007;10:433.

Clozapine

(?)

Brand name: *Clozaril*®
US brands: *Clozaril*®, *Fazalco*®
Australian brands: *Clozaril*®, *Clopine*®

Extra-pyramidal disorders, including tardive dyskinesia, appear to be rare with clozapine and it has little effect on prolactin secretion. It is known to produce sedation and weight gain and there are reports of neutropenia which may progress to a potentially fatal agranulocytosis. Monitoring of white blood cell counts are advised in patients. Clozapine appears to be distributed into breastmilk in relatively high concentrations. Barnas *et al.* (1994) studied one mother taking 50 mg daily who did not breastfeed her baby. Her milk level was measured as 63.5 µg per litre. Dev and Krupp (1995) studied four babies who were breastfed by their mothers who were taking clozapine. He reported one baby experiencing drowsiness and one who developed agranulocytosis possibly due to the drug exposure.

Monitoring of the baby's white blood cell counts is seen to be advisable if breastfeeding is undertaken. other drugs are preferable. The risks of drug exposure through breastmilk should be carefully borne in mind. Relative infant dose quoted as 1.4% (Hale 2012 online access).

> Avoid and use alternatives if possible particularly in immediate post-partum period as may concentrate in colostrum. If using, it is essential monitor baby for sedation and agranulocytosis. Use with extreme care.

References

Barnas C, Bergant A, Hummer M, Saria A, Fleischhacker WW, Clozapine concentrations in maternal and fetal plasma, amniotic fluid, and breastmilk, *Am J Psychiatry*, 1994;151:945.
Dev VJ, Krupp P, Adverse event profile and safety of clozapine, *Rev Contemp Pharmacother*, 1995;6:197–208.

Olanzapine

Brand name: *Zyprexa*®
US brands: *Zyprexa*®
Australian brands: *Zyprexa*®

The most frequent adverse effects in adults with olanzapine are somnolence and weight gain. Hyper-prolactinaemia occurs but rarely presents clinical symptoms. Olanzapine is associated with a low incidence of extra-pyramidal effects. Gardiner *et al.* (2003) studied seven women taking a median dose of 7.5 mg olanzapine. The drug was not detectable in the serum of six infants and no adverse events were noted in any of the infants.

Goldstein *et al.* (2000) reported on two babies whose mothers were taking olanazpine. One developed jaundice and sedation in the immediate post-natal period but it may be assumed that this was not related to the drug as the condition continued when breastfeeding was stopped and formula offered. The second child was first exposed at 2 months of age when its mother took 10 mg daily. No untoward effects were noted. Croke *et al.* (2002) studied five mothers and their babies and took nine milk samples. There were no apparent ill effects in the infants. Theoretical infant dose through breastmilk is quoted as 1.12 µg per kg per day with a relative infant dose quoted as 1.2% (Hale 2012 online access).

Probably compatible with use during breastfeeding, based on two studies and low theoretical infant dose. Be aware of possibility of drowsiness in the baby. Mother should not fall asleep with the baby in bed, on a settee or chair.

References

Croke S, Buist A, Hackett LP, Ilett KF, Norman TR, Burrows GD, Olanzapine excretion in human breastmilk: estimation of infant exposure, *Int J Neuropsychopharmacol*, 2002;5(3):243–47.

Gardiner SJ, Kristensen JH, Begg EJ, Hackett LP, Wilson DA, Ilett KF, Kohan R, Rampono J, Transfer of olanzapine into breastmilk, calculation of infant drug dose, and effect on breast-fed infants, *Am J Psychiatry*, 2003;160:1428–31.

Goldstein DJ, Corbin LA, Fung MC, Olanzapine-exposed pregnancies and lactation: early experience, *J Clin Psychopharmacol*, 2000;20:399–403.

Quetiapine

☺

Brand name: *Seroquel*®
US brands: *Seroquel*®
Australian brands: *Seroquel*®

Quetiapine has been associated with a low incidence of extra-pyramidal symptoms but tardive dyskinesia may occur after long-term treatment. The most frequent adverse effects with quetiapine are somnolence and dizziness. Weight gain, particularly during early treatment, has also been noted. It appears to have a minimal effect on prolactin levels. It is 98% plasma protein bound. The half-life is 6 to 7 hours.

Lee *et al.* (2004) studied one mother taking 200 mg daily throughout pregnancy. Breastfeeding was not initiated in the absence of safety data until measurement of her breastmilk samples were available. Levels measured indicated that an exclusively breastfed baby would normally ingest only 0.09% of the weight adjusted dose (maximum 0.43%). The mother initiated breastfeeding 8 weeks after delivery. Follow up at 4.5 months indicated normal development with no adverse effects.

Misri *et al.* (2006) studied six mothers taking 25 to 400 mg daily together with an anti-depressant. In mothers taking less than 75 mg, milk levels were below the level of detection. One mother taking 400 mg daily had a level of drug in her milk of 101 µg per litre. Misri *et al.* (2006) studied developmental outcomes of 6 babies exposed to quetiapine. Four of the 6 babies scored as being within normal limits whilst 2 showed mild developmental delays. However, when compared to the 4 babies who developed normally the 2 with mild delays did not show higher exposure to medication. The authors concluded this result was due to effects other than exposure to the drug.

Several other case study reports of quetiapine use have been reported with low levels of drug reported in the babies and no adverse reactions directly attributable to the drug identified (Rampono *et al.* 2007; Kruninger *et al.* 2007; Balke 2001; Seppala 2004; Ritz 2005; Gentile 2006). A relative infant dose quoted as 0.070.1% is quoted (Hale 2012 online access).

The BNF recommends that it is present in breastmilk and should be avoided.

> Probably compatible with use during breastfeeding based on limited studies and low theoretical infant dose. Be aware of possibility of drowsiness in the baby. Mother should not fall asleep with the baby in bed, on a settee or chair.

References

Balke LD, Quetiapine effective in the treatment of bipolar affective disorder during pregnancy, *World J Biol Psychiatry*, 2001;2:303S. Abstract P02115.

Gentile S, Quetiapine-fluvoxamine combination during pregnancy and while breastfeeding, *Arch Womens Ment Health*, 2006;9:158–9.

Kruninger U, Meltzer V, Hiemke C *et al.* [Pregnancy and lactation under treatment with quetiapin], *Psychiatr Prax Suppl*, 2007;34:S756.

Lee A, Giesbrecht E, Dunn E, Ito S, Excretion of quetiapine in breastmilk, *Am J Psychiatry*, 2004;161:17156.

Misri S, Corral M, Wardrop AA, Kendrick K. Quetiapine augmentation in lactation: a series of case reports. J Clin Psychopharmacol. 2006;26:508-11.

Rampono J, Kristensen JH, Ilett KF, Hackett LP, Kohan R, Quetiapine and breastfeeding, *Ann Pharmacother*, 2007;41:7114.

Ritz S, Quetiapine monotherapy in post-partum onset bipolar disorder with a mixed affective state, *Eur Neuropsychopharmacol*, 2005;15 (Suppl. 3):S407. Abstract.

Seppala J, Quetiapine ('Seroquel') is effective and well tolerated in the treatment of psychotic depression during breastfeeding, *Int J Neuropsychopharmacol*, 2004;7 (Suppl. 1):S245. Abstract P01.431.

Risperidone

Brand name: Risperdal®
US brands: *Risperdal®*
Australian brands: *Risperdal®*

Risperidone is reported to be less likely to cause sedation or extra-pyramidal effects in the mother but more likely to produce agitation than typical anti-psychotics. Risperidone has been reported to cause raised prolactin levels, gynecomastia and galactorrhea in patients. Hill *et al.* (2000) studied one mother who took 6 mg of risperidone with low levels transferred, equivalent to 4.3% of the weight adjusted maternal dose. Ilett *et al.* (2004) studied three women taking 1.5 mg, 3 mg and 4 mg and reported weight adjusted percentages of 2.3%, 2.8%, and 4.7%. No adverse events were noted in any of the babies and no drug was detected in the plasma of the two babies who were breastfed. Aichhorn *et al.* (2005) studied one baby whose mother was taking 3 mg risperidone, over a 3-month period with no adverse effects noted. Relative infant dose quoted as 2.89.1% (Hale 2012 online access).

The BNF states that it should be used only if potential benefit outweighs risk as small amount is present in milk.

> Probably compatible with use during breastfeeding based on limited studies and low theoretical infant dose. Be aware of possibility of drowsiness in the baby. Mother should not fall asleep with the baby in bed, on a settee or chair.

References

Aichhorn W, Stuppaeck C, Whitworth AB, Risperidone and breastfeeding, *J Psychopharmacol*, 2005;19:21113.

Hill RC, McIvor RJ, Wojnar-Horton RE, Hackett LP, Ilett KF, Risperidone distribution and excretion into human milk: case report and estimated infant exposure during breastfeeding, *J Clin Psychopharmacol*, 2000;20:285–6.

Ilett KF, Hackett LP, Kristensen JH, Vaddadi KS, Gardiner SJ, Begg EJ, Transfer of risperidone and 9-hydroxyrisperidone into human milk, *Ann Pharmacother*, 2004;38:273–6.

Drugs to treat bipolar disorder

Lithium ☹

Brand name: *Priadel®, Camcolit®, Liskonum®*
US brands: *Eskalith®, Lithobid®*
Australian brands: *Lithocarb®, Clopine®*

Lithium is used to treat bipolar disorder. It is also regarded as a mood stabiliser (SIGN guidelines postnatal depression and puerperal psychosis 2012). It has a narrow therapeutic index and needs close monitoring to avoid toxicity. Signs of lithium toxicity include increasing diarrhoea, vomiting, muscle weakness and lethargy. In the UK mothers receiving lithium are generally advised to formula feed their infants. Chaudron and Jefferson (2000) searched databases for data on the use of lithium, valproate, carbamazepine, gabapentin or lamotrigine during lactation. They located 11 cases of lithium use, eight of which reported infant serum levels. Two cases reported symptoms relating to lithium toxicity in the infants. They recommended considering women's individual circumstances when prescribing during lactation. It may be possible for breastfeeding mothers to take lithium and breastfeed their infants if the baby's blood levels are monitored for lithium, thyroid stimulating hormone, creatinine although alternative medication would be preferred (Schou and Amdisen 1973; Schou 1990; Sykes *et al.*1976; Viguera *et al.* 2007). Lithium is generally felt to be a drug which should not be prescribed during lactation due to the risk of toxicity.

If the baby's state of hydration varies e.g. during illness, levels may change rapidly.

Bogen *et al.* (2012) monitored three women treated with lithium for bipolar disorder during pregnancy and lactation. The four infants born to the women had lithium levels measured at 1 month post-partum. Infant levels ranged from 10 to 17% of maternal levels. Two infants experienced early feeding problems which were overcome with breastfeeding support. The authors suggested that women taking lithium can be supported to breastfeed, but that their infants should be followed closely until breastfeeding is well established.

A relative infant dose quoted as 12 to 30.1% has been quoted (Hale 2012 online access).

The BNF advises that lithium is present in milk and there is a risk of toxicity in infant so it should be avoided.

For other mood-modifying agents please see entries for carbamazepine, valproic acid, gabapentin and lamotrigine entries under epilepsy.

> Use alternatives if possible. If used by breastfeeding mother monitor baby closely for signs of toxicity. Monitor mother and baby for lithium, creatinine and thyroid levels and ensure the baby is well hydrated.

References

Bogen DL, Sit D, Genovese A, Wisner KL, Three cases of lithium exposure and exclusive breast-feeding, *Arch Womens Ment Health*, 2012;15(1):6972.

Chaudron LH, Jefferson JW, Mood stabilizers during breastfeeding: a review:, *J Clin Psychiatry*, 2000 Feb;61(2):79–90

Schou M, Amdisen A, Lithium and pregnancy—III, lithium ingestion by children breastfed by women on lithium treatment, *BMJ*, 1973;2:138.

Schou M, Lithium treatment during pregnancy, delivery, and lactation: an update, *J Clin Psychiatry*, 1990;51:410–13.

SIGN guidelines postnatal depression and puerperal psychosis, 2012 (www.sign.ac.uk/guide-lines/fulltext/60/)

Sykes PA, Quarrie J, Alexander FW, Lithium carbonate and breastfeeding, *BMJ*, 1976;2:1299.

Viguera AC, Newport DJ, Ritchie J, Stowe Z, Whitfield T, Mogielnicki J, Baldessarini RJ, Zurick A, Cohen LS, Lithium in breastmilk and nursing infants: clinical implications, *Am J Psychiatry*, 2007;164:3425.

Anti-depressants

It is important that post-natal depression is recognised and treated effectively as it may impair bonding between mother and child and enjoyment of an important period in the relationship. Approximately 80% of women experience post-natal blues while some 10 to 15% experience more severe symptoms and need medication and or counselling. Some mothers may not immediately recognise or accept that they are depressed. Some fathers may recognise the difference in their partners. Others will deny the possibility.

The infants of depressed mothers may not have normal neurobehavioral development at one year. Treatment depends on a risk: benefit assessment for each mother:baby pair. However, it must be borne in mind that many mothers with depression report that breastfeeding is the only part of their life which they feel is under their control and at which they can succeed. Advising a mother to cease breastfeeding in order to administer anti-depressant medication should not be necessary. Should mothers need to be admitted to hospital, it should be in a mother and baby unit allowing her to continue to care for her infant. The use of cognitive counselling together with anti-depressant therapy has been shown to be advantageous.

The symptoms of post-natal depression may include obsessive thoughts often concerning harm to the baby, hyperactivity or lethargy, weight loss, volatility of behaviour and restlessness. Some women will express suicidal tendencies. But many symptoms are non-specific e.g. feeling of tiredness and not wanting to get up, not being able to cope as the day goes on and needing to go to bed early – which could describe the natural effects of caring for a new baby 24 hours a day. Some women, particularly those who are normally natural leaders, may express concern over loss of confidence. Standard depression screening tools should be used if depression is suspected e.g. International Statistical Classification of Diseases and Related Health Problems (ICD), Diagnostic and Statistical Manual of Mental Disorders (DSM-IV), Edinburgh Postnatal Depression Scale.

Most anti-depressants take three to four weeks to exert maximal efficacy and it is important that the mother is informed of this. Many patients stop taking anti-depressant medication within the first four weeks having found no benefit.

> **Antid-epressant of choice in a mother during breastfeeding based on evidence of benefit and safety for the baby:**
>
> **Sertraline or paroxetine (SSRI) or imipramine or nortriptyline (TCA)**

Tricyclic anti-depressants

Tricyclic anti-depressants (TCAs) have been available for a considerable period and much is known of their metabolism, safety and side effects. However, the side effects can be intolerable for some nursing mothers, which include sleepiness, dry mouth, urine retention and constipation.

Amitriptyline

Brand name: *Tryptizol*®
US brands: *Enovil*®
Australian brands: *Endep*®, *Tryptanol*®

Amitriptyline undergoes extensive first-pass metabolism. It is extensively bound to plasma proteins. The levels measured in breastmilk are low, because of this.

Bader and Newman (1980) studied a mother who took amitriptyline 100 mg daily for 6 weeks post-partum. She had breastmilk levels of amitriptyline and its metabolite nortriptyline of 151 and 59 µg per litre, respectively. This was calculated to represent 1.8% of the maternal weight-adjusted dosage. There were no reports of adverse effects on the baby. Misri and Sivertz (1991) followed-up a group of 20 breastfed infants whose mothers were taking a TCA for up to 3 years and found no adverse effects on growth and development even at a dose of 150 mg daily. Brixen-Rasmussen *et al.* (1982) studied a 3-week-old breastfed who had undetectable serum amitriptyline (<5 µg per litre) and nortriptyline (<15 µg per litre) during maternal amitriptyline use of 75 mg daily. Relative infant dose quoted as 1.5% (Hale 2012 online access).

The BNF states that the amount in breastmilk is too small to be harmful.

Compatible during breastfeeding due to extensive plasma protein binding and first-pass metabolism

References

Bader TF, Newman K, Amitriptyline in human breastmilk and the nursing infant's serum, *Am J Psychiatry*, 1980;137(7):85556.

Brixen-Rasmussen L, Halgrener J, Jorgensen A, Amitriptyline and nortriptyline excretion in human breastmilk, *Psychopharmacology*, 1982;76:945.

Misri S, Sivertz K, Tricyclic drugs in pregnancy and lactation: a preliminary report, *Int J Psychiatry Med*, 1991;21:15771.

Clomipramine ☺

Brand name: *Anafranil*®
US brands: *Anafranil*®
Australian brands: *Anafranil*®, *Placil*®

Clomipramine is particularly useful for panic attacks and obsessive, compulsive disorders. It is extensively plasma protein bound and undergoes extensive first-pass metabolism. In one study of four women taking 75 to 125 mg daily, plasma levels of clomipramine in the infants were below the level of detection. No untoward effects were noted in any of the infants (Wisner *et al.* 1995).

Schimmell *et al.* (1991) studied a woman who took a maximum of 150 mg clomipramine and detected a maximum of 624 µg per litre representing 2.2% of the maternal weight-adjusted dosage. Relative infant dose quoted as 2.8% (Hale 2012 online access).

The amount of TCAs secreted into breastmilk is too small to be harmful (BNF).

Compatible with use during breastfeeding due to extensive plasma protein binding and first-pass metabolism.

References

Schimmell MS, Katz EZ, Shaag Y, Pastuszak A, Koren G, Toxic neonatal effects following maternal clomipramine therapy, *Clin Toxicol*, 1991;29:47984.

Wisner KL, Perel JM, Foglia JP, Serum clomipramine and metabolite levels in four nursing mother-infant pairs, *J Clin Psychiatry*, 1995;56(1):1720.

Dosulepin

Brand name: *Prothiaden*®
US brands:
Australian brands: *Dothep*®, *Prothiaden*®

Dosulepin (Dothiepin) is a TCA with more sedative activity. It is extensively metabolised in the liver by first-pass metabolism to an active metabolite which has an elimination half-life of up to 46 hours.

At a maternal dose of 75 mg per day a concentration of 11µg per litre was estimated in breastmilk by Rees (1976). Wisner *et al.* (1996) studied a variety of anti-depressants including dothiepin (dosulepin) and could not find quantifiable amounts in nurslings, and no adverse effects were reported. Ilett *et al.* (1992) studied eight mothers taking 25 to 225 mg per day. No adverse effects were noted in any of the infants. Buist and Janson (1995) retrospectively studied 15 mothers who had taken dothiepin (dosulepin) while breastfeeding. She noted that exposure to the medication through breastmilk did not alter cognitive abilities in the children at 3 to 5 years of age compared with 15 children of mothers who had suffered from depression but not taken dothiepin (dosulepin) and 36 children of non-depressed mothers. Relative infant dose quoted as 0.8–2.2% (Hale 2012 online access).

The amount of TCAs secreted into breastmilk is too small to be harmful (BNF).

> Compatible with use during breastfeeding if alternatives unsuitable, due to first-pass metabolism although it has an active metabolite with a long half-life.

References

Buist A, Janson H, Effect of exposure to dothiepin and northiaden in breastmilk on child development, *Br J Psychiatry*, 1995;167(3):370373.
Ilett KF, Lebedevs TH, Wojnar-Horton RE, Yapp P, Roberts MJ, Dusci LJ, Hackett LP, The excretion of dothiepin and its primary metabolites in breastmilk, *Br J Clin Pharmacol*, 1992;33(6):63539.
Rees JA, Serum and breastmilk concentrations of dotheipin, Practitioner, 1976;217:686.
Wisner KL, Perel JM, Findling RL, Anti-depressant treatment during breastfeeding, *Am J Psychiatry*, 1996;153(9):11327.

Imipramine

Brand name: *Tofranil*®
US brands: *Tofranil*®
Australian brands: *Tofranil*®, *Melipramine*®

Imipramine has an active metabolite, desipramine. It is extensively bound to plasma proteins. Plasma concentrations vary widely between individuals. Imipramine is less sedating than some other TCAs. It would be prudent to observe the baby for sedation although this is unlikely. Ware and DeVane (1990) studied two women taking imipramine 50 mg daily for panic attacks. In one baby levels of impiramine and desipramine, the active metabolite, were 91 and 185 µg per litre, respectively. In the other, only trace levels were detected. Yoshida *et al.* (1997) observed four babies breastfed for up to 18 weeks while the mothers took up to 150 mg imipramine. Infant development up to 30 months of age was normal. The normal dose of imipramine as an anti-depressant is 75 mg daily in divided doses. At therapeutic doses it is estimated that the baby would receive 0.2 mg per litre and no adverse effects have been noted (NICE CG45 2007). It is used to treat nocturnal enuresis in children over the age of 6 years at a dose of 25 mg. Relative infant dose quoted as 0.1–4.4% (Hale 2012 online access).

The amount of TCAs secreted into breastmilk is too small to be harmful (BNF).

> Compatible with use during breastfeeding due to extensive plasma protein binding although it has an active metabolite.

References

NICE Antenatal and Postnatal mental health CG45 2007.

Ware MR, DeVane CL, Imipramine treatment of panic disorder during pregnancy, *J Clin Psychiatry*, 1990;51:4824.

Yoshida K, Smith B, Craggs M, Kumar RC, Investigation of pharmacokinetics and possible adverse effects in infants exposed to tricyclic anti-depressants in breastmilk, *J Affective Disord*, 1997;43:22537.

Lofepramine ☺

Brand name: *Gamanil®*
US brands:
Australian brands:

Although the amount of lofepramine in breastmilk is likely to be too small to present risk to breastfed baby (99% plasma protein bound), there is no data on transfer available.

The amount of TCAs secreted into breastmilk is too small to be harmful (BNF).

> Compatible with use during breastfeeding due to high plasma protein binding although there are no studies of transfer into milk.

Selective serotonin re-uptake inhibitors (SSRIs)

SSRIs have different side effects from TCAs. They include nausea which may be particularly marked in the early weeks of therapy, diarrhoea, headache, insomnia and agitation. They are safer than the tricyclics in overdose.

Fluoxetine ⑦

Brand name: *Prozac*®
US brands: *Prozac*®, *Sarafem*®
Australian brands: *Prozac*®, *Auscap*®, *Fluohexal*®, *Luvan*®, *Fluoxebell*®, *Zactrin*®

Fluoxetine has a long half-life (46 days in long-term use) which may in theory, lead to accumulation and high levels in the infant. It has an active metabolite norfluoxetine with a half-life extending up to 16 days. It is 95% protein bound.

Adverse effects including increased irritability, vomiting, watery diarrhoea and colic have been reported (Epperson *et al.* 2003; Kristensen *et al.* 1999; Isenberg 1990). One anecdotal report linking severe colic with the use of fluoxetine has been published (Lester *et al.* 1993). A 6-week-old baby showed signs of increased crying, decreased sleep, increased vomiting and watery stools when exposed to fluoxetine via breast-milk. The symptoms were reduced when the baby was formula-fed. Lester measured levels of fluoxetine and norfluoxetine as 69 ng per ml and 90 ng per ml, respectively, in breastmilk.

Taddio *et al.* (1996) measured the total dose of fluoxetine and norfluoxetine 0.165 mg in breastmilk, which was equivalent to 10.8% of the maternal dose. No adverse effects were noted.

Similar levels have been reported in other studies without adverse effects noted in the infants (Isenberg 1990; Burch and Wells 1992; Yoshida *et al.* 1998).

Chambers *et al.* (1999) reported reduced weight gain in infants exposed to fluoxe-tine through maternal breastmilk She studied 64 women who had taken fluoxetine during pregnancy 26 of these women breastfed their infants and continued to take the medication; 38 breastfed their infants but did not take the medication. Postnatal weight gain was obtained from medical records, and the frequency of side effects was determined by maternal response to a questionnaire. The infants who were breastfed by mothers taking fluoxetine had a growth curve significantly below that of infants who were breastfed by mothers who did not take the drug. The average deficit in measurements taken between 2 weeks and 6 months of age was 392 g. No mother who breastfed her infant while taking fluoxetine reported any unusual symptoms that could be attributed to the medication. The reduced weight gain did not exceed 2 stan-dard deviations below the mean so may not be of clinical significance in an otherwise well baby. Hendrick *et al.* (2003) used similar methodology to study and found that drug exposure did not affect weight gain but the degree of depression experienced by the mother did.

Hale (2001) reports personal communications that indicate that it can cause exces-sive sedation if used throughout pregnancy and then in subsequent lactation. He has recommended that if it is used in pregnancy that the mother is changed onto another SSRI in the 2 weeks before expected delivery. This may not always be possible depend-ing on the state of mother's mental health. It is suggested that use in mothers of babies more than 6 months old would appear to be compatible with breastfeeding.

The BNF states that it is present in breastmilk and should be avoided.

Compatible with use during breastfeeding in mothers of babies more than 6 weeks of age based on studies. May cause excessive drowsiness after delivery if used during pregnancy. Has been reported to cause irritability or drowsiness in the baby and delayed weight gain.

References

Burch KJ, Wells BG, Fluoxetine/norfluoxetine concentrations in human milk, *Pediatrics*,1992;89:676–7.

Chambers CD, Anderson PO, Thomas RG, Dick LM, Felix RJ, Johnson KA, Jones KL, Weight gain in infants breastfed by mothers who take fluoxetine, *Pediatrics*, 1999;104(5):e61.

Epperson CN, Jatlow PI, Czarkowski K, Anderson GM, Maternal fluoxetine treatment in the post-partum period: effects on platelet serotonin and plasma drug levels in breastfeeding mother-infant pairs, *Pediatrics*, 2003;112:e4259.

Hale TW, Shum S, Grossberg M, Fluoxetine toxicity in a breastfed infant, *Clin Pediatr*, 2001;40:6814.

Hendrick V, Smith LM, Hwang S, Altshuler LL, Haynes D, Weight gain in breastfed infants of mothers taking anti-depressant medications, *J Clin Psychiatry*, 2003;64:41012.

Isenberg KE, Excretion of fluoxetine in human breastmilk, *J Clin Psychiatry*, 1990;51:169. Letter.

Kristensen JH, Ilett KF, Hackett LP, Yapp P, Paech M, Begg EJ, Distribution and excretion of fluoxetine and norfluoxetine in human milk, *Br J Clin Pharmacol*, 1999;48:5217.

Lester BM, *et al*. Possible association between fluoxetine hydrochloride and colic in an infant, *J Am Acad Child Adolesc Psychiatry*, 1993;32:1253–5.

Taddio A, Ito S, Koren G, Excretion of fluoxetine and its metabolite, norfluoxetine, in human breastmilk, *J Clin Pharmacol*, 1996;36:42–7.

Yoshida K, Smith B, Craggs M, Kumar RC, Fluoxetine in breastmilk and developmental outcome of breastfed infants, *Br J Psychiatry*, 1998;172:175–9.

Sertraline ☺

Brand name: *Lustral*®
US brands: *Zoloft*®
Australian brands: *Zoloft*®, *Xydep*®

Sertraline has a long half-life metabolite which is only marginally active, unlike that in fluoxetine, and hence is unlikely to cause effects in the baby. It undergoes extensive first-pass metabolism and is 98% plasma bound.

Altshuler *et al.* (1995) studied one woman at 3 weeks and 7 weeks after delivery. Lowest levels of sertraline and its metabolite were found immediately before the daily medication as might be expected and highest levels 5 to 9 hours after the dose. Drug levels were undetectable in the infant's serum and no adverse effects were noted.

Hendrick *et al.*(2001) studied 30 mothers and babies and found detectable levels in 24% of samples. This was more likely with younger babies and those exposed to 100 mg or more daily. She noted no adverse events. Kristensen *et al.* (1998) studied eight women and their babies (average age 5.7 months) and could not detect any drug in the serum of four babies. No adverse events were noted and all babies reached their developmental milestones. She deduced a m/p ratio of 1.93 for sertraline and 1.64 for the metabolite N-desmethylsertraline. Stowe *et al.* (2003) studied 26 women taking 25 to 200 mg sertraline daily, fifteen of whom supplied breastmilk samples. He found widely varying milk plasma ratios 0.42 to 4.81 and that maternal daily dose, duration of medication exposure, and infant age and weight at sampling did not correlate with either detectability. No adverse events were documented. There are multiple published studies on infants with no untoward effects noted. In almost all cases little, if any, of the drug has been detected in the infant plasma. There is one report of an infant developing benign neonatal sleep at 4 months, which resolved at 6 months. It is unclear whether this bears any relationship with the maternal use of sertraline (Mammen *et al.* 1997). Rohan (1997) reported a case of agitation which resolved spontaneously. Relative infant dose quoted as 0.4 to 2.2% (Hale 2012 online access).

The BNF states that it is not known to be harmful but consider discontinuing breastfeeding.

> Compatible with use during breastfeeding and anti-depressant of choice during breastfeeding because it is highly plasma protein bound and has an inactive metabolite.

References

Altshuler LL, Burt VK, McMullen M, Hendrick V, Breastfeeding and sertraline: a 24-hour analysis, *J Clin Psychiatry,* 1995;56:243–5.

Hendrick V, Fukuchi A, Altshuler L, Widawski M, Wertheimer A, Brunhuber MV, Use of sertraline, paroxetine and fluvoxamine by nursing women, *Br J Psychiatry,* 2001;179:163–6.

Kristensen JH, Ilett KF, Dusci LJ, Hackett LP, Yapp P, Wojnar-Horton RE, Roberts MJ, Paech M, Distribution and excretion of sertraline and N-desmethylsertraline in human milk, *Br J Clin Pharmacol,* 1998;45:453–7.

Mammen OK, Perel JM, Rudolph G, Foglia JP, Wheeler SB, Sertraline and norsertraline levels in three breastfed infants, *J Clin Psychiatry,* 1997;58:1003.

Rohan A, Drug distribution in human milk, *Aust Prescriber,* 1997;20:84.

Stowe ZN, Hostetter AL, Owens MJ, Ritchie JC, Sternberg K, Cohen LS, Nemeroff CB, The pharmacokinetics of sertraline excretion into human breastmilk: determinants of infant serum concentrations, *J Clin Psychiatry,* 2003;64:73–80.

Citalopram

Brand name: *Cipramil®*
US brands: *Celexa®*
Australian brands: *Celapram®, Ciazil®, Cipramil®, Talam®, Talohexal®*

Citalopram has a lower plasma protein binding of less than 80% than sertraline. The metabolite enters breastmilk in low levels.

There is one report of an infant exhibiting 'uneasy' sleep patterns on a maternal dose of 40 mg per day (Schmidt *et al.* 2000) that resolved when the mother's dose was reduced and partial substitution with artificial formula undertaken. The manufacturer reports cases of excessive somnolence, decreased feeding and weight loss in breastfed infants have been reported according to Hale (online access 2012). Spigsett *et al.* (1997) studied two patients and estimated the absolute dose to the infant during steady-state conditions would be 0.7 to 5.9% of the weight-adjusted maternal dose. Berle's study (2004) of 25 women taking SSRI antidreprssants (nine taking citalopram) noted no adverse effects on the babies were noted. The infant serum levels of citalopram were undetectable in four infants and low in the remaining six. Lee *et al.* (2004) conducted a prospective, observational study of 31 mothers suffering from depression and taking citalopram with 12 mothers with depression but not taking citalopram and 31 healthy control women and babies. Mothers were taking up to 60 mg citalopram daily. There were numerically more reports of adverse events in the trial group 3 per 31 (depressed and taking citalopram group) compared with 1 per 31 (control group) and 0 per 12 (depressed but not taking citalopram group) but this was not a statistically significant difference. Infants of the mothers in the group exposed to citalopram reported colic, decreased feeding and irritability.

Heikkinen *et al.* (2002) studied 11 mother and baby pairs with matched controls, for up to 2 months after delivery. The neurodevelopment of the children was monitored for up to 1 year. The levels in infant plasma were very low or undetectable. The delivery outcomes and development were normal. Relative infant dose quoted as 3.6% (Hale 2012 online access).

The BNF states that it is present in breastmilk and should be used with caution.

> Compatible with use during breastfeeding from studies and low relative infant dose. Be aware of the risk of colic, decreased feeding and irritability.

References

Berle JØ, Steen VM, Aamo TO, Breilid H, Zahlsen K, Spigset O, Breastfeeding during maternal anti-depressant treatment with serotonin reuptake inhibitors: infant exposure, clinical symptoms, and cytochrome P450 genotypes, *J Clin Psychiatry,* 2004;65:122834.

Heikkinen T, Ekblad U, Kero P, Ekblad S, Laine K, Citalopram in pregnancy and lactation, *Clin Pharmacol Ther*, 2002;72: 184–91

Lee A, Woo J, Ito S, Frequency of infant adverse events that are associated with citalopram use during breastfeeding, *Am J Obstet Gynecol*, 2004;190(1):21821.

Schmidt K, Oleson OV, Jensen PN, Citalopram and breastfeeding: serum concentration and side effects in the infant, *Biol Psychiatry*, 2000;47:1645.

Spigset O, Carieborg L, Ohman R, Norstrom A, Excretion of citalopram in breastmilk, *Br J Clin Pharmacol*, 1997;44(3):2958.

Escitalopram

Brand name: *Cipralex*®
US brands: *Lexapro*®
Australian brands: *Lexapro*®

Escitalopram is the *S*-enantiomer of citalopram. Its mechanism of action is similar but it is claimed to have a faster onset of action. Rampono *et al.* (2006) studied eight mothers taking escitalopram for post-natal depression. Results showed that the total relative infant dose for escitalopram plus its demethyl metabolite was 5.3%. All of the infants in the study met normal developmental milestones and no adverse effects were seen. Side-effect profile may be expected to be lower than those of citalopram as dose is smaller reflecting use of the active enantiomer. Relative infant dose quoted as 5.2 to 8% (Hale 2012 online access).

The BNF states that it is present in breastmilk and use should be avoided.

> Compatible with use during breastfeeding from one study. As the enantiomer of citalopram profile might be expected to be similar.

Reference

Rampono J, Hackett LP, Kristensen JH, Kohan R, Page-Sharp M, Ilett KF, Transfer of escitalopram and its metabolite demethylescitalopram into breastmilk, *Br J Clin Pharmacol*. 2006;62(3):31622.

Paroxetine

Brand name: *Seroxat*®
US brands: *Paxil*®, *Pexeva*®
Australian brands: *Aropax*®, *Oxetine*®, *Paxtine*®

Paroxetine is 95% plasma protein bound and undergoes extensive first-pass metabolism in the liver. Although Begg (1999) detected levels of paroxetine in two studies of a total 10 mother and baby pairs The drug was not detected in the plasma of seven of the infants studied and was detected but not quantifiable (<4 µg per litre) in one infant and no adverse effects were observed in any of the infants. The mean dose of paroxetine received by the infants in the second study (four babies) was 1.25% (range 0.38 to 2.24) of the weight-adjusted maternal dose. The mean m/p ratio calculated was 0.96. Similarly Öhman *et al.* (1999) measured mean milk: serum concentration ratios in six subjects as ranging from 0.39 to 1.11 and the mean estimated dose to the infants ranging from 0.7% to 2.9% of the weight-adjusted maternal dose. Hendrick *et al.* (2001) found no detectable medication was present in any of the 16 infants she studied exposed to paroxetine. Merlob *et al.* (2004) carried out a prospective observational study on weight gain as well as reported adverse events of 27 mothers taking paroxetine and breastfeeding, 19 who did not breastfeed and did not take paroxetine and 27 mothers who breastfed but took no medication. There were no statistically significant differences between the paroxetine group and control groups in mean infant weight at ages 6 and 12 months. The usual developmental milestones were reached in all groups. One mother reported irritability in her breastfed infant. The authors concluded it was a reasonable choice of SSRI during lactation.

There are reports of neonatal withdrawal syndrome in newborns exposed to paroxetine *in utero*. Symptoms include jitteriness, vomiting, irritability and hypoglycaemia (Stiskal *et al.* 2001). There is some discussion on whether this is withdrawal or serotonin toxicity exacerbated by the use of opiates in the delivery room (Isbister *et al.* 2001). Relative infant dose quoted as 1.2 to 2.8% (Hale 2012 online access).

It is present in breastmilk but at levels too small to be harmful (BNF).

> Compatible with use during breastfeeding due to high plasma protein binding and extensive first-pass metabolism. Observe for symptoms of jittery behaviour immediately after birth.

References

Begg EJ, Duffull SB, Saunders DA, Buttimore RC, Ilett KF, Hackett LP, Yapp P, Wilson DA, Paroxetine in human milk, *Br J Clin Pharmacol*, 1999;48:142–7.

Hendrick V, Fukuchi A, Altshuler L, Widawski M, Wertheimer A, Brunhuber MV, Use of sertraline, paroxetine and fluvoxamine by nursing women, *Br J Psychiatry*, 2001;179:1636.

Isbister GK, Dawson A, Whyte IM, Prior FH, Clancy C, Smith AJ, Neonatal paroxetine withdrawal syndrome or actually serotonin syndrome?, *Arch Dis Child Fetal Neonatal Ed*, 2001;85(2):F147F148.

Merlob P, Stahl B, Sulkes J, Paroxetine during breastfeeding: infant weight gain and maternal adherence to counsel, *Eur J Pediatr*, 2004;163:135–9.

Ohman R, Hägg S, Carleborg L, Spigset O, Excretion of paroxetine into breastmilk, *J Clin Psychiatry*, 1999;60:519–23.

Stiskal JA, Kulin N, Koren G, Ho T, Ito S, Neonatal paroxetine withdrawal syndrome, *Arch Dis Child Fetal Neonatal Ed*, 2001;84:F134F135.

Venlafaxine ☺

Brand name: *Efexor*®
US brands: *Effexor*®
Australian brands: *Efexor*®

Venlafaxine is 27% plasma protein bound and its metabolite 30%. The dose transferred to the infant is relatively high and although no adverse reports have been reported it may be wise to use this drug with caution. However, as it has a high rate of discontinuation problems, stopping the drug should be regarded as unlikely and breastfeeding monitored and not a contraindication.

De Moor *et al.* (2003) reported withdrawal symptoms in a baby delivered to a mother who had taken venlafaxine throughout pregnancy. The symptoms were restlessness, hypertonia, jitteriness, irritability and poor feeding. Administration of a 1 mg dose directly to the child temporarily reduced symptoms which resolved spontaneously after 8 days. Ilett *et al.* (2002) studied three mothers and babies and estimated that the mean total infant dose of venlafaxine was 7.6% (range 4.7 to 9.2%) of the maternal weight-adjusted dose. No adverse effects were noted. He further studied seven mothers and babies with a mean child age of 7 months whose mothers were taking 225 to 300 mg venlafaxine per day. Venlafaxine was detected in the plasma of one out of seven infants studied and the metabolite in four. The concentrations of venlafaxine and the metabolite O-desmethyl venlafaxine in breastmilk were 2.5 and 2.7 times those in maternal plasma. Ilett *et al.* reported the mean total drug exposure of the breastfed infants was 6.4% (5.5 to 7.3%). There were no adverse effects in any of the infants and the authors suggested that the data support the use of venlafaxine in breastfeeding. Relative infant dose quoted as 6.8 to 8.1% (Hale 2012 online access).

It is present in breastmilk and should be avoided (BNF).

> Although not a drug of choice, probably compatible with use during breastfeeding although a relatively large amount is transferred into breastmilk, effects noted in babies are relatively uncommon in studies. Observe for symptoms of jittery behaviour and discontinuation syndrome when breastfeeding ceases.

References

de Moor RA, Mourad L, ter Haar J, Egberts AC, Withdrawal symptoms in a neonate following exposure to venlafaxine during pregnancy, *Ned Tijdschr Geneeskd*, 2003;147:1370–72.

Ilett KF, Kristensen JH, Hackett LP, Paech M, Kohan R, Rampono J, Distribution of venlafaxine and its O-desmethyl metabolite in human milk and their effects in breastfed infants, *Br J Clin Pharmacol*, 2002;53(1):17–22.

Progesterone injections and pessaries

It has been suggested that post-natal depression and pre-menstrual disorder may be linked to low progesterone levels. Dalton and Holton (2001) advocated the use of progesterone injections for the first 10 days after birth followed by the use of progesterone (*Cyclogest®*) as a suppository or pessary 400 mg twice a day until periods return and for the last 14 days of the cycle thereafter. This is compatible with lactation but should be accompanied by adequate carbohydrate consumption (every two hours by day) according to Dalton and Holton. This treatment has not been proved by double-blind trials and is now somewhat controversial. However, if the mother does not wish to take anti-depressant medication it may provide some support, if only at a placebo level.

> Compatible with use during breastfeeding as absorption into breastmilk is low.

Reference

Dalton K, Holton W, *Depression after Childbirth: How to Recognize, Treat, and Prevent Postnatal Depression (4th Ed)*, Oxford University Press, 2001.

Anti-obesity drugs

The prevalence of obesity is increasing in developed countries. It results from an imbalance of energy intake and expenditure particularly from high-fat, high-sugar and high-protein convenience foods. Obesity brings with it increased risks of cardiovascular disease, diabetes and some cancers. Behavioural modification should be the mainstay of obesity treatment but may be difficult for some individuals. Mothers should be reminded that breastfeeding utilises calories stored during pregnancy and that accompanied by exercise and sensible eating patterns leads to a gradual weight loss. Weight loss in pregnancy guidelines were produced by NICE in 2010 (PH27). Earlier guidelines suggest that mothers should not actively strive to reduce weight during pregnancy (NICE PH11 2008).

The use of medication to facilitate weight loss has become increasingly popular. In April 2009, Orlistat became available as an OTC drug at a strength of 5 mg under the brand name Alli®. Anti-obesity drugs are recommended where the individual body mass index (BMI) exceeds 30. Use during lactation should be carefully considered. In the absence of safety data, healthy lifestyle encouragement and continued lactation is a preferable option to medication. Mothers who have had bariatric surgery can still breastfeed so long as they are consuming 1800 calories a day and their weight is stable (*Breastfeeding Answer Book* 2012). It is advisable that the mother takes vitamin B12, iron, calcium in a multivitamin and mineral supplement.

> **Anti-obesity drug of choice in a mother during breastfeeding based on evidence of benefit and safety for the baby:**
>
> **No evidence of safety**
> **Follow a low-fat diet and increased exercise for weight loss**

References

NICE, PH27 Weight loss before, during and after pregnancy, 2010.

Orlistat

Brand name: Xenical®, Alli®
US brands: Xenical®
Australian brands: Xenical®

Orlistat is a lipase inhibitor and reduces the absorption of dietary fat. It is used in conjunction with a hypocalorific diet with a low fat level. Orlistat may reduce the absorption of fat-soluble vitamins. There is no information on its use in lactation although it is reported to be minimally absorbed after oral doses (Martindale 2007). In the absence of safety data, lifestyle advice and support may be preferable. No information is available and it should be avoided (BNF).

> Avoid as no information on passage into breastmilk.

Drugs used to treat nausea and vertigo

Nausea can be triggered by a variety of factors including food poisoning, motion sickness, labarynthitis, vertigo, pregnancy, migraine or as a symptom of other underlying conditions e.g. IBD.

Travel sickness is caused by a contradictory set of signals from the eyes and the inner ear balance mechanism, which is why reading in a car may trigger symptoms for many people. Treatment may be achieved by simple remedies such as avoiding heavy meals, fresh air, acupressure bands and ginger or peppermint. However, some mothers may need medication if their symptoms are severe or prolonged e.g. a long flight or sea crossing. It may be important that the mother is not made drowsy by the remedy if she has to care for the child during the journey. Frequently travel sickness remedies are based on anti-histamines e.g. promethazine (*Avomine®*, *Phenergan®*), although the passage of these sedating remedies may produce some drowsiness in the baby, in the short term this is unlikely to cause major difficulties with milk supply and may assist the journey by sedating the baby. If the baby is excessively drowsy it may need to be woken and prompted to feed to prevent dehydration.

Other remedies rely on the anti-muscarinic action of hyoscine and may make the mother thirsty but less drowsy e.g. *Kwells®*.

> **Anti-nauseant of choice in a mother during breastfeeding based on evidence of benefit and safety for the baby:**
>
> **Travel sickness – short term according to preference**
> **Vertigo – prochlorperazine**
> **Nausea – domperidone**

Cinnarazine

Brand name: *Stugeron®*
US brands:
Australian brands:

Cinnarazine is used for symptomatic treatment of nausea and vertigo caused by Ménière's disease as well as prevention of travel sickness. There is no data on transfer into breastmilk but it is licensed for use in children.

The BNF states that although not known to be harmful, the manufacturer advises it should be avoided by breastfeeding mothers.

> Probably compatible with use during breastfeeding. Although there is no data on transfer into breastmilk, it is licensed for use in children.

Prochlorperazine

Brand names: *Stemetil®*, *Buccastem®*
US brands: *Compazine®*, *Compro®*
Australian brands: *Stemetil®*, *Stemzine®*

Prochlorperazine is used to treat vertigo, labarynthitis, migraine or drug-induced emesis. It can be administered as a buccal tablet for rapid onset of action or where severe vomiting is a problem. Its oral bio-availability is low due to high first-pass metabolism, but like all phenothiazines, has many metabolites, some active. It is not generally used in travel sickness prophylaxis. It is a member of the phenothiazine family to which children are particularly sensitive. Long-term use should be avoided in breastfeeding where possible, particularly with very young babies where there is a potential risk of apnoea. However, short-term acute use probably poses few risks as it is licensed for use in children over 10 kg.

Phenothiazine derivatives are sometimes used in breastfeeding women for short-term treatment of nausea and vomiting (BNF).

> Probably compatible with use during breastfeeding if used short term. Avoid long term or where child is at risk of apnoea.

Domperidone

Brand name: *Motilium®, Motilium 10®*
US brands:
Australian brands: *Motilium®*

Domperidone acts at the chemoreceptor trigger zone. It is used for nausea and vomiting associated with chemotherapy. It stimulates gastric emptying – hence its OTC licence in the UK for 'over full and bloated feelings' under the brand name *Motilim 10®*. It causes fewer central effects such as sedation and dystonia (although there are still reports of these) because it does not cross the blood–brain barrier. Its dopamine antagonist activity stimulates prolactin release, which makes it useful as a galactagogue. There have been no reports of adverse events in babies who have been breastfed by mothers while taking this drug (see section on drugs to increase lactation).

Domperidone is metabolised by cytochrome P450 so care should be taken with potential interactions. It is more than 90% bound to plasma proteins and has a low bio-availability on an empty stomach (15%) when taking orally due to first-pass hepatic and intestinal metabolism. Mean serum levels of domperidone measured in babies through maternal use of 10 mg three times daily was only 1.2 ng per ml. The total amount of the drug that would be ingested by the infant (Da Silva *et al.* 2001) would be extremely small (about 180 ng per kg daily, assuming a daily milk intake of 150 ml per kg). Relative infant dose quoted as 0.01 to 0.04% (Hale 2012 online access).

The BNF states that the amount secreted into breastmilk is probably too small to be harmful.

Doses of more than 60 mg per day have been associated with sudden cardiac death although reports have been predominantly in the elderly and in those receiving intravenous doses (FDA 2004, Joss *et al.* 1982, Giaccone *et al.* 1984, Weaving 1984, Roussak 1984, Osborne *et al.* 1985, manufacturers information 2012).

> Compatible with use during breastfeeding due to extensive plasma protein binding. See also information as a galactogogues.

References

Da Silva OP, Knopper t DC, Angelini MM, Forret PA, Effect of domperidone on milk production in mothers of premature newborns: a randomized, double-blind, placebo-controlled trial, *CMAJ* 2001;164(1):17–21.

FDA warns against women using unapproved drug, domperidone, to increase milk production (7 June 2004). Available online: www.fda.gov/bbs/topics/ANSWERS/2004/ ANS01292.html

Giaccone G, Bertetto O, Calciati A, Two sudden deaths during prophylactic antiemetic treatment with high doses of domperidone and methylprednisolone, *Lancet*, 1984;ii:1336–7.

Joss RA, Goldhirsch A, Brunner KW, Galeazzi RL, Sudden death in cancer patient on high-dose domperidone, *Lancet*, 1982;i:1019.

Osborne RJ, Slevin ML, Hunter RW, Hamer J, Cardiotoxicity of intravenous domperidone, *Lancet*, 1985;2:385.

Roussak JB, Carey P, Parry H, Cardiac arrest after treatment with intravenous domperidone, *BMJ*, 1984;289:1579.

Weaving A, Bezwoda WR, Derman DP, Seizures after antiemetic treatment with high dose domperidone: report of four cases, *BMJ*, 1984;288:1728.

Metoclopramide ☺

Brands as anti-emetic: *Maxolon*®
Anti-migraine preparations: *Migravess*®, *Paramax*®
US brands: *Reglan*®, *Octamide*®, *Reclomide*®
Australian brands: *Maxolon*®, *Pramin*®

Metoclopramide is a dopamine antagonist and can cause extra-pyramidal side effects in particular acute dystonia. This adverse effect is most commonly seen in children and young adults, especially females, so it is not a drug of choice in lactating mothers who generally fall into this age group. It may also precipitate hypotension and depression. Other side effects reported include headache, diarrhoea, dry mouth and change in appetite (Ingram *et al.* 2011). It stimulates prolactin secretion and has been used as a galactogogue but has now been superseded by domperidone because of the latter does not cross the blood–brain barrier (Ingram *et al.* 2011). The bio-availability of oral metoclopramide is about 75% but varies widely between patients due to its hepatic first-pass metabolism. Concentrations higher than those in maternal plasma may be reached in breastmilk particularly in the early puerperium, although these decrease with increased maturity.

Metoclopramide has pro-kinetic and anti-emetic properties and acts directly on the gastro-intestinal tract without altering acid secretion. It may be used in combination with analgesics to treat migraine symptoms. In the UK its use is restricted for children below 20 years of age unless they have severe intractable vomiting of known cause, due to vomiting of radiotherapy or cytotoxics.

It is more frequently used in the US where domperidone is not available. Relative infant dose quoted as 4.7 to 14.3% (Hale 2012 online access). The BNF states that only a small amount is present in breastmilk but should be avoided.

> Compatible with use during breastfeeding but avoid if possible due to risk of extra-pyramidal effects and link with depression. Use domperidone as an alternative.

References

Ingram J, Taylor H, Churchill C, Pike A, Greenwood R, Metoclopramide or domperidone for increasing maternal breastmilk output: a randomised controlled trial, *Arch Dis Child Fetal Neonatal Ed*, 2012;97(4):F241–5.

Cyclizine

Brand name: *Valoid®* and in *Migril®* (for migraines)
US brands: *Marazine®* (for travel sickness)
Australian brands: In *Migril®* (for migraines)

Cyclizine is an anti-emetic used to treat nausea and vomiting including motion sickness, post-operative nausea and vomiting, after radiotherapy, and in drug- induced situations. It is also included in *Migril®* tablets which are used to treat migraine but this product is contra-indicated in breastfeeding due to its ergotamine content. There are no reports of levels entering breastmilk (BNF) or data on which to base conclusions. There is an unlicensed dose for children aged over 6 years.

> Avoid if possible as no information on passage into breastmilk although if use considered essential unlikely to produce adverse effects if used short term. Long-term use may cause drowsiness in baby and consequent weight loss.

Hyoscine

Brand names: *Joy Rides®, Kwells®, Buscopan®, Scopoderm TTS®* and in *Feminax®*
US brands: *Transderm Scop®*
Australian brands: *Kwells®, Buscopan®, Setacol®, Travacalm HO®*

Hyoscine produces a reduction in salivation as well as some sedation. It is commonly used to prevent travel sickness as well as other types of nausea, either as an oral tablet or as a patch. It is readily absorbed through the skin (*Scopoderm TTS®*). Hyoscine butylbromide is also used in conditions associated with smooth muscle spasm of the gut (*Buscopan®*). It is also included in a product available over the counter to treat dysmenorrhoea (*Feminax®*). It is believed to pass into breastmilk but no studies report the amounts. No reports of adverse effects appear to have been made and it appears compatible with breastfeeding, particularly to prevent travel sickness. Long-term use could decrease lactation.

BNF suggests that the amount in breastmilk is too small to be harmful.

> Safe to use during breastfeeding to prevent travel sickness. No studies on passage into breastmilk but no adverse events reported so safety presumed as used in paediatric doses.

Ondansetron

Brand name: *Zofran*®
US brands: *Zofran*®
Australian brands: *Ondaz*®, *Zofran*®

This drug is a 5-HT$_3$ antagonist with antiemetic activity. It is used in the management of nausea and vomiting induced by cytotoxic chemotherapy and radiotherapy. It is also used for the prevention and treatment of post-operative nausea and vomiting that have not responded to other antiemetic agents. It is licensed for use in children from two years of age. It is 60% orally bio-available and 70 to 75% plasma protein bound. The terminal half-life is 3 hours after oral doses. There are no studies on transfer into breastmilk although it has been found in *animal* studies (BNF).

> Avoid if possible as no information on passage into breastmilk but licensed for use in children > 2 years.

Analgesics

There are a wide variety of commercially available painkillers available OTC and on prescription. The breastfeeding mother should check with the pharmacist before purchasing a brand to ensure that it does not contain aspirin.

> **Analgesic of choice in a mother during breastfeeding based on evidence of benefit and safety for the baby:**
>
> **Paracetamol or NSAID e.g. ibuprofen or diclofenac**

OTC preparations

Preparations containing paracetamol (acetaminophen) are suitable, as are those containing ibuprofen. Aspirin as a painkiller should be avoided (although 75 mg taken as a blood thinning agent is acceptable) because of the link with Reye's syndrome. The amount transferring is a very small level but as it has good alternatives, it is best avoided. Codeine has been reported to cause sedation particularly if the baby is immature. There are four cases of neonatal apnoea following a dose of 60 mg given to breastfeeding mothers. One death has been reported in a mother who was an ultra-rapid metabolizer. Although codeine was not detected in the serum of the babies, symptoms resolved when the drug was discontinued.

   The most widely used analgesics are listed below. However, there are many combinations used.

Paracetamol

Plasma protein binding is negligible at usual therapeutic concentrations and the elimination half-life of paracetamol is between 1 and 3 hours.

Berlin *et al.* (1980) studied 12 mothers given 650 mg oral paracetamol: saliva, plasma and urine samples were taken at defined intervals the authors concluded that the infants would ingest 0.28 to 1.51 mg of drug, a maximum of 2% of the maternal adjusted dose. Peak levels of 10 to 15 micrograms per ml were measured and a m/p ratio of approximately 1. Infant urine samples were all negative for drug levels. Bitzén *et al.* (1981) studied three lactating women and determined that less than 0.1% of the maternal dose would be present in 100 ml milk. Matheson *et al.* (1985) reported a single case of a baby whose mother took 1 g of paracetamol at bedtime for 2 nights. The 2-month-old infant developed a maculopapular rash on the upper trunk and face. The rash subsided when the drug was discontinued but re-occured on rechallenge.

The Ito *et al.* study (1993) did not find any adverse reports from the follow-up telephone study. A study (Notarianni *et al.* 1987) of the breastmilk of mothers who had taken paracetamol suggests that infants will receive 0.9 mg per kg per day with a maternal dose of 1 g four times daily compared with a therapeutic dose for a 1 to 3-month-old baby of 60 mg per kg per day. The level of drug secreted into breastmilk does not preclude the use of oral paracetamol suspension in the infant while the mother is taking regular doses herself as the drug has a wide therapeutic index.

Relative infant dose quoted as 8.8 to 24.2% (Hale 2012 online access).

Amount secreted into breastmilk too small to be harmful (BNF).

> Compatible with use during breastfeeding even if the baby needs paracetamol liquid directly as well.

References

Berlin CM Jr, Yaffe SJ, Ragni M, Disposition of acetaminophen in milk, saliva, and plasma of lactating women, *Pediatr Pharmacol*, 1980;1:135–41.

Bitzén PO, Gustafsson B, Jostell KG, Melander A, Wåhlin-Boll E, Excretion of paracetamol in human breastmilk, *Eur J Clin Pharmacol*, 1981;20(2):123–25.

Ito S, Blajchman A, Stephenson M, Prospective follow-up of adverse reactions in breastfed infants exposed to maternal medication, *Am J Obstet Gynecol*, 1993;168:1393–9.

Matheson I, Lunde PKM, Notarianni L, Infant rash caused by paracetamol in breastmilk?, *Pediatrics*, 1985;76:651–2. Letter.

Notarianni LJ, Oldham HG, Bennett PN, Passage of paracetamol into breastmilk and its subsequent metabolism by the neonate, *Br J Clin Pharmacol*, 1987;24(1):63–7.

Aspirin

Aspirin is not generally recommended to be used by lactating women due to the link between aspirin and Reye's sundrome.

Aspirin is 80 to 90% bound to plasma proteins. Erickson and Oppenheim (1979) found that even at a dose of 4 g per day the levels of salicylate measured in one mother suffering from rheumatoid arthritis were below the level of detection. Findlay *et al.* (1981) studied two mothers exposed to 454 mg aspirin. They found that salicylic acid penetrated poorly into milk, with peak levels of only 1.12 to 1.60 µg per ml, and estimated that about 0.1% of the mothers' total dose would appear in breastmilk.

While it is unlikely that an anti-platelet dose of 75 mg per day will significantly increase the risk of Reye's syndrome particularly if the baby is afebrile, Glasgow (2006) suggests that some of the evidence points to a dose relation with the severity of the illness and that in the presence of a viral infection no dose of aspirin can be considered safe.

Accidental consumption of a single dose of aspirin by a lactating mother need not lead to expressing and discarding of her breastmilk. Theoretical infant dose through breastmilk is quoted as 0.25 mg per kg per day with a relative infant dose quoted as 2.5 to 10.8% (Hale 2012 online access).

The BNF states: 'Avoid—possible risk of Reye's syndrome; regular use of high doses could impair platelet function and produce hypoprothrombinaemia in infant if neonatal vitamin K stores low'. Vitamin K is secreted in breastmilk and is added to formula.

Use alternative analgesics If taken accidentally no evidence that continuing to breastfeed after single dose is harmful.

References

Erickson SH, Oppenheim GL, Aspirin in breastmilk, *J Fam Pract*, 1979;8(1):189–90.
Findlay JW, DeAngelis RL, Kearney MF, Welch RM, Findlay J, Analgesic drugs in breastmilk and plasma, *Clin Pharmacol Ther*, 1981;29:625–33.
Glasgow JF, Reye's syndrome: the case for a causal link with aspirin, *Drug Saf*, 2006;29(12):1111–21.

Reye's syndrome

This is a rare syndrome, characterized by acute encephalopathy and fatty degeneration of the liver, usually after a viral illness or chickenpox. The incidence is falling but sporadic cases are still reported. It was often associated with the use of aspirin during the prodromal illness. Few cases occur in white children under 1 year although it is more common in black infants in this age group. Many children retrospectively examined show an underlying inborn error of metabolism.

Codeine (see also entry under gastro-intestinal drugs)

Codeine combinations have formed the mainstay of many analgesics used, particularly in the early post-partum period. Its painkilling action is caused by metabolites which include morphine. A case report of the death of a baby whose mother took codeine phosphate 30/500 mg has recently caused much debate as to whether codeine is compatible with lactation (Koren *et al.* 2006). The baby was born healthy at term after a vaginal delivery. His mother took codeine 30 mg with paracetamol for episiotomy pain for 2 weeks. On day 7 he became lethargic and had intermittent periods of difficulty in breastfeeding and lethargy. On day 11 he was taken to a paediatrician because he was described as grey in colour and was feeding poorly. He had regained his birthweight but the following day he was found cyanotic by an ambulance team and despite resuscitation attempts was pronounced dead. At postmortem he was found to have very high levels of morphine in his blood (86 ng per ml compared to an expected level in a neonate exposed to codeine through breastmilk of 2.2 ng per ml. The mother had initially taken two tablets every six hours (four times a day) but had halved the dose when she suffered constipation and somnolence. She was subsequently found to have multiple copies of the gene which metabolises codeine into morphine. In adults this has been shown to result in severe opioid toxicity, demonstrated by this mother by her sensitivity to the drug and the side effects experienced. This genotype occurs in approximately 1% of people in Finland, Denmark, Greece, Portugal and other Caucasians, but 29% of Ethiopians and 10% of southern Europeans.

Should a breastfeeding mother take codeine, she should be warned to discontinue if her baby exhibits excessive drowsiness and poor feeding. It might be wise to limit the dose of codeine to 15 mg or less (co-codamol 8/500) and if the baby is suspected of having received an overdose of morphine, administration of the antidote naloxone might be tried. Relative infant dose quoted as 8.1% (Hale 2012 online access).

Many women across the world are prescribed codeine routinely for post-natal pain without any ensuing problems. The side effects, particularly of constipation, may not be welcome to women. The use of simple paracetamol and non-steroidal anti-inflammatories may be considered a safer option (Spigset and Hagg 2000).

The BNF states that the amount in breastmilk is usually too small to be harmful; however, mothers vary considerably in their capacity to metabolise codeine—risk of morphine overdose in infant (BNF).

> Avoid if possible. Use for a short a time as possible. Observe baby for drowsiness. If baby becomes drowsy stop drug immediately and seek medical advice.

References

Koren G, Cairns J, Chitayat D, Gaedigk A, Leeder SJ, Pharmacogenetics of morphine poisoning in a breastfed neonate of a codeine-prescribed mother, *Lancet*, 2006;368(9536):704.

Spigset O, Hagg S, Analgesics and breastfeeding: safety considerations, *Paediatric Drugs*, 2000;2(3):223–38.

Compound codeine preparations

The combination of the analgesics and opiate is intended to produce more effective analgesia.

Co-codamol – paracetamol 500 mg and codeine 8 mg or 30 mg per tablet
Co-dydramol – paracetamol 500 mg and dihydrocodeine 10mg

> Avoid if possible. Use for a short a time as possible. Observe baby for drowsiness. If baby becomes drowsy stop drug immediately and seek medical advice

Tramadol

Brand name: *Zydol®, Zamadol®*
US brands: *Ultram®*
Australian brands: *Tramahexal®, Tramal®, Zydol®*

Tramadol is an opiate analgesic used for moderate to severe pain. Its use would appear to have increased as a result of concern over codeine preparations. It is subject to first-pass metabolism. It has an elimination half-life of 6 hours. Tramadol inhibits the reuptake of noradrenaline and serotonin and may potentiate the action of other drugs with similar action e.g. SSRI anti-depressants.

Ilett *et al.* (2008) studied 75 breastfeeding mothers who were given 100 mg tramadol post-caesarian section on days 2 to 4. He collected milk and plasma samples of four or more doses to reflect steady state. Additionally he observed the infants together with matched controls not exposed to tramadol. He determined a relative infant dose quoted as 2.24% for tramadol and 0.64% for its metabolite. No difference was noted in the behaviours of the infants exposed compared with the controls and the authors therefore concluded that short-term maternal use of tramadol is compatible with breastfeeding.

As with other opiates, exposure of premature infants should be undertaken with caution because of the risk of apnoea and sedation.

Amount probably too small to be harmful, but manufacturer advises avoidance (BNF).

> Avoid if possible although the amount in breastmilk is probably too small to be harmful. Use for a short a time as possible. Observe baby for drowsiness. If baby becomes drowsy stop drug immediately and seek medical advice.

References

Ilett KF, Paech MJ, Page-Sharp M, Sy SK, Kristensen JH, Goy R, Chua S, Christmas T, Scott KL, Use of a sparse sampling study design to assess transfer of tramadol and its o-desmethyl metabolite into transitional breastmilk. *Br J Clin Pharmacol*, 2008;65(5):661–6..

Opiate analgesics

Morphine

Therapeutic doses of morphine in the breastfeeding mother are unlikely to be harmful to baby in short term e.g. post-operatively. Infants under 4 weeks of age have a prolonged elimination half-life and clearance does not approach adult levels until 2 months of age. Respiratory difficulties may be important to be aware of with premature babies or others at risk of apnoea.

Robieux *et al.* (1990) reported a single case of an infant who was breastfed while his mother was receiving low doses of morphine. Morphine concentration in his serum was in the analgesic range (4 ng per ml), while concentrations in the milk varied substantially from 10 to 100 ng per ml. The authors calculated that the baby had received 0.8 to 12% of maternal dose. Oberlander *et al.* (2000) studied one baby born to a mother who received morphine intra-thecally during and after pregnancy. Minimal levels were determined in breastmilk over 7 weeks and the infant's development and feeding up to 7 months were normal. Baka *et al.* (2002) also studied women receiving patient controlled analgesia post-caesarian section and noted that the concentrations of morphine in breastmilk were very small (<1 to 274 ng per ml) with a m/p ratio <1. Relative infant dose quoted as 9.1% (Hale 2012 online access).

Therapeutic doses unlikely to affect infant (BNF).

> Compatible with use short term during breastfeeding. Observe baby for sedation and poor feeding.

References

Ilett KF, Paech MJ, Page-Sharp M, Sy SK, Kristensen JH, Goy R, Chua S, Christmas T, Scott KL, Colostrum morphine concentrations during postcesarean intravenous patient-controlled analgesia, *Anesth Analg*, 2002;94:184–7.

Oberlander TF, Robeson P, Ward V, Huckin RS, Kamani A, Harpur A, McDonald W, Prenatal and breastmilk morphine exposure following maternal intrathecal morphine treatment, *J Hum Lact*, 2000;16:137–42.

Robieux I, Koren G, Vandenbergh H, Schneiderman J, Morphine excretion in breastmilk and resultant exposure of a nursing infant, *J Toxicol Clin Toxicol* 1990;28:365–70.

Diamorphine (heroin)

When used short-term post-operatively is suitable for use by breastfeeding mothers and is frequently used post-caesarean section. It is converted in the body to morphine. The baby may be sedated, restless or vomit. It may exhibit withdrawal symptoms from placental transfer. See section on drugs of misuse.

Klenka (1986) studied 25 babies born to 23 drug-abusing mothers, most of whom were smoking heroin. Nineteen of the babies developed withdrawal symptoms and 12 needed treatment. He found that withdrawal symptoms were short lasting and often self-limiting, and no evidence of adverse effects on post-natal growth and development were found. Only four of the mothers established breastfeeding, although all were supported and encouraged to do so. Measurements of drug levels were not made. Mothers should be encouraged to join a detoxification programme during pregnancy and to avoid street drugs which may be adulterated. If mothers continue to use heroin intermittently and breastfeed, the baby may also experience repeated withdrawal. Few users are successful at breastfeeding.

Therapeutic doses unlikely to affect infant; withdrawal symptoms in infants of dependent mothers; breastfeeding not best method of treating dependence in offspring (BNF).

Avoid as substance of misuse. Probably compatible short term for post-operative analgesia.

References

Klenka HM, Babies born in a district general hospital to mothers taking heroin, *BMJ*, 1986;293:745–6.

Pethidine

According to research carried out by the National Birthday Trust in 1993 (Chamberlain *et al.* 1993), 36.9% of women in labour received pethidine as an analgesic in labour. This compared with 60% using entenox and 34% receiving no pain relief (Steer 1993). The limitation to its use is known to be respiratory depression in the infant resulting from accumulation in the neonate. Rajan (1994) concluded that, apart from general anaesthesia, 'pethidine proved to be the most inhibiting drug to breastfeeding'. She attributed this to sleepiness induced in the baby and to a lesser extent the mother.

Freeborn *et al.* (1980) showed that breastfed babies continue to show an increase in saliva levels of pethidine on the first day after birth, followed by a subsequent, gradual reduction in the following 24 hours. They deduced that pethidine continued to be excreted through breastmilk, although the half-life in the mother is normally believed to be less than 4 hours. The baby may be at risk of hypoglycaemia due to infrequent feeds and the mother may lose confidence in her ability to breastfeed.

Pethidine undergoes rapid first-pass clearance by the liver but it is cleared very much more slowly by infants less than 3 months because of hepatic immaturity. The active metabolite norpethidine is excreted by the kidneys and may also accumulate in neonates who have inherently low kidney function. The average half-life in young babies is estimated to be 11 hours but can range from 3 to 60 hours.

Pethidine hydrochloride is absorbed from the gastro-intestinal tract, but only about 50% of the drug reaches the blood because of first-pass metabolism. Obstetrically it is more likely to be given by intramuscular injection. Peak plasma concentrations have been reported 1 to 2 hours after oral doses. It is about 60 to 80% bound to plasma proteins. Its elimination half-life is about 3 to 6 hours and that of its metabolite norpethidine 20 hours. However, Hogg *et al.* (1977) found that if given late in labour placental transferred pethidine might take 2 to 3 days to be eliminated. The impact of pethidine on breastfeeding cannot be ignored (Chamberlain *et al.* 1993).

With repeated doses, the metabolite of pethidine can accumulate in both the mother and infant (Mander 1997).

Compatible with use during breastfeeding other than in immediate neo-natal period. Use late in labour may produce excessive drowsiness in the baby.

References

Chamberlain G, Wraight A, Steer P (eds.), *Pain and its relief in childbirth – the results of a national survey conducted by the National Birthday Trust*, Edinburgh: Churchill Livingstone, 1993.

Freeborn SF, Calvert RT, Black P, Saliva and blood pethidine concentrations in the mother and the newborn baby, *Br J Obst & Gynecol*, 1980;87:966–9.

Hogg MI, Wiener PC, Rosen M, Mapleson WW, Urinary excretion and metabolism of pethidine and norpethidine in the newborn, *Br J Anaesth*, 1977;49(9):891–99.

Mander R, Pethidine in childbirth, *MIDIRS Midwifery Digest*, 1997:202–4.

Rajan L, The impact of obstetric procedures and analgesia/anaesthesia during labour and delivery on breastfeeding, *Midwifery*, 1994;10(2):87–103.

Steer P, *Pain and its relief in childbirth – the results of a national survey conducted by the National Birthday Trust*, Edinburgh: Churchill Livingstone, 1993;49–68.

Epilepsy

> **Anti-epileptic drug of choice in a mother during breastfeeding based on evidence of benefit and safety for the baby:**
>
> **According to patient needs. Multiple drug regimens are more likely to lead to adverse reactions There is no reason to discourage breastfeeding**

There is no reason why women who have taken anti-epileptic medication throughout their pregnancy should not be encouraged to breastfeed their baby. However, women should be counselled on the signs of risk to be aware of, in particular excessive somnolence and poor weight gain. The risks increase with multiple drug regimens.

Women taking anti-epileptic monotherapy should generally be encouraged to breastfeed. If a woman is on combination therapy or if there are other risk factors, such as premature birth, specialist advice should be sought. All infants should be observed for sedation, feeding difficulties, adequate weight gain and developmental milestones. Infants should also be monitored for adverse effects associated with the specific anti-epileptic drug particularly if the anti-epileptic is readily transferred into breastmilk causing high infant serum–drug concentrations (e.g. ethosuximide, lamotrigine, primidone and zonisamide), or if slower metabolism in the infant causes drugs to accumulate (e.g. phenobarbital and lamotrigine). A serum–drug concentration sometimes should be obtained in breastfed infants if suspected adverse reactions develop. If toxicity develops it may be necessary to introduce formula feeds to limit the infant's drug exposure, or to wean the infant off breastmilk altogether. Primidone, phenobarbital and the benzodiazepines are associated with an established risk of drowsiness in breastfed babies and caution is required. Withdrawal effects may occur in infants if a mother suddenly stops breastfeeding, particularly if she is taking phenobarbital, primidone or lamotrigine (BNF).

Phenytoin

Brand name: *Epanutin*®
US brands: *Phenytek*®, *Dilantin*®
Australian brands: *Dilantin*®

All studies of phenytoin show levels in breastmilk to be too low to cause difficulties for breastfed infants (Bar-Oz *et al.* 2000, Meador *et al.* 2010, SIGN). Much is known about the transfer of this drug and it can be used safely in lactation. It is rapidly metabolised in the liver to inactive metabolites. It is widely used to treat neonates. Phenytoin is extensively bound to plasma proteins (90%) but it is subject to interactions resulting from displacement, particularly if used in combination with other anti-epileptics and is subject to many interactions. There is one reported case of a baby who developed methemoglobinaemia and extreme sedation when exposed to 390 mg phenobarbital daily and phenytoin 400 mg daily (Finch and Lorber 1954). Discontinuation of breastfeeding resolved symptoms but they reoccurred at each rechallenge. Relative infant dose quoted as 0.6 to 7.7% (Hale 2012 online access).

BNF information on safety in breastfeeding as above, licensed in children from 1 month according to response but at maximum of 7.5 mg per kg twice daily. Small amounts present in milk, but not known to be harmful.

Compatible with use during breastfeeding.

References

Bar-Oz B, Nulman I, Koren G, Ito S, Anticonvulsants and breastfeeding: a critical review, *Paediatr Drugs*, 2000;2:113–26.
Finch E, Lorber J, Methaemoglobinaemia in the newborn. Probably due to phenytoin excreted in human milk, *J Obstet Gynaecol Br Emp*, 1954;61:833–4.
Meador KJ, Baker GA, Browning N, Clayton-Smith J, Combs-Cantrell DT, Cohen M, Kalayjian LA, Kanner A, Liporace JD, Pennell PB, Privitera M, Loring DW; NEAD Study Group, Effects of breastfeeding in children of women taking antiepileptic drugs, *Neurology*, 2010;75:1954–60.
SIGN guideline 70 www.sign.ac.uk

Sodium valproate

Brand name: *Epilim*®, *Orlept*®, *Depakote*®
US brands: *Depacon*®, *Depakene*®, *Depakote*®
Australian brands: *Epilim*®, *Valpro*®

Low levels are found in breastmilk but theoretically it is recommended that the baby should be monitored for jaundice and liver damage.

One case of thrombocytopaenia, anaemia and reticulocytosis has been reported in a baby whose mother was treated with valproic acid which may or may not be linked with mother's medication. This is a recognised adverse effect of valproic acid and when the mother stopped breastfeeding, the infant recovered (Stahl *et al.* 1997).

Piontek *et al.* (2000) noted low levels and no adverse events in a study of six women. von Unruh *et al.* (1984) measured valproic acid levels in 36 random breast-milk samples from 16 patients and found 0.4 to 3.9 µg per ml. Relative infant dose quoted as 1.4 to 1.7% (Hale 2012 online access).

BNF safety information in breastfeeding as above; used in babies from one month at usual maintenance dose 25 to 30 mg per kg daily in two divided doses. Amount too small to be harmful (BNFC).

> Compatible with use during breastfeeding.

References

Piontek CM, Baab S, Peindl KS, Wisner KL, Serum valproate levels in 6 breastfeeding mother-infant pairs, *J Clin Psychiatry*, 2000;61:170–72.

Stahl MM, Neiderud J, Vinge E, Thrombocytopenic purpura and anemia in a breastfed infant whose mother was treated with valproic acid, *J Pediatr*, 1997;130:1001–3.

von Unruh GE, Froescher W, Hoffmann F, Niesen M, Valproic acid in breastmilk: how much is really there?, *Ther Drug Monit*, 1984;6:272–6.

Carbamazepine ☺

Brand name: *Tegretol*®
US brands: *Carbatrol*®, *Epitol*®, *Equetro*®, *Tegretol*®, *Teril*®
Australian brands: *Tegretol*®, *Teril*®

Carbamazepine is also used to treat manic depression and trigeminal neuralgia. It reaches measurably detectable levels in infant serum but below the therapeutic range. The infant should be monitored for jaundice, drowsiness and adequate weight gain as sedation, poor sucking and hepatic dysfunction have been reported although rarely. In case of concern monitoring infant serum levels may reassure (see below). It is 75% bound to plasma proteins and has active metabolites. It induces its own metabolism and metabolism is induced by other hepatic enzyme inducers so the plasma half-life is variable. It is widely used in children. Most studies of levels in breastmilk include other drugs as well which may interact with carbamazepine.

Drowsiness, poor sucking and elevated liver enzymes have been reported. No absolute causality to carbamazepine has been shown but the risk should not be disregarded. Relative infant dose quoted as 3.8 to 5.9% (Hale 2012 online access).

BNF safety of breastmilk as above but licensed in children up to a year at dose of 100 to 200 mg daily. Amount probably too small to be harmful but monitor infant for possible adverse reactions (BNFC).

> Compatible with use during breastfeeding. Observe for sedation.

Lamotrigine (?)

Brand name: *Lamictal*®
US brands: *Lamictal*®
Australian brands: *Lamictal*®, *Elmendos*®, *Lamitrin*®

Relatively high plasma levels have been reported in breastfed babies whose mothers are taking this drug, Neonates are particularly susceptible due to their inability to metabolise the drug if the dosage is not reduced to the pre-pregnancy dosage in the immediate post-partum period. If lamotrigine is required by the mother, it is not necessarily a reason to discontinue breastfeeding, because no adverse reactions have been reported and concerns are theoretical. It is 55% bound to plasma proteins and is metabolised by the liver where it slightly induces its own metabolism.

Liporace *et al.* (2004) studied four breastfed infants and found that serum concentrations of the drug 10 days after birth were about <1.0 to 2.0 µg per ml – three babies had levels >1 µg per ml – this represented average levels of approximately 30% of maternal levels; the drug was undetectable in the fourth. The authors concluded that serum concentrations of lamotrigine in breastfed children were higher than expected, in some cases reaching 'therapeutic' ranges. These high levels may be explained by poor neonatal drug elimination due to inefficient glucuronidation. Page-Sharp *et al.* (2006) reported on six breastfeeding women taking a mean dose of 400 mg per day lamotrigine. Five of the babies were exclusively breastfed and the remaining one fed with half breastmilk and half artificial milk feeds. They determined a relative infant dose quoted as 7.6%, representing 0.45 mg per kg per day (compared with adjunctive therapy maintenance dose with valproate of 1 to 5 mg per kg). No adverse events were noted in any of the infants. Breastfed infants should be carefully monitored for side effects such as rash, drowsiness or poor sucking. In case of concern monitoring of infant serum levels may reassure professionals and parents. If an infant rash occurs, breastfeeding should be discontinued until the cause can be established (Tomson *et al.* 1997; Öhman *et al.* 2000).

Relative infant dose quoted as 9.2 to 18.3% (Hale 2012 online access). This is above the upper level of the safe range of 10% and should be used with caution.

BNF suggests that women taking antiepileptic monotherapy should generally be encouraged to breastfeed, if a woman is on combination therapy or if there are other risk factors, such as premature birth, specialist advice should be sought.

All infants should be monitored for sedation, feeding difficulties, adequate weight gain and developmental milestones. Infants should also be monitored for adverse effects associated with the anti-epileptic drug particularly with newer anti-epileptics, if the anti-epileptic is readily transferred into breastmilk causing high infant serum–drug concentrations (e.g. ethosuximide, lamotrigine, primidone and zonisamide), or if slower metabolism in the infant causes drugs to accumulate (e.g. phenobarbital and lamotrigine). Serum–drug concentration monitoring should be undertaken in breastfed infants if suspected adverse reactions develop; if toxicity develops it may be necessary to introduce formula feeds to limit the infant's drug exposure, or to wean the infant off breastmilk altogether.

The BNFC states that lamotrigine is present in milk, but limited data suggest no harmful effect on infant.

> Probably compatible with use during breastfeeding. Observe for sedation, poor feeding and rash.

References

Liporace J, Kao A, D'Abreu A, Concerns regarding lamotrigine and breastfeeding, *Epilepsy Behav*, 2004;5:102–5.

Öhman I, Vitols S, Tomson T, Lamotrigine in pregnancy: pharmacokinetics during delivery, in the neonate, and during lactation, *Epilepsia*, 2000;41(6):709–13.

Page-Sharp M, Kristensen JH, Hackett LP, Beran RG, Rampono J, Hale TW, Kohan R, Ilett KF, Transfer of lamotrigine into breastmilk, *Ann Pharmacother*, 2006;40:1470–1. Letter.

Tomson T, Ohman I, Vitols S, Lamotrigine in pregnancy and lactation: a case report, *Epilepsia*, 1997;38:1039–41.

Topiramate

Brand name: *Topamax*®
US brands: *Topamax*®
Australian brands: *Topamax*®

Initial reports suggest that maternal doses of topiramate up to 200 mg daily produce low levels in infant serum despite the fact that transfer into breastmilk reaches significant levels (Öhman *et al.* 2002). Topiramate is only 9 to 17% protein bound and metabolism may be affected by other enzyme inducing drugs, including other anti-epileptic agents. It has been linked to cleft lip with or without cleft palate following first trimester use (Margulis *et al.* 2012).

Öhman observed five babies at delivery and followed three of them through lactation. Two to three weeks after delivery two of the breastfed infants had detectable but unquantifiable levels of topiramate and one had an undetectable concentration; m/p ratios of around 0.86 were determined throughout the study period and no adverse events noted.

One infant whose mother was taking 100 mg of topiramate daily developed watery, slimy stools with up to ten bowel movements daily at 40 days of age (Westergren *et al.* 2009). Topiramate levels in breastmilk were of 5.5 mg per litre. Breastfeeding was discontinued two weeks later. Within 24 hours, the stool frequency declined to two to three times daily, which were more solid and the colour and odour normalised. Topiramate was the reported to be the probable cause of the diarrhoea in the infant.

Gentile (2009) reported a single case study of a mother who took 300 mg topiramate daily throughout pregnancy and breastfed for 8 months. Neither adverse drug effects nor neurodevelopmental delay were noted by the baby's pediatrician.

The infant exposed to topiramate through breastmilk, should be monitored for drowsiness, diarrhoea and adequate weight gain particularly if the mother is receiving a multiple drug therapy regimen. It is used as an adjunctive treatment in children from

2 years of age at 2.5 to 4.5 mg per kg twice daily. Relative infant dose quoted as 24.5% (Hale 2012 online access). This is above the upper level of the safe range of 10% and should be used with caution.

BNF states that manufacturer advises avoid as it is present in milk.

> Probably compatible with use during breastfeeding. Observe for sedation, poor feeding and diarrhoea

References

Gentile S, Topiramate in pregnancy and breastfeeding, *Clin Drug Investig*, 2009;29:139–41.
Margulis AV, Mitchell AA, Gilboa SM, Werler MM, Mittleman MA, Glynn RJ, Hernandez-Diaz S; National Birth Defects Prevention Study, Use of topiramate in pregnancy and risks of oral clefts, *Am J Obstet Gynecol*, 2012 ;207(5):405.e1–7.
Ohman I, Vitols S, Luef G, Söderfeldt B, Tomson T, Topiramate kinetics during delivery, lactation, and in the neonate: preliminary observations, *Epilepsia*, 2002;43:1157–60.
Westergren T, Hjelmeland K, Kristoffersen B *et al.* Topiramate-induced diarrhoea in a 2-month-old breastfed child, *Drug Saf*, 2009;32:38. Abstract.

Phenobarbital

This is now rarely used to control epilepsy unless as a therapeutic adjunct. It is, however, frequently used to control neonatal seizures. It has a long half-life and levels in breastmilk can lead to accumulation. It is very likely to cause sedation in the baby producing poor weight gain as a consequence In case of concern, monitor infant serum levels and observe the baby for sedation. Mothers taking phenobarbital should not co-sleep with their infants as their natural instincts may be dulled. Relative infant dose quoted as 24% (Hale 2012 online access).

> Avoid during breastfeeding.

Levetiracetam

Brand name: *Keppra®*
US brands: *Keppra®*
Australian brands: *Keppra®*

Kramer *et al.* (2002) studied one baby born at 36 weeks and unstable at birth. Following maternal intake of levetiracetam on day 7 the baby became hypotonic and fed poorly. The mother was taking multiple medications to control her epilepsy and the link with any one drug is difficult to confirm. Johannessen *et al.* (2005) studied eight women with maternal doses of levetiracetam up to 3.5 g daily which produced low levels in milk and no adverse effects in their breastfed infants. The babies of mothers taking levetiracetam should be monitored for drowsiness and adequate weight gain particularly if the mother is receiving a multiple drug therapy regimen. Relative infant dose quoted as 3.4 to 7.8% (Hale 2012 online access).

BNF Relative safety as above. Manufacturer advises avoid – present in milk (BNFC).

> Probably compatible with use during breastfeeding. Observe for sedation, poor feeding.

References

Johannessen SI, Helde G, Brodtkorb E, Levetiracetam concentrations in serum and in breast-milk at birth and during lactation, *Epilepsia*, 2005;46:775–7.

Kramer G, Hosli I, Glanzmann R, Holzgreve W, Levetiracetam accumulation in human breast-milk, *Epilepsia*, 2002;43(Suppl. 7):105.

Gabapentin

Brand name: *Neurontin®*
US brands: *Gabarone®, Neurontin®*
Australian brands: *Neurontin®, Gantrin®, Nupentin®, Pendine®*

Limited information indicates that maternal doses of gabapentin up to 2.1 g daily produce relatively low levels in infant serum (Goa and Sorkin 1993). No adverse effects on the children have been noted in several studies and infant plasma levels have been low to undetectable (Ramsay 1994; Dichter and Brodie 1996). Minimal plasma protein binding is apparent with gabapentin. Öhman *et al.* (2005) studied six women taking 0.9 to 3.2 g gabapentin and their babies. The infant dose of gabapentin was estimated to be 0.2 to 1.3 mg per kg per day. No adverse effects were observed. The plasma concentrations in the breastfed infants were approximately 12% of the mother's plasma levels. Kristensen *et al.* (2006) studied one mother and baby pair and determined a m/p ratio of 0.86 and a relative infant dose of 2.34%. No adverse effects were noted in the baby. The baby should be monitored for drowsiness and adequate weight gain particularly if the mother is receiving a multiple drug therapy regime. Relative infant dose quoted as 6.6% (Hale 2012 online access).

BNF relative safety in breastfeeding as above. Present in milk – manufacturer advises use only if potential benefit outweighs risk (BNFC).

> Probably compatible with use during breastfeeding. Observe for sedation, poor feeding.

References

Dichter MA, Brodie MJ, New antiepileptic drugs, *N Engl J Med*, 1996;334(24):1583–90.

Goa KL, Sorkin EM, Gabapentin. A review of its pharmacological properties and clinical potential in epilepsy, *Drugs*, 1993;46(3):409–27.

Kristensen JH, Ilett KF, Hackett LP, Kohan R, Gabapentin and breastfeeding: a case report, *J Hum Lact*, 2006;22:426–8.

Öhman I, Vitols S, Tomson T, Pharmacokinetics of gabapentin during delivery, in the neonatal period, and lactation: does a fetal accumulation occur during pregnancy?, *Epilepsia*, 2005;46:1621–4.

Ramsay RE, Clinical efficacy and safety of gabapentin, *Neurology*, 1994;44(6 Suppl. 5):S23–S30.

Vigabatrin ☺

Brand name: *Sabril*®
US brands:
Australian brands: *Sabril*®

This drug is used where control of seizures has not been achieved. It is not significantly bound to plasma proteins. Tran *et al.* (1998) studied two mother and baby pairs. He estimated the maximum amount of R and S enantiomers of vigabatrin that a suckling infant would ingest in a day is 3.6% and 1% of the weight-adjusted daily dose respectively. There is little evidence from studies on transfer into breastmilk (Dichter and Brodie 1996). It irreversibly inactivates gamma-aminobutyric acid (GABA) and the effect of this on neonatal brains is unknown. However, it is used directly to control infant spasms.

BNF states that the manufacturer advises it is avoided as it is present in milk.

Probably compatible with use during breastfeeding. Observe for sedation, poor feeding.

References

Dichter MA, Brodie MJ, New antiepileptic drugs, *N Engl J Med*, 1996;334(24):1583–90.

Tran A, O'Mahoney T, Rey E, Mai J, Mumford JP, Olive G, Vigabatrin: placental transfer in vivo and excretion into breastmilk of the enantiomers, *Br J Clin Pharmacol*, 1998;45:409–11.

Drugs of abuse

Use of illicit drugs during breastfeeding is unconscionable
Mothers have the right to information on the safety of any substance they have used and to be able to understand any reasons for interruption of breastfeeding

Gauging from calls to the Drugs in Breastmilk Helpline there is anecdotal evidence that mothers who breastfeed may also use illicit drugs either regularly or on an occasional social level. There have also been instances where mothers have had their drinks spiked by friends or strangers. Other mothers may plan in advance that they will use a drug e.g. cocaine on a specific occasion and may seek information on the time they need to discontinue breastfeeding. In this section the social drugs alcohol and nicotine have been included as they have an effect on the breastfed baby.

It is difficult to develop guidelines on the use of drugs of abuse as each mother and baby is an individual situation. Treated empathetically mothers (and their partners) may decide to enter a detox programme for the sake of their baby. Babies in households where there is drug use may benefit from breastmilk in protection from infections. Use of street drugs should be heavily discouraged due to the risks of unknown contaminants. Wherever possible mothers should be encouraged to enter supported drug programmes and use prescribed methadone and buprenorphine in a controlled manner.

Long-term effects of breastfeeding in the presence of illicit drugs is largely unknown and of concern particularly with regard to cannabis smoking which appears to have become widespread and normal within some areas of the community.

Alcohol

Social drinking by the mother is unlikely to pose a risk to the breastfed baby. However, alcohol passes freely into breastmilk. Chronic exposure to more than 2 units per day consumed by the mother, may have an effect on the baby's development. Maternal blood levels have to reach 300 mg per 100 ml before mild sedation is reached in the baby (this compares with a level of 80 mg per 100 ml needed to fail the police breath test in the UK).

Temporary reduction of let down is reported when the mother drinks heavily (Mennella 2001). Peak levels in the milk appear 30 to 90 minutes after the mother has consumed alcohol. Binge drinking may reduce the ability of the mother to be aware of her baby's needs.

Mothers who have drunk alcohol heavily should not take their baby into bed with them as they are at risk of overlaying and suffocating the infant.

Excess levels of alcohol in milk may lead to drowsiness, deep sleep, weakness and long term decreased growth in the infant.

To reduce exposure of the baby to alcohol the mother should avoid breastfeeding for 2 to 3 hours per drink after drinking. Chronic consumption of alcohol is more likely to cause harm than occasional modest level social drinking. Teenage mothers, in particular, may perceive advice that they should not drink alcohol if they intend to breastfeed as too restrictive to their lifestyles and become a factor in their choice to formula feed their infants. Thus 'ideal' advice may need to be tempered with an understanding of difficulties and strategies to reduce risk to the baby recommended.

Alcohol, particularly Guiness and stout, has in the past been recommended to increase milk production. It is hypothesised that polysaccharides derived from barley and hops are responsible for the prolactin-stimulating effect (Koletzko and Lehner 2000).

It is not necessary to pump breastmilk off to clear it of alcohol, as the mother's blood levels fall, the level of alcohol in the breastmilk will decrease. In general mothers should avoid breastfeeding for 2 hours for every unit of alcohol consumed to limit exposure of the infant (Ho et al. 2001). This does, however, vary somewhat with the weight of the mother (Palmquist et al. 2005). If indulging in 'binge drinking' – defined as consuming more than 5 units of alcohol in one session – it is essential that the baby is cared for by a sober adult.

Once the mother is able to recognise the needs of her child and feel reasonably sober then the amount of alcohol in her breastmilk is likely to be low. Relative infant dose quoted as 16% (Hale 2012 online access).

Occasional social drinking when mother remains sober is acceptable. Beware regular consumption and binge drinking

References

Carlson HE, Wasser HL, Reidelberger RD, Beer-induced prolactin secretion: a clinical and laboratory study of the role of salsolinol, *J Clin Endocrinol Metab*, 1985;60:673–7.

Ho E, Collantes A, Kapur BM, Moretti M, Koren G, Alcohol and breast feeding: calculation of time to zero level in milk, *Biol Neonate*, 2001;80(3):219–22.

Koletzko B, Lehner F, Beer and breastfeeding, *Adv Exp Med Biol*, 2000;478:23–8.

Mennella JA, Infants' suckling responses to the flavour of alcohol in mothers' milk, *Alcohol Clin Exp Res*, 1997;21:581–5.

Mennella JA, Regulation of milk intake after exposure to alcohol in mothers' milk, *Alcohol Clin Exp Res*, 2001;25:590–93.

Palmquist M, Grainger D, Frazier L, Topolinski A, Studts P, Nipper HC, Elimination of alcohol from breastmilk: Establishing guidelines for resumption of breastfeeding after alcohol consumption, *Fertil Steril*, 2005;84:S415.

Amphetamine

Steiner *et al.* (1984) studied one woman receiving 20 mg of dexamphetamine daily for narcolepsy. The urine of her infant contained small amounts of amphetamine. The infant had no adverse effects and developed normally up to 2 years of age. although the drug appeared to concentrate in breastmilk.

High doses of amphetamines suppress prolactin secretion in patients with hyperprolactinaemia (De Leo *et al.* 1997) therefore, there is a possibility it may suppress lactation although this has not been recorded so far. Ilett *et al.* (2007) studied four women taking amphetamine (range 15 to 45 mg per day) for attention deficit disorder. They found a relative infant dose quoted as less than 10% with no adverse events seen. Because of the lack of clinical data, women should be discouraged from using amphetamine recreationally. Therapeutic dosing seems to be relatively compatible with breastfeeding below 45 mg daily but data is limited. Relative infant dose quoted as 1.8 to 6.9% (Hale 2012 online access).

The BNF states that a significant amount is present in breastmilk and it should therefore be avoided.

Therapeutic use appears acceptable with caution but illicit use should be discouraged.

References

De Leo V, Cella S, Camanni F, Genazzani AR, Müller EE, Prolactin lowering effect of amphetamine in noroprolactinaemia. In: Willis S, *Drugs of Abuse*, The Pharmaceutical Press: London, 1997.

Ilett KF, Hackett LP, Kristensen JH, Kohan R, Transfer of dexamphetamine into breastmilk during treatment for attention deficit hyperactivity disorder, *Br J Clin Pharmacol*, 2007;63(3):371–5.

Steiner E, Villén T, Hallberg M, Rane A, Amphetamine secretion in breastmilk, *Eur J Clin Pharmacol*, 1984;27(1):123–4.

Cocaine

Cocaine is a naturally occurring alkaloid, which acts as a local anaesthetic and a powerful central nervous system stimulant. It is well absorbed from all locations including the stomach, nasal passages, lungs and even via eye drops. Adverse effects include agitation, nervousness, restlessness, hallucination, tremors, seizures and irregular heart beats. The pharmacological effects are relatively brief (20 to 30 minutes) but cocaine is only slowly metabolised and excreted over a prolonged period. Infants do not possess the enzyme necessary to metabolise cocaine and are therefore at an increased risk of its effects.

Acute symptoms of cocaine withdrawal will depend on foetal maturity and may be delayed 1 to 2 days especially in the pre-term infant. Studies on breastfed infants where the mothers are known to have used cocaine are limited in number.

Cocaine intoxication has been reported in a 14-day-old infant where the mother had snorted (in Hale 2012 online access and LactMed) approximately 0.5 mg of cocaine over 4 hours and nursed the infant five times during this period (Chasnoff *et al.* 1987). Within 3 hours the infant had developed clinical signs of cocaine intoxication: tachycardia, tachypnea, hypertension, irritability and tremulousness. The infant improved and all symptoms resolved over 72 hours. In an unusual case, a mother applied cocaine powder to her sore nipples and the 11-day-old infant was found gasping, choking and blue, 3 hours after feeding. The physical and neurological examination on the infant did not return to normal for 5 days (Chaney *et al.* 1988). Breastfeeding in a cocaine-using mother is not recommended. Hale (2012 online access) recommends a minimum period to pump and dump of 24 hours (half-life of cocaine 0.8 hours).

> Avoid during breastfeeding. If mother uses she should pump and discard her milk for a minimum of 24 hours to 48 hours – a breastfed infant may still have positive urine test results due to the transfer of inactive metabolites.

References

Chaney NE, Franke J, Wadlington WB, Cocaine convulsions in a breastfeeding baby, *J Pediatr*, 1988;112(1):134–5.

Chasnoff I, Lewis D, Squires L, Cocaine intoxication in a breastfed infant, *Paediatrics*, 1987;80:836–8.

Ecstasy

There does not appear to be any available information but the action could probably be similar to the effects of amphetamine use to which it is related.

> Avoid during breastfeeding. If mother uses she should pump and discard her milk for a minimum of 24 to 48 hours due to lack of information on the amount passing into breastmilk.

Lysergic acid diethylamide

Lysergic acid dethylamide (LSD) is a powerful hallucinogenic drug. There is no data available on transfer into breastmilk. This drug is contra-indicated while breastfeeding. Maternal urine remains positive for up to 120 hours after use (Hale 2012 online access).

> Avoid during breastfeeding.

Marijuana

The main ingredient of marijuana is delta-9 tetrahydrocannabinol or THC which is rapidly distributed to the brain and adipose tissue, it is stored in fat tissue for long periods and may accumulate with ongoing use. Small to moderate secretion into breastmilk has been documented. In 27 infants evaluated at 1 year of age who were exposed to marijuana via breastmilk, compared with 35 non-exposed infants, no significant difference was found in age at weaning, growth and mental and motor development (Tennes *et al.* 1985). Occasional and chronic use may need to be differentiated together with the risk to the infant of inhaling second-hand smoke containing marijuana be that from the mother or other significant adults in the infant's life.

In addition the mother's ability to respond appropriately to her child's needs may be questioned if she is a regular, heavy user. In chronic users, the half-life of marijuana may be 4 days because of storage in body fat, which can be detected for up to a month after last use. It is excreted in urine and feces over a prolonged period (Djulus *et al.* 2005).

Klonoff-Cohen *et al.* studied 239 infants who died of SIDS in southern California from 1989 to 1992, and compared them with a matched group of healthy infants. After adjusting for confounding factors, maternal dose was not associated with SIDS. However, there were statistically significant differences between the cases and controls in terms of marijuana use around conception and post-natally and the risk of SIDS.

Astley and Little (1990) studied 68 infants exposed to marijuana via maternal milk and 68 matched controls. They found a decrease in infant motor development at one year associated with maternal use during the first month post-partum.

In a study comparing THC concentrations in breastmilk and plasma of two women who were long-term users and had breastfed for 7 to 8 months, there was a marked difference between the two samples (Perez-Reges and Wall 1985). The difference in THC between the two samples was thought to be due to the amount of marijuana smoked and the interval between smoking and collection of samples. There were high levels of metabolites found in faecal samples from the infants which the author interpreted as individual differences in the infants' absorption and metabolism of THC. Both infants were developing normally.

In adults THC may impair perception, judgement, motor skills, short-term memory and learning and is strongly associated with symptoms of paranoia. The longer-term effects of THC in breastmilk exposure are unknown (effect on children entering teens) in addition to exposure via passive smoking. Smoking marijuana and breastfeeding, or using near children should not be undertaken until more data are available on long-term effects especially the risk of psychosis in later life.

> Occasional recreational use **may not** be detrimental but regular use should be **strongly** discouraged.

References

Astley SJ, Little RE, Maternal marijuana use during lactation and infant development at one year, *Neurotoxicol Teratol*, 1990;12:161–8.

Djulus J, Moretti M, Koren G, Marijuana use and breastfeeding, *Can Fam Physician*, 2005;51(3):349–50.

Klonoff-Cohen H, Lam-Kruglick P, Maternal and paternal recreational drug use and sudden infant death syndrome, *Arch Pediatr Adolesc Med*, 2001;155:765-70

Perez–Reyes M, Wall ME, Presence of tetrahydrocannabinol in human milk, *N Engl J Med*, 1982;307:818–20.

Tennes K, Avitable N, Blackard C, Boyles C, Hassoun B, Holmes L, Kreye M, Marijuana: prenatal and postnatal exposure in the human, *NIDA Res Monogr*, 1985;59:48–60.

Diamorphine

Diamorphine (heroin) is a pro-drug which is rapidly converted to 6-acetylmorphine and more slowly to morphine.

The effect on the breastfed baby of maternal chronic administration of large doses of opioids is not known but monitoring the infant for signs of sedation and respiratory depression are needed. There are some reports that breastfeeding can be one method of treating the addicted infant (Cobrinik *et al.* 1959). When breastfeeding stops or is delayed for any time, then it is possible that the infant may display signs and symptoms of drug withdrawal. Addicts use large doses to maintain their habit and in this situation may best be advised not to attempt breastfeeding. The mother may not be responsive to her infant's needs, due to the effects of the drug and the safety of the child may need to be considered.

Cobrinik *et al.* reported on the outcomes of 22 infants born to narcotic-using mothers. The mothers had taken heroin and morphine. The infants exhibited signs of tremors, excessive crying, sleeplessness, restlessness or hyper-irritability. Vomiting and poor feeding were observed in ten infants, diarrhoea in six, yawning and sneezing in six, fever in four and convulsions in one. There appeared to be a correlation between the severity of the infant's symptoms and the maternal narcotic dosage. There was complete recovery of all the newborn infants. The withdrawal was due to placental transfer not the effect of the drug passage from breastmilk. The study reported withdrawal in the first 4 days but shows how hard it may be to establish breastfeeding after maternal abuse of diamorphine.

Klenka (1986) studied 25 babies born to 23 drug-abusing mothers, most of whom were smoking heroin. Nineteen of the babies developed withdrawal symptoms and 12 needed treatment. He found that withdrawal symptoms were short lasting and often self-limiting, and no evidence of adverse effect on postnatal growth and development was found. Only 4 of the mothers established breastfeeding, although all were supported and encouraged to do so. Measurements of drug levels were not made. Mothers should be encouraged to join a detoxification programme during pregnancy and to avoid street drugs which may be adulterated. If mothers continue to use heroin intermittently and breastfeed, the baby may also experience repeated withdrawal. Few users are successful at breastfeeding.

Therapeutic doses unlikely to affect infant withdrawal symptoms in infants of dependent mothers; breastfeeding not best method of treating dependence in offspring (BNF).

> Avoid as a drug of abuse during breastfeeding. The risk of adulterants used to cut the drug as well as the risk of HIV/AIDS increases the risk to the baby. Encourage enrolment in a methadone programme.

References

Cobrinik R, Hood R, Chusid E, The effects of maternal narcotic addiction on the newborn infant, *Paediatrics*, 1959;24:288–304.

Klenka HM, Babies born in a district general hospital to mothers taking heroin, *BMJ*, 1986;293:745–6.

Substance dependence

> **Mothers who are using medication instead of illicit drugs should be supported to breastfeed if possible**
> **They need to be aware of the risks for their baby if they use street drugs while breastfeeding**

Buprenorphine   (?)

Brand name: *Subutex*®
US brands: *Subutex*®
Australian brands: *Subutex*®

Buprenorphine is a potent opioid analgesic classified as an agonist and antagonist. It can be used as an alternative to methadone as well as being used to treat moderate to severe pain. It has a prolonged duration of action particularly following sublingual doses. Buprenorphine is subject to considerable first-pass metabolism after oral doses and the terminal elimination half-life after sublingual doses is 20 to 25 hours. It has an active metabolite norbuprenorphine. Oral bio-availability is generally poor.

In a study of one mother (Marquet *et al.* 1997) using 4 mg per day to facilitate withdrawal from adictive opioid medication, the amount of drug transferred into breastmilk was only 3.28 µg per day. This was determined by the authors, to be a clinically insignificant amount. The baby exhibited a degree of withdrawal on the second day after delivery from which it recovered rapidly. Later interruption of breastfeeding did not precipitate withdrawal symptoms. No other adverse effects were noted in the baby. A study of four mothers (Jernite *et al.* 1999) taking 0.4, 2, 4 or 6 mg of oral buprenorphine maintenance once daily during pregnancy and lactation had milk levels measured. Levels of buprenorphine and the metabolite were undetectable in the mother on the lowest dose. It was estimated that an exclusively breastfed infant would receive less than 1% of the maternal weight-adjusted dosage. It has been suggested (Hirose *et al.* 1997) that buprenorphine may reduce breastmilk production and infant weight gain in a study of continuous epidural administration post-caesarian. The infants of ten mothers given the drug for 3 days to relieve post-operative pain were monitored. At 11 days they exhibited lower weight gain and milk intake than those whose mothers who had an extradural bupivacane anaesthetic only and no buprenorphine. The relevance to oral use is unclear. Ilett *et al.* (2011) studied seven pregnant opioid-dependent women who proposed to breastfeed. The dose of buprenorphine ranged from 2.4 to 24 mg daily. Milk samples were taken over a 24-hour period once lactation had been established. The mean relative infant dose of norbuprenorphine was 0.18 and of buprenorphine was 0.38. All infants developed normally and no adverse effects were noted.

Infants exposed to buprenorphine through breastmilk should be monitored for sedation and weight gain as a precaution.

Relative infant dose quoted as 1.9% (Hale 2012 online access).

Buprenorphine is excreted in low concentrations in breastmilk and has low oral bio-availability; however, neonates should be monitored for drowsiness, adequate weight gain and developmental milestones. Increased sleepiness, breathing difficulties or limpness in breastfed babies of mothers taking opioid substitutes should be reported urgently to a healthcare professional (BNF).

Generally appears compatible but monitor baby for sedation and weight gain.

References

Hirose M, Hosokawa T, Tanaka Y, Extradural buprenorphine suppresses breastfeeding after cesarean section, *Br J Anaesth*, 1997;79:120–21.

Ilett KF, Hackett LP, Gower S, Doherty DA, Hamilton D, Bartu AE, Estimated dose exposure of the neonate to buprenorphine and its metabolite norbuprenorphine via breastmilk during maternal buprenorphine substitution treatment, *Breastfeed Med*, 2012 ;7:269–74.

Jernite M, Diemunsch P, Kintz P, Buprenorphine excretion in breastmilk. *Anesthesiology*, 1999;91:A1095. Abstract.

Marquet P, Chevrel J, Lavignasse P, Merle L, Lachâtre G, Buprenorphine withdrawal syndrome in a newborn, *Clin Pharmacol Ther*, 1997;62:569–71.

Methadone

Methadone enters the breastmilk in low concentrations and may help to prevent withdrawal symptoms in addicted infants. Support for the neonate may still be necessary. Methadone is extensively plasma protein bound and has a long elimination half-life. It has high bio-availability following oral dosage.

Arletta *et al.* (2005) studied 86 babies born to mothers enrolled on a methadone maintenance programme in pregnancy. They found that babies were more likely to be born prematurely, to be at risk of intra-uterine growth retardation and had a higher incidence of micrencephaly then normal births. Pharmaceutical treatment was required by 62% to relieve abstinence syndrome. Of the babies studied 42% were removed from their mothers and placed in care as part of a child protection service.

Blinick *et al.* (1975) studied ten mothers between 3 and 10 days post-partum taking maintenance methadone doses between 10 and 80 mg daily. Milk samples had methadone levels between 50 and 570 µg per litre equivalent to an infant exposure of a maximum of 86 µg per kg, 6% of the maternal weight-adjusted dosage. Jansson *et al.* (2008) monitored eight breastfed and eight formula-fed infants born to methadone using mothers taking between 50 and 105 mg methadone daily. No differences in neobehavioral behaviours were noted between the two groups but fewer infants in the breastfed group required pharmacotherapy for neonatal abstinence syndrome although this did not reach statistical significance. Similar results were found by Sharpe *et al.* (1975) who studied 16 breastfed babies of mothers taking up to 100 mg oral methadone and the babies of a matched group who had chosen to artificially feed. He found the breastfed babies needed less treatment for withdrawal and needed a shorter duration of hospital stay. Newman *et al.* (1975) collected breastmilk and plasma samples from 3 to 10 days after delivery from 10 women taking 10 to 80 mg methadone. The average m/p ratio was 0.83. Another study on two women ingesting 60 to 73 mg of methadone daily showed a m/p ratio that varied from 0.52 to 1.53 (Geraghty *et al.* 1997). Increased methadone levels generally resulted in higher breastmilk levels but this rise was not linear. At least one death has possibly been attributed to methadone obtained through breastfeeding (Smalek *et al.* 1997) although this infant had several pre-existing severe congenital defects and the methadone level in the infant's blood was not high by adult standards.

Williams (1990) describes how if women who are long-time drug users converted to methadone and stayed closely monitored were encouraged to breastfeed in the post-natal period and the women responded very positively to this care. Any methadone medication is best taken immediately after a breastfeed. This avoids peak levels of the drug passage into the breastmilk after 0.5 to 1 hours. Methadone has a long half-life in adults so there is the possibility of an accumulation of the drug in the baby. Mothers should be encouraged to monitor their infant for signs of sedation.

When breastfeeding stops there is a possibility that the infant may experience withdrawal signs and symptoms particularly if the mother was on high-dose therapy. If the baby shows signs of increased sleepiness difficulty breastfeeding, breathing difficulties or limpness, medical help should be sought immediately. Relative infant dose quoted as 1.9 to 6.5% (Hale 2012 online access).

Babies exposed to methadone in utero will be more tolerant to the drug than those whose mothers initiate it post-natally.

The dose of methadone should be kept as low as possible in breastfeeding mothers and the infant should be monitored for sedation (high doses of methadone carry an increased risk of sedation and respiratory depression in the neonate). Increased sleepiness, breathing difficulties or limpness in breastfed babies of mothers taking opioid substitutes should be reported urgently to a healthcare professional (BNF).

> Generally appears compatible but monitor baby for sedation, breathing difficulties and weight gain level of arousal. Ensure the daily methadone bottles are kept well out of the reach of children to prevent accidental dosage

References

Blinick G, Inturrisi CE, Jerez E, Wallach RC, Methadone assays in pregnant women and progeny, *Am J Obstet Gynecol*, 1975;121:617–21.

Geraghty B, Graham E, Logan B, Weiss E, Methadone levels in breastmilk, *J Hum Lact*, 1997;13(3):227–30.

Jansson LM, Choo R, Velez ML, Lowe R, Huestis MA, Methadone maintenance and breastfeeding in the neonatal period, *Pediatrics*, 2008;121:106–14.

Newman R, Bashkow S, Calko D, The results of 313 consecutive live births of infants delivered to patients in New York methadone maintenance programme, *Am J Obstet Gynecol*, 1975;121:233–7.

Sharpe C, Kuschel C, Outcomes of infants born to mothers receiving methadone for pain management in pregnancy, *Arch Dis Child Fetal Neonatal Ed*, 2004;89:F33-6.

Smalek J, Montforte J, Aronow R, Spitz W, Methadone deaths in children – a continuing problem, *JAMA*, 1997;238:2516–17.

Williams A, Reproductive concerns of women at risk of HIV infection, *J Nurse Midwifery*, 1990;35:292–8.

Arlettaz R, Kashiwagi M, Das-Kundu S, Fauchère JC, Lang A, Bucher HU, Methadone maintenance program in pregnancy in a Swiss perinatal center (II): neonatal outcome and social resources, Acta Obstet Gynecol Scand, 2005;84(2):145–50.

Nicotine replacement therapy

Smoking is the single most important cause of preventable illness and premature death in the UK and USA: it is estimated that around one in five deaths are due to smoking-related illnesses. Any products which help smokers to quit should be encouraged. This includes lactating mothers. There are a variety of nicotine replacement (NRT) preparations available. They include patches gum, lozenge, tablets, nasal spray and inhalator.

> **NRT form of choice in a mother during breastfeeding based on evidence of benefit and safety for the baby:**
>
> **According to patient wishes. Whatever form of NRT helps a mother to quit is beneficial to her baby's long-term health.**

NRT helps to stave withdrawal symptoms from nicotine by gradual reduction in nicotine levels while the smokers breaks the habits associated with smoking. Product choice is individual and no one method has been shown to be superior although patches do produce a continuous level of nicotine so that the patient no longer suffers peaks and troughs of nicotine levels associated with cravings. Use of NRT has been shown to double the chances of a successful quit attempt, whether or not it is supported by behavioural change support. Ilett *et al.* (2003) studied 15 women who used patches ranging from 21 to 7 mg per 24 hours as they stopped smoking. The authors conclude that the absolute dose of nicotine and its metabolite decrease by 70% from smoking or using the 21 mg patch to when the mothers were using the 7 mg patch. The nicotine patch had no significant influence on the milk intake by the breastfed infants. NRT products are licensed for use in breastfeeding.

Nicotine is present in milk; however, the amount to which the infant is exposed is small and less hazardous than second-hand smoke. Intermittent therapy is preferred (BNF).

> Compatible with breastfeeding as level of nicotine reaching baby is likely to be lower than that passed on through smoking.

References

Ilett KF, TW, Page-Sharp M, Kristensen JH, Kohan R, Hackett LP, Use of nicotine patches in breastfeeding mothers: transfer of nicotine and cotinine into human milk, *Clin Pharmacol Ther*, 2003;74(6):516–24.

Bupropion

Brand name: *Zyban*®
US brands: *Zyban*®
Australian brands: *Clorpax*®, *Zyban*®

Bupropion was originally developed as an anti-depressant but is rarely used as such in the UK currently. It is, however, used to support smoking cessation attempts. Its use is contra-indicated in patients with a history of seizure and use by mothers whose baby has suffered any form of seizure is best avoided. Bupropion undergoes extensive first-pass metabolism, it has several active metabolites with long half-lives. It is 80% plasma protein bound. It is given as a modified-release preparation in smoking cessation at an initial dose of 150 mg once daily for 6 days, increasing to 150 mg twice daily on day 7. Treatment is started about 1 to 2 weeks before an agreed quit date, to allow steady-state blood levels of bupropion to be reached, and therapy normally continues up to 12 weeks. There is a case report of a 6-month-old baby who suffered seizures 3 days after the mother initiated 150 mg per day dose of bupropion (Chaudron and Schoenecker 2004). The mother discontinued the drug and no further adverse events were noted.

Haas *et al.* (2004) studied ten women whose babies had an average age of 12 months. The mothers had to agree not to breastfeed for the duration of the study and were provided with breastpumps and information on maintaining their supply. They were given sustained release bupropion 150 mg daily for 3 days, then 300 mg daily for 4 days. On the seventh day samples of breastmilk, plasma, urine and saliva were taken. The average m/p ratio was 2.8. The authors estimated that the infants would consume an average of 6.75 µg per kg per day of bupropion via breastmilk and concluded that that bupropion taken by a breastfeeding mother should not present a concern for most infants. Although the drug appears to concentrate in breastmilk the relative infant dose remains low and use should not be precluded if the mother is breastfeeding. Individual risk:benefit assessments should be undertaken with neonates and other forms of NRT tried first with behavioural support. Relative infant dose quoted as 0.2 to 2% (Hale 2012 online access). The BNF reports that it is present in breastmilk and recommends it is avoided.

Limited data on use as an agent for smoking cessation. Use only if no other method has been successful and the baby has no previous history of seizure.

References

Chaudron LH, Schoenecker CJ, Bupropion and breastfeeding: a case of possible infant seizure, *J Clin Psychiatry*, 2004:64(6):881–2. Letter.

Haas JS, Kaplan CP, Barenboim D, Jacob P 3rd, Benowitz NL, Bupropion in breastmilk: an exposure assessment for potential treatment to prevent post-partum tobacco use, *Tob Control*, 2004;13:52–6.

Varenicline ☹

Brand name: *Champix®*
US brands: *Chantrix®*
Australian brands:

Varenicline is a recently developed drug for smoking cessation. There are currently no data on transfer into breastmilk. As there are alternatives whose safety has been determined, the use of this drug should be restricted. The BNF notes that it is present in milk in animal studies and should be avoided.

Avoid during breastfeeding due to lack of any data on passage into breastmilk. Other methods of smoking cessation should be used.

Cigarettes and smoking

Nicotine is found in breastmilk. The flavour of breastmilk collected 30 to 60 minutes after smoking has been identified as tasting more like cigarettes than samples taken at any other time. The levels of cotinine (metabolite of nicotine) in the urine of breast-fed babies whose mothers smoked were ten times higher than those of formula-fed babies of smoking mothers. Thus levels are due to passage through breastmilk not passive absorption. Babies of mothers who smoke are more likely to suffer from colic. (Matheson *et al.* 1989). Smoking appears to lower breastmilk production and more women who smoke believe they have insufficient milk. (Hopkinson *et al.* 1992). Mothers who smoke are likely to breastfeed for a shorter length of time. Passive smoking is related to early onset of wheezing. However, many women continue to smoke while breastfeeding perceiving it as stress relieving, reducing tiredness and helping to reduce appetite promoting faster weight loss. As with alcohol consumption, the reality of life with new baby influences habits. Some women stop smoking when pregnant only to restart as soon as they deliver when they perceive the activity to be less dangerous to the baby. Maternal smoking in pregnancy is associated with low birthweight infants and increased risk of abortion, stillbirth and neonatal death. Nicotine is present in breastmilk in concentrations between 1.5 to 3 times the maternal plasma concentration.

Mothers may believe that smoking away from the baby limits exposure although we know that this is not true. Lactating mothers (and their formula-feeding counterparts) should be encouraged not to smoke both for their own and their children's health. However, the breastmilk of a mother who smokes still retains many benefits and retains the majority of benefits over formula. One study reported that the incidence of acute respiratory illness in infants whose mothers smoked was decreased in those who were breastfed when compared with those infants who were bottle fed (Woodward *et al.* 1990).

Dahlstrom *et al.* (2004) measured nicotine levels in breastmilk and urine of 40 women (20 non-smokers, 20 smoking between two and 18 cigarettes per day and two snuff users). Two women who were non-smoking, non-snuff using mothers had measurable nicotine in their breastmilk. They had smoking partners. The shorter the interval between smoking and breastfeeding the more nicotine transferred into breastmilk.

> Cigarette smoking has many disadvantages for mother and child. Mothers, fathers and other adults in close contact with the baby should be encouraged to give up. The baby should not be exposed to second-hand smoke from any adult. However, breastmilk from a smoking mother still has advantages over formula milk.

References

Dahlstrom A, Ebersjo C, Lundell B, Nicotine exposure in breastfed infants, *Acta Paediatr*, 2004;93(6):810–16.

Hopkinson JM, Schanler RJ, Fraley JK, Garza C, Milk production by mothers of premature infants: influence of cigarette smoking, Pediatrics, 1992;90(6):934–8.

Matheson I, Rivrud GN, The effect of smoking on lactation and infantile colic, *JAMA*, 1989;261(1):42–3.

Woodward A, Douglas RM, Graham NM, Miles H, Acute respiratory illness in Adelaide children: breastfeeding modifies the effect of passive smoking, *J Epidemiol Community Health*, 1990;44:224–30.

Infections

Antibiotics

Antibiotics are acknowledged to be overused which is one of the reasons that multiply resistant *Staphylococcus aureus* (MRSA) and *Clostridium difficile* have become more widespread. It is sensible to consider whether a mother needs to be treated with antibiotics before exposing both her and her breastfed baby. Babies exposed to antibiotics via their mother's breastmilk may develop symptoms of colic, abdominal discomfort and diarrhoea. These are an inconvenience and not a reason to suspend breastfeeding.

Research undertaken in Canada in 1993 (Ito *et al.* 1993) showed that 15% of women prescribed antibiotics chose not to take the medicine and continue to breastfeed, rather than expose their baby to a risk which they had been assured was minimal. By contrast, 7% stopped breastfeeding during therapy despite reassurance. The research team also examined the reporting of adverse effects by mothers made aware of potential diarrhoea in the child with antibiotics passing through breastmilk. Although more women warned of side effects reported clinical effects which they had noted and judged to be due to the medication, than those not made aware, the difference is not statistically significant (87% compared with 68%). No difference in compliance with the antibiotic regimen or breastfeeding pattern, were noted between the two groups (Taddio *et al.* 1995).

Wherever possible, local and national guidelines should be followed on the selection of the most effective antibiotic to treat the bacterial infection, following wherever possible, sensitivity testing. Delayed prescriptions for antibiotics may be useful in minimising exposure of mother and child. These follow recommendations from the doctor that the 'infection' may be self-limiting but if symptoms develop further or fail to resolve in the following 48 hours, then the course of antibiotics should be taken. Little *et al.* have suggested restricting the use in the treatment of otitis media, upper respiratory infection and sore throat ((Little 2002; 2005; 1997) beginning the public health message about reducing the use of antibiotics.

References

Ito S, Koren G, Einarson TR, Maternal non compliance with antibiotics during breastfeeding, *Ann Pharmacother*, 1993;27(1):40–42.

Little P, Williamson I, Warner G, Gould C, Gantley M, Kinmonth AL, Open randomised trial of prescribing strategies in managing sore throat, *BMJ*, 1997;314:722.

Little P, Delayed prescribing of antibiotics for upper respiratory tract infection, *BMJ*, 2005;331(7512):301.

Little P, Gould C, Moore M, Warner G, Dunleavey J, Williamson I, Predictors of poor outcome and benefits from antibiotics in children with acute otitis media: pragmatic randomised trial, *BMJ*, 2002;325(7354):22.

Taddio A, Ito S, Einarson TR, Leeder JS, Koren G, Effect of counselling on maternal reporting of adverse effects in nursing infants exposed to antibiotics through breastmilk, *Reprod Toxicol*, 1995;9(2):153–7.

Penicillins

This group of drugs is bactericidal and interferes with cell wall synthesis. Allergic reactions are reported to occur in up to 10% of the population, normally evident as rashes. However, an anaphylactic reaction is possible in 0.05% of patients. Those with a previous reaction are more at risk. A child exposed to penicillin for the first time through its mother's milk is highly unlikely to react but may do so subsequently having been sensitised. It is also possible that a reaction will occur the first time the child receives its own dose of medication.

Phenoxymethylpenicillin

Phenoxymethypenicillin (penicillin V) is licensed to be used in children at a dose of 62.5 mg four times a day. Matheson *et al.* (1988) have estimated that a baby would receive between 20 and 90 µg per kg per day following a single maternal dose of 1320 mg. There are reports of sore buttocks and diarrhoea in some babies in this study and one case of stains of blood in the stool although this has been reported before the drug was initiated (Matheson *et al.* 1988).

The BNF reports that there are trace amount in breastmilk but that it is appropriate to use in breastfeeding mothers.

Compatible with use during breastfeeding.

References

Matheson I, Samseth M, Løberg R, Faegri A, Prentice A, Milk transfer of phenoxymethylpenicillin during puerperal mastitis, *Br J Clin Pharmacol*, 1988;25:33–40.

Flucloxacillin

Brand name: *Floxapen*®
US brands:
Australian brands: *Flopen*®, *Floxapen*®, *Floxsig*®, *Flubiclox*®, *Flucil*®, *Staphylex*®

Flucloxacillin is bactericidal and resistant to staphylococcal penicillinase. Absorption is reduced by food in the gut so should be taken on an empty stomach. It is extensively plasma protein bound (95%). It is effective in treating skin infections and is also the initial drug of choice for mastitis so long as the mother is not allergic to penicillins. It is given to children under 2 years at one quarter the adult dose and it has a wide therapeutic index. It can be given to breastfeeding mothers.

The BNF reports that there are trace amount in breastmilk but that it is appropriate to use in breastfeeding mothers.

Compatible with use during breastfeeding.

Amoxycillin

Brand name: *Amoxil*®
US brands: *Amoxil*®, *Trimox*®
Australian brands: *Alphamox*®, *Amohexal*®, *Amoxil*®, *Ibiamox*®, *Maxamox*®, *Moxacin*®

Amoxycillin is a derivative of ampicillin which was the original broad spectrum penicillin. It is only 20% bound to plasma proteins. It is effective against Gram-positive and -negative organisms but is inactivated by beta lactamases. It is not inactivated by gastric acid and is not affected by the presence of food in the stomach. In infants less than 3 months old, the maximum dose should be 30 mg per kg daily in divided doses every 12 hours. But older babies are given 125 mg four times a day as the drug has a wide therapeutic index. Levels passing through breastmilk are very small and amoxycillin can be given to a breastfeeding mother. Using Kafetzis *et al.*'s data (1981), an exclusively breastfed infant would be expected to receive a maximum of about 0.1 mg per kg daily of amoxicillin with a maternal dose of 500 mg three times daily. Relative infant dose quoted as 1% (Hale 2012 online access).

The BNF reports that there are trace amount in breastmilk but that it is appropriate to use in breastfeeding mothers.

Compatible with use during breastfeeding.

References

Kafetzis DA, Siafas CA, Georgakopoulos PA, Papadatos CJ, Passage of cephalosporins and amoxicillin into the breastmilk, *Acta Paediatr Scand*, 1981;70:285–8.

Co-amoxiclav

Brand name: *Augmentin*®
US brands: *Amoclan*®, *Timentin*®, *Augmentin*®
Australian brands: *Augmentin*®, *Ausclav*®, *Clamoxyl*®, *Clavulin*®, *Curam*® *Timentin*®

Co-amoxiclav is the combination amoxicillin with clavulanic acid designed to extend the spectrum of activity. The UK CSM, Medicines Control Agency (1997) recommends that this drug should be reserved for bacterial infections likely to be caused by amoxicillin-resistant beta-lactamase-producing strains and that treatment should not usually exceed 14 days because of the risk of cholestatic jaundice although the risk is highest in males over the age of 65 years.

Benyamini *et al.* (2005) studied 67 women who called a drug consultation centre for information about the potential risks of amoxicillin/clavulanic acid. These were matched with a control group of mothers taking antibiotics known to be safe in lactation. Fifteen infants in the group (22.3%) experienced adverse effects that increased, with increased dosage. This was significantly higher than in the amoxycllin-treated group who reported adverse events in 3% of cases. All adverse effects were minor, self-limiting and did not necessitate interruption of breastfeeding. It is licensed for use in infants. Relative infant dose quoted as 0.95% (Hale 2012 online access).

The BNF reports that there are trace amount in breastmilk but that it is appropriate to use in breastfeeding mothers.

Compatible with use during breastfeeding.

References

Benyamini L, Merlob P, Stahl B, Braunstein R, Bortnik O, Bulkowstein M, Zimmerman D, Berkovitch M, The safety of amoxicillin/clavulanic acid and cefuroxime during lactation, *Ther Drug Monit*, 2005;27:499–502.

Committee on Safety of Medicines, Medicines Control Agency. Revised indications for co-amoxiclav (Augmentin). Current Problems. Also available online www.mhra.gov.uk), 1997;23:8.

Co-fluampicil

Brand name: *Magnapen*®
US brands:
Australian brands:

Co-fluampicil is a combination of flucloxacillin and ampicillin often used to treat infections involving streptococci or staphylococci e.g. cellulitis. Both ingredients and the combination are compatible with breastfeeding. The BNF reports that there are trace amount in breastmilk but that it is appropriate to use in breastfeeding mothers.

Compatible with use during breastfeeding.

Cephalosporins

These antibiotics are bactericidal and act by inhibiting synthesis of the bacterial cell wall. Pharmacologically they are very similar to the penicillins. Approximately 10% of patients allergic to penicillin will be allergic to cephalosporins (BNF).

Cefaclor

Brand name: *Distaclor*®, *Distaclor MR*®, *Keftid*®, *Bacticlor*®
US brands: *Ceclor*®, *Raniclor*®
Australian brands: *Aclor*®, *Ceclor*®, *Cefklor*®, *Karlor*®, *Keflor*®

Cefaclor is well absorbed from the GI tract, although the presence of food may delay absorption. Takase *et al.* (1979) studied two breastfeeding mothers given a single dose of 250 mg cefaclor – in one mother the level was undetectable; in the other the maximum achieved was 0.19 mg per litre. He also studied five mothers who took single doses of 500 mg cefaclor and determined an average peak level of 0.21 mg per litre. Relative infant dose quoted as 0.4 to 0.8% (Hale 2012 online access).

The BNF states that it is present in breastmilk in low concentrations but that it is appropriate to use in breastfeeding mothers. The drug is given directly to babies over 1 month old (BNFC).

Compatible with use during breastfeeding.

References

Takase Z, Shirafuji H, Uchida M, Clinical and laboratory studies of cefaclor in the field of obstetrics and gynecology, *Chemotherapy (Tokyo)*, 1979;27(Suppl. 7):666–72.

Cefalexin

Brand name: *Keflex®, Ceporex®*
US brands: *Biocef®, Cefanex®, Keflex®*
Australian brands: *Cilex®, Ialex®, Ibilex®, Keflex®, Sporahexal®*

Cefalexin (cephalexin) is a first-generation cephalosporin antibacterial. Kafetzis *et al.* (1981) gave a single 1 g oral dose of cephalexin to six women in the immediate postpartum period. The maximum levels achieved in breastmilk were measured as 0.51 mg per litre. In Ito *et al.*'s prospective study (1993) one of 11 women who took cephalexin reported diarrhoea in her infant which she attributed to exposure to the drug through breastmilk. Cephalexin is given directly to babies one month of age at a dose of 125 mg twice daily. Relative infant dose quoted as 0.5% (Hale 2012 online access).

The BNF states that it is present in breastmilk in low concentrations but that it is appropriate to use in breastfeeding mothers.

Compatible with use during breastfeeding.

References

Ito S, Blajchman A, Stephenson M, Prospective follow-up of adverse reactions in breastfed infants exposed to maternal medication, *Am J Obstet Gynecol*, 1993;168:1393–9.
Kafetzis DA, Siafas CA, Georgakopoulos PA, Papadatos CJ, Passage of cephalosporins and amoxicillin into the breastmilk, *Acta Paediatr Scand*, 1981;70:285–8.

Cefadroxil

Brand name: *Baxan®*
US brands: *Duricef®*
Australian brands:

Although higher concentrations of cefadroxil were reported in breastmilk compared with cefalexin, no adverse events have been reported as the dose received by the baby is still considerably smaller than the level licensed to be given directly (25 mg per kg per day) (Kafetzis *et al.* 1981). Relative infant dose quoted as 0.8 to 1.3% (Hale 2012 online access). The BNF states that it is present in breastmilk in low concentrations but that it is appropriate to use in breastfeeding mothers.

> Compatible with use during breastfeeding.

References

Kafetzis DA, Siafas CA, Georgakopoulos PA, Papadatos CJ, Passage of cephalosporins and amoxicillin into the breastmilk, *Acta Paediatr Scand*, 1981;70:285–8.

Cefradine

Brand name: Velosef®
US brands:
Australian brands:

Cefradine is less protein bound than the other cephalosporins (8 to 12%) but still has low levels in breastmilk with an average milk level of 1 mg per litre compared with a licensed paediatric dose of 25 to 50 mg per day so is compatible with breastfeeding (Kafetzis *et al.* 1981; Mischler *et al.* 1972; Mischler *et al.* 1978).

The BNF states that it is present in breastmilk in low concentrations but that it is appropriate to use in breastfeeding mothers.

> Compatible with use during breastfeeding.

References

Kafetzis DA, Siafas CA, Georgakopoulos PA, Papadatos CJ, Passage of cephalosporins and amoxicillin into the breastmilk, *Acta Paediatr Scand*, 1981;70:285–8.
Mischler TW, Corson SL, Larranaga A, Bolognese RJ, Neiss ES, Vukovich RA, Presence of cephradine in body fluids of lactating and pregnant women, *Clin Pharmacol Ther*, 1972;15:214.
Mischler TW, Corson SL, Larranaga A, Bolognese RJ, Neiss ES, Vukovich RA, Cephradine and epicillin in body fluids of lactating and pregnant women, *J Reprod Med*, 1978;21:130–6.

Cefuroxime

Brand name: *Zinnat®*, *Zinacef®*
US brands: *Zinacef®*, *Ceftin®*
Australian brands: *Zinnat®*

Cefuroxime is a second-generation cephalosporin which is less susceptible to inactivation by beta lactamases. It is 50% plasma protein bound. No levels in breastmilk have been published on oral use but it has a paediatric licence dose of 125 mg twice daily for babies over 3 months. It would be very unlikely that levels in breastmilk would approach this. The BNF states that it is present in breastmilk in low concentrations but that it is appropriate to use in breastfeeding mothers.

Compatible with use during breastfeeding.

Tetracyclines

This group of antibacterials are bacteriostatic. Their value is declining due to adverse effects and resistance. Use in children under the age of 12, and pregnant women, is discouraged due to deposition in growing bones and teeth brought about by binding onto calcium. However, as there are high levels of calcium in milk it is likely absorption from the GI tract will be inhibited and that short courses in lactation are not contra-indicated. The long-term use in acne should, however, be discouraged due to lack of research.

Tetracycline

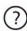

Tetracycline is secreted into breastmilk in extremely small quantities. In one study, five women were given 2 g per day doses for 3 days and the milk concentration measured was 0.43 to 2.58 mg per litre, however, serum levels in their breastfed infants were below the level of detection (Posner *et al.* 1955). Relative infant dose quoted as 0.6% (Hale 2012 online access).

The BNF recommends that tetracyclines should **not** be given to women who are breastfeeding, although absorption and therefore discoloration of teeth in the infant is probably prevented by chelation with calcium in milk.

Compatible with use during breastfeeding in short courses. Avoid in durations >7 days due to theoretical risk of tooth staining in baby

References

Posner AC, Prigot A, Konicoff NG, Further observations on the use of tetracycline hydrochloride in prophylaxis and treatment of obstetric infections, *Antibiot Annu 1954–1955*, 1955;594–8.

Doxycycline

Brand name: *Vibramycin*®
US brands: *Vibramycin*®, *Adoxa*®, *Monodox*®
Australian brands: *Vibramycin*®, *Doxyhexal*®

Doxycycline can cause oesophageal ulceration if capsules are taken with insufficient fluid or with the patient lying down: it should be taken with at least half a glass of water, in an upright position, and well before retiring to bed. Doxycycline is used to treat sinusitis and acne as well as a prophylactic for malaria in some areas. It has a longer half-life and is generally only taken once daily. Various studies have demonstrated low milk transfer but levels in the baby's serum have not been reported.

Morganti *et al.* (1968) studied 15 mothers whose infants were aged 15 to 30 days. They were given 200 mg doxycycline and a further 100 mg 12 hours later. Milk levels were measured as 0.77 mg per litre after 3 hours and 0.38 mg per litre 24 hours after the second dose.

Lutziger (1969) gave 100 mg doxycycline to ten mothers over two days. As Morganti did, he measured milk levels 3 and 24 hours after the second dose and determined levels of 0.82 mg per litre and 0.46 mg per litre which he concluded represented 6% of the maternal weight-adjusted dosage. Tokuda *et al.* (1969) studied doses of doxycycline 100 mg twice daily over 5 days and found breastmilk levels of 3.6 mg per litre. Similarly Borderon *et al.* (1975) measured peak levels of 0.6 mg per litre with the 100 mg dose in three women, and 1.1 mg per litre in a further 11 women who received 200 mg daily.

Doxycycline has a lower affinity for binding with calcium than many tetracyclines. However, for the same reason doxycycline has a lower propensity to bind to calcium in the teeth so the risk of staining remains low. Relative infant dose quoted as 4.2 to 13.3% (Hale 2012 online access). The BNF recommends that tetracyclines should **not** be given to women who are breastfeeding (although absorption and therefore discoloration of teeth in the infant is probably usually prevented by chelation with calcium in milk).

> Compatible with use during breastfeeding in short courses. Avoid in durations >7 days due to theoretical risk of tooth staining in baby.

References

Borderon E, Soutoul JH *et al.* [Excretion of antibiotics in human milk], *Med Mal Infect*, 1975;5:373–6.

Lutziger H, Konzentrationsbestimmungen und klinisch wirksamkeit von doxycyclin (Vibramycin) in uterus, adnexen und muttermilch, *Ther Umsch*, 1969;26:476–80.

Morganti G, Ceccarelli G, Ciaffi G, Comparative concentrations of a tetracycline antibiotic in serum and maternal milk, *Antibiotica*, 1968;6:216–23.

Tokuda G, Yuasa M, Mihara S *et al.* [Clinical study of doxycycline in obstetrical and gynecological fields], *Chemotherapy (Tokyo)*, 1969;17:339–44.

Lymecycline

Brand name: *Tetralysal*®
US brands:
Australian brands:

Lymecycline is a tetracycline derivative with similar properties to tetracycline. It is frequently used to treat acne. There is no data available on transfer into milk. The long-term use of oral tetracyclines to treat acne is probably not advisable.

The BNF recommends that tetracyclines should **not** be given to women who are breastfeeding (although absorption and therefore discoloration of teeth in the infant is probably usually prevented by chelation with calcium in milk).

> Compatible with use during breastfeeding in short courses. Avoid in durations >7 days due to theoretical risk of tooth staining in baby.

Minocycline

Brand name: *Minocin*®
US brands: *Minocin*®, *Arestin*®, *Dynacin*®, *Myrac*®
Australian brands: *Akamin*®, *Minomycin*®

Minocycline should also be taken with a full glass of water while remaining upright in order to avoid oesophageal ulceration. A black chaelate of minocycline has been found in the breastmilk of two women causing the production of black milk, this may also be involved in skin pigmentation which is associated with minocycline (Basler and Lynch 1985; Hunt *et al.* 1996). A study of two patients given a single dose of minocycline 200 mg peak milk levels of 0.8 mg per litre were measured at 6 hours after the dose (Mizuno *et al.* 1969). The most frequent use of minocycline is to treat acne vulgaris. Although milk levels may be low, the risk of dental staining cannot be quantified so the drug should be avoided other than in short courses. Relative infant dose quoted as 0.2 to 1.4% (Hale 2012 online access). The BNF recommends that tetracyclines should **not** be given to women who are breastfeeding (although absorption and therefore discoloration of teeth in the infant is probably usually prevented by chelation with calcium in milk).

> Compatible with use during breastfeeding in short courses. Avoid in durations >7 days due to theoretical risk of tooth staining in baby.

References

Basler RSW, Lynch PJ, Black galactorrhea as a consequence of minocycline and phenothiazine therapy, Arch Dermatol, 1985;121:417–18.

Hunt MJ, Salisbury ELC, Grace J, Armati R, Black breastmilk due to minocycline therapy, *Br J Dermatol*, 1996;134:943–4.

Mizuno S, Takata M, Sano S, Ueyama T, Minocycline, *Jpn J Antibiot*, 1969;22:473–9.

Oxytetracycline

Oxytetracycline has similar activity and safety to tetracycline. It is widely used to treat acne and rosacea in dose of 1 g daily. No adverse effects were noted in an unspecified number of breastfed infants whose mothers were taking oral oxytetracycline 1.5 or 2 g daily for 3 days (Gruner 1955). Milk levels were measured as 3 mg per litre but no long-term outcome data on tooth staining was reported. Borderon *et al.* (1975) studied two mothers who were given 1.5 g daily of oxytetracycline. Milk levels ranged from 0.7 to 1.1 mg per litre. The authors estimated that a breastfed infant would receive 300 µg daily of oxytetracycline in milk.

The BNF recommends that tetracyclines should **not** be given to women who are breastfeeding (although absorption and therefore discoloration of teeth in the infant is probably usually prevented by chelation with calcium in milk).

> Compatible with use during breastfeeding in short courses. Avoid in durations >7 days due to theoretical risk of tooth staining in baby.

References

Borderon E, Soutoul JH *et al.* Excretion of antibiotics in human milk, *Med Mal Infect*, 1975;5:373–6.

Gruner JM, The excretion of terramycin and tetracycline in human milk, *Geburtshilfe Frauenheilkd*, 1955;15:354–60.

Aminoglycosides

This group of drugs is poorly absorbed from the gastro-intestinal tract, although well distributed after parenteral dosage. Aminoglycosides should in general only be used for the treatment of serious infections because of their potential toxicity. Dosages are generally monitored to maintain them in a limited therapeutic range.

Gentamicin

A study involving 10 mothers given prophylactic gentamicin 80 mg intramuscularly three times a day for 5 days post-partum, found measurable gentamicin concentrations in the serum of five of the ten neonates (averaged 410 µg per litre), indicating that gastro-intestinal absorption had occurred. It was, however, considered that these low concentrations would not cause clinical effects. Levels of gentamicin were undetectable in the serum of the other five infants (Celiloglu *et al.* 1994). Oral absorption has been demonstrated in premature neonates (Nelson and McCracken 1972; Testa *et al.* 2007) due to poor clearance in neonates and particularly premature babies. Due to the large inter-cellular gaps in the first few days after delivery, large molecules are able to penetrate into breastmilk. Therapeutic drug level monitoring of the infant as well as the mother may be advisable. Celiloglu estimated a daily ingestion of 307 µg from breastmilk produced by mothers who were given 80 mg by intramuscular injection three times a day for 5 days, compared with a neonatal licensed dose of 3 mg per kg twice daily.

Relative infant dose quoted as 2.1% (Hale 2012 online access); however, due to poor bio-availability older infants will not be able absorb much of the drug although gut flora disruption is possible.

The BNF makes no recommendation on breastfeeding.

Compatible with use during breastfeeding in short courses due to poor oral bio-availability.

References

Celiloglu M, Celiker S, Guven H, Tuncok Y, Demir N, Erten O, Gentamicin excretion excretion and uptake from breastmilk by nursing infants, *Obstet Gynecol*, 1994;84:263–5.

Nelson JD, McCracken GH, Jr, The current status of gentamicin for the neonate and young infant, *Am J Dis Child*, 1972;124(1):13–14.

Testa M, Fanos V, Martinelli V, Stronati M, Mussap M, Del Zompo M, Therapeutic drug monitoring of gentamicin in neonatal intensive care unit: experience in 68 newborns, *J Chemother*, 2007;19 Suppl. 2:39–41.

Gentamycin eye and ear drops

Brand name: *Genticin®, Gentisone HC®*
US brands: Gentacidin®, *Genoptic®, Gentasol®, Ocu-mycin®*
Australian brands: *Genoptic®*

Maternal use of ear or eye drop containing gentamicin presents little or no risk for the breastfed infant (Niebyl 1992).

Compatible with use during breastfeeding.

References

Niebyl JR, Use of antibiotics for ear, nose, and throat disorders in pregnancy and lactation, *Am J Otolaryngol*, 1992;13:187–92.

Neomycin

Neomycin is used for bowel sterilistion before surgery – it is considered too toxic for systemic use as it has potent nephrotoxic and ototoxic properties. It is poorly absorbed from the GI tract. The BNF makes no recommendation on use in breast-feeding.

Oral use compatible with use during breastfeeding.

Neomycin eye and ear drops

Brand names: *Betnesol N®, Vista methasone N®, Neo-cortef®, Otosporin®, Predsol N®, Tri-adcortyl otic®, Otomize®, Otosporin®*
US brands: *Neo-cortef®, Neosporin®, Cortisporin®*
Australian brands: *Neopt®, Neosporin®*

It is frequently used topically in eye and ear drops from which there is little potential for toxicity (Niebyl 1992; Leachman and Reed 2006).

Compatible with use during breastfeeding.

References

Leachman SA, Reed BR, The use of dermatologic drugs in pregnancy and lactation, *Dermatol Clin*, 2006;24:167–97.
Niebyl JR, Use of antibiotics for ear, nose, and throat disorders in pregnancy and lactation, *Am J Otolaryngol*, 1992;13:187–92.

Macrolides

The properties of macrolides are very similar to each other and in general they have low toxicity and a similar spectrum of antimicrobial activity with cross-resistance occurring between individual members of the group. The macrolides are bacteriostatic or bactericidal, depending on the concentration and the type of micro-organism, and they are thought to interfere with bacterial protein synthesis.

Erythromycin

Brand name: *Erythroped®, Erythrocin®, Erymax®*
US brands: Eramycin®, *Eryped®, Erythrocin®*
Australian brands: *Eryhexal®, Erythrocin®*

Erythromycin is destroyed by gastric acid and must therefore be given as enteric-coated formulations or as one of its more stable salts or esters such as the stearate or ethyl succinate. Erythromycin is used as an alternative to penicillin in many infections, especially in patients who are allergic to penicillin. It can cause nausea and diarrhoea in some patients probably because of its stimulant action on the gut. Allergic reaction can occur in around 0.5% of patients. A case report in 1986 linked erythromycin with pyloric stenosis (Stang 1986). A cohort study in Denmark comparing 1166 women prescribed macrolides in the early post-natal period with 34, 690 controls confirms the link between use of a macrolide and the risk of hypertrophic pyloric stenosis (Sorensen *et al.* 2003). Affected infants were 2.3 to 3 times more likely to have a mother taking a macrolide antibiotic during the 90 days after delivery with the odds ratio being higher for female babies. However, Goldstein *et al.* did not note a correlation between macrolides (erythromycin, azithromycin, clarithromycin and roxithromycin) and pyloric stenosis. He studied 55 infants exposed to macrolides and 36 exposed to amoxycillin. The infants exposed to macrolides experienced rash, diarrhoea, loss of appetite and somnolence, whereas the infants exposed to amoxicillin experienced only rashes and somnolence.

The use of this drug during the first three months should be considered against the possible risk of pyloric stenosis. Relative infant dose quoted as 1.4 to 1.7% (Hale 2012 online access).

The BNF reports that only small amounts are present in breastmilk and are not known to be harmful.

Compatible with use during breastfeeding. Avoid if possible in mothers of babies <3 months due to small risk of pyloric stenosis.

References

Goldstein LH, Berlin M, Tsur L, Bortnik O, Binyamini L, Berkovitch M, The safety of macrolides during lactation, *Breastfeed Med*, 2009;4(4):197–200.

Sørensen HT, Skriver MV, Pedersen L, Larsen H, Ebbesen F, Schønheyder HC, Risk of infantile hypertrophic pyloric stenosis after maternal postnatal use of macrolides, *Scand J Infect Dis*, 2003;35:104–6.

Stang H, Pyloric stenosis associated with erythromycin ingested through breastmilk, *Minn Med*, 1986;69:669–70, 682.

Azithromycin

Brand name: *Zithromax*®
US brands: *Zithromax*®, *Zmax*®
Australian brands: *Zithromax*®

Gastro-intestinal disturbances are generally less severe with azithromycin than with erythromycin and the drug is given once daily. There is a licensed paediatric dose of 10 mg per kg for a baby over 6 months of age. Goldstein *et al.* did not note a correlation between macrolides (erythromycin, azithromycin, clarithromycin and roxithromycin) and pyloric stenosis. He studied 55 infants exposed to macrolides and 36 exposed to amoxycillin. The infants exposed to macrolides experienced rash, diarrhoea, loss of appetite and somnolence, whereas the infants exposed to amoxicillin experienced only rashes and somnolence.

Relative infant dose quoted as 5.9% (Hale 2012 online access).

The BNF reports that it is present in breastmilk and should only be used if there are no suitable alternatives.

Compatible with use during breastfeeding.

References

Goldstein LH, Berlin M, Tsur L, Bortnik O, Binyamini L, Berkovitch M, The safety of macrolides during lactation, *Breastfeed Med*, 2009;4(4):197–200.

Sørensen HT, Skriver MV, Pedersen L, Larsen H, Ebbesen F, Schønheyder HC, Risk of infantile hypertrophic pyloric stenosis after maternal postnatal use of macrolides, *Scand J Infect Dis*, 2003;35:104–6.

Clarithromycin

Brand name: *Klaricid®*
US brands: *Biaxin®*
Australian brands: *Clarac®, Kalixocin®, Klacid®*

Clarithromycin is known to transfer into animal milk. Sedlmayr *et al.* (1993) studied 12 women with puerperal infections who were given 250 mg clarithromycin for 6 days. The mean peak concentrations of clarithromycin and 14-hydroxy-clarithromycin in breastmilk were about 25% and 75%, respectively, of the corresponding serum concentrations but there are no studies on human transfer.

It is commonly used in paediatrics at a dose of 7.5 mg per kg, a dose unlikely to be exceeded through breastmilk. It is largely given to treat respiratory tract infections including otitis media.

The BNF reports that the manufacturer advises it should be avoided unless potential benefit outweighs riskas it is present in milk.

Probably compatible with use during breastfeeding.

References

Sedlmayr T, Peters F, Raasch W, Kees F, Clarithromycin, a new macrolide antibiotic. Effectiveness in puerperal infections and pharmacokinetics in breastmilk, *Geburtshilfe Frauenheilkd*, 1993;53:488–91.

Other antibiotics

Clindamycin

Brand name: Dalacin C®
Topical clindamycin solution: Dalacin®
US brands: Cleocin®, Cleocin T(topical)
Australian brands: Cleocin®, Dalacin C®, Dalacin T® (topical)

Clindamycin is rarely used as an oral antibiotic because of serious side effects, particularly antibiotic-associated colitis, with which it is associated more frequently than other antibiotics. It is being used more to counteract MRSA. If diarrhoea develops (reported in 20% of cases following systemic use). The drug should be discontinued immediately and medical help sought. Hypersensitivity reactions such as urticaria are seen in 10% of cases.

It has a licensed paediatric dose but is only used in severe infections. Wherever possible, use should be avoided in preference for an alternative drug.

The BNF states that the amount secreted into breastmilk is probably too small to be harmful but that one infant developed bloody diarrhoea.

Compatible with use during breastfeeding but beware if infant develops bloody diarhoea.

Topical Clindamycin solution should not pose any threat to breastfeeding as absorption through the skin is very low.

Compatible with use during breastfeeding as topical absorption is very low.

Trimethoprim

Trimethoprim can be used to treat urinary tract or respiratory infections. It has in the past been used in combination with a sulphonamide as co-trimoxazole. This product is now rarely used in the UK except in very specific circumstances because of increasing bacterial resistance. It can be used prophylactically in babies from one month with renal problems at a dose of 4 mg per kg twice a day. Low levels are excreted into breastmilk and it is compatible with use during breastfeeding. The amount passing into breastmilk measured in a study of 50 women (Miller and Salter 1973) was estimated as 2 mg per litre, which represented an insignificant amount in the opinion of the authors. This agreed with research by Arnauld *et al.* (1972) who measured 1.8 mg per litre and no reported adverse effects in the babies. Ito *et al.* (1993) identified 12 mothers who took co-trimoxazole while breastfeeding, two reported poor feeding but none reported diarrhoea. The BNF notes that it is present in breastmilk but that short-term use is not known to be harmful.

Compatible with use during breastfeeding as licensed for use in neonates and babies.

References

Arnauld R, Soutoul JH, Gallier J, Borderon JC, Borderon E, A study of the passage of trimethoprim into the maternal milk, *Quest Med*, 1972;25:959–64.

Ito S, Blajchman A, Stephenson M, Eliopoulos C, Koren G, Prospective follow-up of adverse reactions in breastfed infants exposed to maternal medication, *Am J Obstet* Gynecol, 1993;168:1393–9.

Miller RD, Salter AJ, The passage of trimethoprim/sulphamethoxazole into breastmilk and its significance. In: Daikos GK (ed.) Progress in Chemotherapy, Proceedings of the Eighth International Congress of Chemotherapy, Athens, *Hellenic Soc Chemother*, 1974;1:687–691.

Nitrofurantoin

Nitrofurantoin is frequently given for uncomplicated urinary tract infections, and colours the urine yellow. The amount passing into breastmilk is small but could theoretically be sufficient to produce haemolysis in G6PD-deficient infants and should be avoided in these circumstances and where the baby is less than one month of age. Gert detected an average milk concentration of 0.2 mg per kg per day, after a single 100 mg dose given to four women. The authors hypothesise an active transport of the drug into milk but the amount of drug to which the babies were exposed was lower than the 5 to 7 mg per kg per day given directly to babies. Hale 2012 online access reports a relative infant dose quoted as 6.8%. In the Ito *et al.* study (1993) one mother reported a perceived decrease in milk supply. This has not been reported in any studies.

The BNF recommends that it should be avoided, although only small amounts are present in milk they could be enough to produce haemolysis in G6PD-deficient infants.

> Compatible with use during breastfeeding as licensed for use in babies >3 months. Use with care in G6PD deficient infants

References

Gerk PM, Kuhn RJ, Desai NS, McNamara PJ, Active transport of nitrofurantoin into human milk, *Pharmacotherapy*, 2001;21:669–75.

Ito S, Blajchman A, Stephenson M, Eliopoulos C, Koren G, Prospective follow-up of adverse reactions in breastfed infants exposed to maternal medication, *Am J Obstet* Gynecol, 1993;168:1393–9.

Pons G, Rey E, Richard MO, Vauzelle F, Francoual C, Moran C, d'Athis P, Badoual J, Olive G, Nitrofurantoin excretion in human milk, *Dev Pharmacol Ther*, 1990;14:148–52.

Anti-fungals

Imidazole antifungals – clotrimazole, econazole, ketoconazole and tioconazole – are mainly used in the treatment of vaginal candidiasis and dermatophyte infections.

Triazole antifungals, including fluconazole and itraconazole, inhibit cytochrome P450-dependent enzymes in sensitive fungi including *Candida* and other dermatophyte infections. Ideally antifungal treatment should be chosen after the infecting organism has been identified but this is not always possible in primary care.

> Anti-fungal drug of choice in a mother during breastfeeding based on evidence of benefit and safety for the baby:
>
> According to patient needs

Amphotericin (amphoteracin B)

Amphotericin may be given as a lozenge for oral infections. It may also be given parenterally to treat systemic fungal infections. It is toxic and generally only used in life-threatening situations. There is no data available on transfer into breastmilk (BNF) but its low oral bio-availability (<9%) makes transfer probably low.

Probably compatible with use during breastfeeding due to low bio-availability but no studies are available.

Fluconazole

Brand name *Diflucan®, Canesten Once®*
US brands: *Diflucan®*
Australian brands: *Diflucan®*

Fluconazole is widely used to treat *Candida* species vaginally, on the mucosa, tinea pedis and dermal candidiasis and invasive *Candida* infections. It has been used in pre-term infants. Steady-state concentrations are reached in 5 to 10 days but may be attained on day 2 if a loading dose is given. It is only 12% plasma protein bound, The elimination half-life of fluconazole is about 30 hours. It is well absorbed with an oral bio-availability of 90%. Concentrations in breastmilk, joint fluid, saliva, sputum, vaginal fluids and peritoneal fluid are similar to those achieved in plasma.

Force (1995) studied one 12-week post-partum woman who was given a single oral dose of fluconazole 150 mg. The highest milk levels were 2.9 and 2.7 mg per litre at 2 and 5 hours after the dose. Milk fluconazole levels were 1.8 and 1 mg per litre at 24 and 48 hours after the dose, respectively. Schilling *et al.* (1993) also presented a case report of one mother 20 days post-partum who took fluconazole 200 mg orally once daily for 18 days. She was found to have a peak milk level of 4.1 mg per litre 2 hours after the dose on day 20 post-partum. Bodley and Powers (1997) studied one woman who presented with candidiasis of the nipple and who was treated with fluconazole (100 mg increased to 200 mg daily after 15 days) for 6 weeks, neither mother or baby's liver function tests changed significantly and no adverse effects were noted.

There are many other case reports of use of fluconazole to treat candidiasis of the nipple and breast. To date, no large trials have been undertaken to confirm the link between symptoms and culture of *Candida*. Treatment remains controversial in some sources but if breastfeeding position and attachment are optimised, treatment appears to be effective (Jones *et al.* 2006).

There is a children's dose of 3 to 12 mg per kg per day (given every 72 hours in neonates up to 2 weeks old and every 48 hours in neonates 2 to 4 weeks old (BNFC). Relative infant dose is 16% (Hale 2012 online access).

The BNF states that it is present in breastmilk but in levels too small to be harmful.

Compatible with use during breastfeeding.

References

Bodley V, Powers D, Long-term treatment of a breastfeeding mother with fluconazole-resolved nipple pain caused by yeast: a case study, *J Hum Lact*, 1997;13:307–11.

Force RW, Fluconazole concentrations in breastmilk, *Pediatr Infect Dis J*, 1995;14:235–6.

Jones W, Sachs M, Buchanan P, Is candida of the breast being correctly diagnosed and treated?, *MIDIRS Midwifery Digest*, 2006;16(3):381–6.

Schilling CG, Seay RE, Larson TA *et al*. Excretion of fluconazole in human breastmilk, *Pharmacotherapy*, 1993;13:287. Abstract.

Itraconazole

Brand name: *Sporanox*®
US brands: *Sporanox*®
Australian brands: *Sporanox*®

Itraconazole can produce hepatotoxicity and liver function should be monitored and patients counselled on the recognition of warnings e.g. anorexia, nausea, vomiting, fatigue, abdominal pain, yellow sclera or dark urine. The elimination half-life of a single dose is 20 hours and this increases up to 40 hours with multiple doses. Itraconazole is highly protein bound with only 0.2% present as free drug and available to pass into breastmilk. As the drug requires an acid pH environment for optimal absorption levels achieved from breastmilk would be predicted to be low. It may interfere with other drugs metabolised by cytochrome P450. There are no studies on passage into breastmilk. Relative infant dose quoted as 0.2% (Hale 2012 online access). The manufacturers advise that it should be avoided as the small amounts present in breastmilk may accumulate (BNF).

> Use with caution during breastfeeding, due to limited studies. However, this drug is highly plasma protein bound and has a limited theoretical infant dose but has an extended half life.

Ketoconazole

Brand name: Nizoral®
US brands: Nizoral®
Australian brands: Fungoral®, Nizoral®

Ketoconazole is associated with gastro-intestinal side effects, with 3% of patients reporting nausea and vomiting. Hepatic adverse reactions to oral ketoconazole are well known and have resulted in fatalities (BNF). Transient minor elevations of liver enzymes without clinical signs or symptoms of hepatic disease occur in about 10% of patients and may occur at any stage of treatment. Ketoconazole is excreted in breastmilk and the manufacturers state that its oral use should be avoided during breastfeeding. However, no adverse effects were seen in a breastfed infant one month of age whose mother was receiving ketoconazole 200 mg daily for 10 days (Moretti *et al.* 1995). The authors calculated that the infant was exposed to about 0.01 mg per kg daily, a maximum of 0.033 mg per kg daily which is equivalent to 0.4% of the usual therapeutic dose of ketoconazole for this age group. Relative infant dose quoted as 0.3% (Hale 2012 online access).

> Use orally with extreme caution during breastfeeding, due to limited studies and potential risk of hepatotoxicity.
> Topical preparations are unlikely to produce significant levels in breastmilk.

References

Moretti ME, Ito S, Koren G, Disposition of maternal ketoconazole in breastmilk, *Am J Obstet Gynecol*, 1995;173:1625-6.

Nystatin

Brand name: *Nystan®*
US brands: *Mycostatin®, Nilstat®*
Australian brands: *Mycostatin®, Nilstat®*

Nystatin is used vaginally to treat candidiasis and orally to treat intestinal infection. It is poorly absorbed from the gastro-intestinal tract. It is not absorbed through the skin or mucous membranes when applied topically. It is also used to treat oral lesions using suspension or pastilles. Avoidance of food or drink for one hour after administration is advised to maintain contact with the oral mucosa for as long as possible. It has poor bio-availability and so passage into breastmilk is unlikely. The BNF states that absorption from the gastro-intestinal tract is negligible although no levels have been measured in breastmilk.

> Compatible with use during breastfeeding.

Terbinafine

Brand name: *Lamisil®*
US brands: *Lamisil®*
Australian brands: *Lamisil®*

Terbinafine is used to treat dermatophyte infection of the nails and ringworm infections. The most frequent adverse effects after oral use of terbinafine hydrochloride are gastro-intestinal disturbances such as nausea, diarrhoea and mild abdominal pain. Loss or disturbance of taste may occur and occasionally may be severe enough to lead to anorexia and weight loss. Terbinafine hydrochloride is well absorbed from the GI tract. The bio-availability is about 40% because of first-pass hepatic metabolism. Treatment generally lasts for a maximum of 3 months although this may be longer in toenail infections.

Topical absorption is minimal (Leachman and Reed 2006). Oral terbinafine is extensively bound to plasma proteins so passage into breastmilk might be expected to be low. The only research refers to two women given a single dose of 500 mg; the total level of terbinafine mesasure in breastmilk during the 72-hour post-dosing period was 0.65 mg in one mother and 0.15 mg in another. Neither woman was breastfeeding, but both were producing some breastmilk (218 ml and 41 ml, repectively). After 18 hours, the levels of terbinafine were below the level of detection. The volume of milk being produced by the mothers makes this study questionable as an evidence base. However, the authors suggested that using the average milk concentration values over the 24-hour period in the two subjects, an exclusively breastfed infant would receive 3.8% of the maternal weight-adjusted dosage of terbinafine.

Although unlicensed terbinafine has been used to treat tinea capitis in children (Gupta *et al.* 2003).

The BNF reports that manufacturer advises avoidance as it is present in milk, but less than 5% of the dose is absorbed after topical application of terbinafine; avoid application to mother's chest.

The use of the oral drug during breastfeeding should be delayed until cessation of breastfeeding if possible, due to the tolerability of the drug for adults and lack of information.

Avoid use during breastfeeding due to lack of information.

References

Leachman SA, Reed BR, The use of dermatologic drugs in pregnancy and lactation, *Dermatol Clin*, 2006;24:167–97.

Gupta AK, Adamiak A, Cooper EA, The efficacy and safety of terbinafine in children, *J Eur Acad Dermatol Venereol*, 2003;17:627–40.

Thieme G, Peuckert U, Report on a pharmacokinetic study of SF 86-327 in healthy females in the ablactation period. Sandoz document number 303-019. 1986 (information taken from report in Lactmed and Hale 2012 online access).

Anti-virals

Most viral infections resolve without treatment. However, there are specific anti-viral treatments available.

HIV infection

HIV-infected women in developed countries are advised not to breastfeed in the light of transmission of the virus through breastmilk. Babies born to HIV-positive mothers are generally delivered by caesarian section and given anti-retroviral drugs. Drug treatment in lactation for HIV-positive mothers will not be discussed here as wide-ranging support and expert advice outside of the scope of this book should be sought.

Factors that increase the risk of transmission of HIV from mother to child are:

- Recent maternal infection with HIV;
- A mother who develops AIDS;
- Infection with sexually transmitted diseases;
- Vitamin A deficiency;
- Breast trauma or mastitis; and
- Duration of feeding.

The Department of Health have a policy on HIV and Infant Feeding (November 2004), which states: 'In the UK, avoidance of all breastfeeding by HIV-infected women is recommended to prevent breastfeeding transmission of HIV.' The policy recognises that some women will choose to breastfeed: 'When an HIV-infected woman chooses to breastfeed, exclusive breastfeeding should be encouraged and the woman supported to make it achievable.'

The British HIV Association and Children's HIV Association Position Statement 2010 on HIV and infant feeding states that mothers known to be HIV infected regardless of maternal viral load and anti-retroviral therapy should refrain from breastfeeding from birth and be supported to formula feed (BHVA 2010).

Further information is available from the World Health Orginazation (WHO) HIV and Infant Feeding Technical Consultation: Held on behalf of the Inter-agency Task Team (IATT) on Prevention of HIV: Infections in Pregnant Women, Mothers and their Infants, Geneva, October 25–27, 2006. Consensus statement (WHO).

References

British HIV Association and Children's HIV Association Position Statement (www.bhiva.org/documents/Publications/InfantFeeding10.pdf).

Department of Health (www.dh.gov.uk/prod_consum_dh/groups/dh_digitalassets/@dh/@en/documents/digitalasset/dh_4089893.pdf).

World Health Organization (http:who.intreproductive-health/stis/mtct/ infantfeedingconsensusstatement.pdf).

Herpes simplex and varicella zoster infections

Treatment with anti-viral drugs should begin as soon as possible after diagnosis. Infection of the lips with the herpes virus (cold sore) should be treated with topical preparations e.g. aciclovir. In herepes zoster (shingles) systemic antiviral therapy can reduce the severity and duration of pain. Treatment should begin within 72 hours of the rash appearing.

> **Anti-viral drug of choice in a mother during breastfeeding based on evidence of benefit and safety for the baby:**
>
> **Aciclovir – topical or oral**

Aciclovir

☺

Brand name: Zovirax®
US brands: Zovirax®
Australian brands: Acihexal®, Lovir®, Zovir®

Aciclovir can be given during lactation as it achieves less than 1% of the paediatric licensed dose. Oral bio-availability of aciclovir is limited. Aciclovir is widely used to treat neonates and its safety is well established. Frenkel *et al.* (1991) reported on one mother who had taken oral aciclovir 400 mg 3 times daily for 3 days in the neonatal period. Her breastmilk level of aciclovir was 54 µg per litre 5 days after her last dose. Taddio *et al.* (1994) studied a mother with a 7-month-old infant. She was taking 800 mg of aciclovir five times a day. Milk levels on days 5 and 6 of therapy ranged from 4.2 to 5.8 mg per litre. The authors estimated that a fully breastfed infant would receive 0.73 mg per kg per day of drug equivalent to relative infant dose of 1%. The BNF states that significant amounts are found in breastmilk after systemic administration. Although it is not known to be harmful, the manufacturer advises it should not be used. It is given directly to children aged more than one month at half the adult dose.

Compatible with use during breastfeeding.

References

Lau RJ, Emery MG, Galinsky RE, Unexpected accumulation of acyclovir in breastmilk with estimation of infant exposure, *Obstet Gynecol*, 1987;69:468–71.
Frenkel LM, Brown ZA, Bryson YJ, Corey L, Unadkat JD, Hensleigh PA, Arvin AM, Prober CG, Connor JD, Pharmacokinetics of acyclovir in the term human pregnancy and neonate, *Am J Obstet Gynecol*, 1991;164:569–76.
Meyer LJ, de Miranda P, Sheth N, Spruance S, Acyclovir in human breastmilk, *Am J Obstet Gynecol*, 1988;158:586–8.
Taddio A, Klein J, Koren G, Acyclovir excretion in human breastmilk, *Ann Pharmacother*, 1994;28:585–7.

Famciclovir

Brand name: *Famvir*®
US brands: *Famvir*®
Australian brands: *Famvir*®

Famciclovir is rapidly metabolised to penciclovir. It has greater bio-availability than aciclovir but data are not available on its transfer into breastmilk. It has no particular benefits over aciclovir and is more expensive so unless there are compelling reasons why this drug should be used, aciclovir would be preferred during lactation. The BNF states that it is present in milk in animal studies. It is not used in children.

No data on transfer into breastmilk so use of aciclovir as alternative is recommended.

Neuraminidase inhibitors to treat influenza (H1N1/H5N1)

Swine flu (H1N1) is the common name given to a relatively new strain of influenza (flu) that caused a influenza pandemic in 2009 to 2010. H5N1 is the term given to Asian influenza. The evidence for the effectiveness of neuramidase inhibitors is limited but with the number of patients in high-risk groups, and particularly pregnant women, dying during the pandemic, their use as treatment or prophylaxis was widespread.

Zanamivir

Brand name: *Relenza®*
US brands: *Relenza®*
Australian brands: *Relenza®*

Zanamivir is a neuraminidase inhibitor. It is poorly absorbed and has an oral bio-availability of approximately 2% (Aoki and Hayden 1999). It is administered by inhalation to relieve symptoms of influenza, particularly H1N1 (swine flu) or H5N1 (Asian flu).

If an infant being breastfed by the mother receiving oseltamivir or zanamivir needs direct treatment, the recommended dose of zanamivir for infants should be given (UKMI 2011) It is given by inhalation in a dose of 10 mg twice daily for 5 days, starting as soon as possible (within 48 hours) after the onset of symptoms.

There is no study data on the amount of zanamivir passing through breastmilk. However, absorption of a significant amount by a breastfed infant is unlikely because of the limited oral bio-availability. It is therefore recommended that the benefits of continued breastfeeding exceed any theoretical risk (UKMI 2011).

The BNF reports that the amount present in breatmilk is probably too small to be harmful but it should be used only if potential bentefit outweighs risk (e.g. during a pandemic).

> Compatible with use during breastfeeding due to poor bio-availability.

References

Aoki FY, Hayden FG (eds), The pharmacokinetics of zanamivir: a new inhaled antiviral for influenza, *Clin Pharmacokinet*, 1999;36(Suppl. 1):1–58.

Tanaka T, Nakajima K, Murashima A, Garcia-Bournissen F, Koren G, Ito S, Safety of neuraminidase inhibitors against novel influenza A (H1N1) in pregnant and breastfeeding women, *CMAJ*, 2009;181:55–8.

UKMI Q&A 179.3. Oseltamivir or zanamivir – Can mothers breastfeed after treatment for influenza? 2011.

Oseltamivir ☺

Brand name: *Tamiflu®*
US brands: *Tamiflu®*
Australian brands: *Tamiflu®*

Oseltamivir is a neuraminidase inhibitor. It is taken to relieve symptoms of influenza, particularly influenza H1N1 (swine flu) or H5N1 (Asian flu). The most commonly reported adverse effects associated with it are nausea, vomiting and diarrhoea, abdominal pain, bronchitis, insomnia, vertigo/dizziness, headache, cough and fatigue. It is difficult to differentiate adverse effects from symptoms of influenza.

Oseltamivir is readily absorbed from the GI tract and has an active metabolite oseltamivir carboxylate. Plasma protein binding is 3% for the carboxylate and 42% for oseltamivir. Oseltamivir has a half-life of 1 to 3 hours.

Oseltamivir and oseltamivir carboxylate, are excreted into human breastmilk in very small amounts. Limited data suggest that adverse effects in a breastfed infant are unlikely. It is licensed for use in chilren with a dose of 30 mg twice daily for babies under 16 kg compared with 75 mg twice daily in adults and children over 40 kg.

Wentges-van Holthe *et al.* (2008) studied one mother whose baby was 9 months old. The authors calculated that at most the infant would receive 0.012 mg per kg daily with a maternal dose of 75 mg twice daily. This is significantly less than the licensed dose of 4 mg per kg per day. The dose in milk corresponded to 0.5% of the mother's weight-adjusted dosage.

Greer (2011) studied donated breastmilk from seven mothers who were bottle feeding their babies while taking 75 mg of oseltamivir daily. The peak milk level of the active metabolite was 41.9 μg per litre 18.9 hours after the medication was taken.

The BNF reports that the amount present in breastmilk is probably too small to be harmful but it should be used only if potential bentefit outweighs risk (e.g. during a pandemic).

The Department of Health 2009 recommended that:

Women who are breastfeeding and have symptoms of influenza should be treated with an antiviral medicine. The preferred medicine is Tamiflu, as for other adults. However, if a woman's baby is born and breastfeeding is started while the woman is taking Relenza, she should complete the course of Relenza; it is not necessary to switch to Tamiflu. If it is decided that a woman who is breastfeeding requires prophylaxis because of family or other contact with a novel pandemic virus strain, the preferred antiviral medicine is Tamiflu.

Compatible with use during breastfeeding.

References

Department of Health. Pandemic Influenza: Recommendations on the use of antiviral medicines for pregnant women, women who are breastfeeding and children under the age of one year. Updated September 2009.

Greer LG, Leff RD, Rogers VL *et al*. Pharmacokinetics of oseltamivir in breastmilk and maternal plasma, *Am J Obstet Gynecol*, 2011;204:524.e1–4.

Tanaka T, Nakajima K, Murashima A, Garcia-Bournissen F, Koren G, Ito S, Safety of neuraminidase inhibitors against novel influenza A (H1N1) in pregnant and breastfeeding women, *CMAJ*, 2009;181:55–8.

UKMI Q&A 179.3. Oseltamivir or zanamivir – Can mothers breastfeed after treatment for influenza? 2011.

Wentges-van Holthe N, van Eijkeren M, van der Laan JW, Oseltamivir and breastfeeding, *Int J Infect Dis*, 2008;12:451.

Malarial prophylaxis

The choice of drug to prevent infection of malaria takes into account:

- The risk of exposure to malaria;
- The extent of drug resistance;
- The efficacy of drugs;
- Side effects of drugs; and
- Patient-related factors e.g. renal and hepatic impairment.

Thus drug choice varies with the area to be visited. Prophylaxis should normally begin at least one week before entering an endemic area and continued for 4 weeks after leaving.

For information on choice of drug consult:

Clinical Knowledge Summary (www.cks.nhs.uk/malariaprophylaxis) or the Health Protection Agency (www.hpa.org.uk).

Chloroquine ☺

Brand name: Avloclor®, *Nivaquine®*
US brands: *Aralen®*
Australian brands: *Chlorquin®, Nivaquine®*

Chloroquine is used alone and with proguanil. The levels passing through breastmilk are insufficient to protect the infant who should receive his/her own medication to protect against malaria. In seven women given a 5 mg per kg intramuscular dose of chloroquine, milk levels of milk chloroquine levels averaged 227 µg per litre while the therapeutic dose for prophylaxis in a baby below 12 weeks of age is 37.5 mg weekly (Akintonwa *et al*. 1988). Ogunbona *et al*. (1987) studied 11 lactating women treated with 600 mg chloroquine daily to treat malaria. The levels in breastmilk were measured as 0.7% of the 600 mg maternal start dose of the drug in malaria chemotherapy. The authors suggested that it is also acceptable for mothers to breastfeed their infants when undergoing treatment for malaria with chloroquine. Relative infant dose quoted as 0.6 to 21.1% (Hale 2012 online access).

The BNF states that although it is present in breastmilk the risk to the infant is minimal. Although all antimalarials are present in breastmilk the amounts reached are inadequate to provide adequate prophylaxis and the infant should receive its own medication.

Compatible with use during breastfeeding.

References

Akintonwa A, Gbajumo SA, Mabadeje AF, Placental and milk transfer of chloroquine in humans, *Ther Drug Monit*, 1988;10:147–9.

Ogunbona FA, Onyeji CO, Bolaji OO, Torimiro SE, Excretion of chloroquine and desethylchloroquine in human milk, *Br J Clin Pharmacol*, 1987;23:473–6.

Chloroquine with proguanil

Brand name: *Paludrine Avloclor Travel Pack®*

Compatible with use during breastfeeding.

Proguanil

Brand name: *Paludrine®*
US brands:
Australian brands: *Paludrine®*

Proguanil is metabolised in the body to the active antimalarial drug cycloguanil. Its use is becoming limited due to the development of resistance. It is licensed in paediatric formulations with babies under 6.0 kg (0 to 12 weeks of age) being recommended to be given one-eighth the adult dose. The BNF states that although it is present in breastmilk the risk to the infant is minimal. Although all antimalarials are present in breastmilk the amounts reached are inadequate to provide adequate prophylaxis and the infant should receive its own medication.

The BNF reports that the amount in breastmilk is too small to be harmful when used as an antimalarial.

Compatible with use during breastfeeding.

Proguanil with atovaquone

Brand name: Malarone®
US brands: *Malarone*®
Australian brands: *Malarone*®

The BNF recommends that it is used only if there is no suitable alternative.

Presumed compatible with use during breastfeeding but use only if essential.

Atovaquone

Atovaquone is more than 99% bound to plasma proteins and has a long plasma half-life of 2 to 3 days, thought to be due to enterohepatic recycling. There is no data available on the passage into breastmilk but a paediatric formulation exists.

Presumed compatible with use during breastfeeding because of its high plasma protein binding.

Mefloquine

Brand name: *Lariam*®
US brands: *Lariam*®
Australian brands: *Lariam*®

Mefloquine has a long elimination half-life; adverse effects may occur or persist up to several weeks after the last dose. The most frequent adverse effects of mefloquine are nausea, diarrhoea, vomiting, abdominal pain, anorexia, headache, dizziness, loss of balance, somnolence and sleep disorders, notably insomnia and abnormal dreams. Neurological or psychiatric disturbances have also been reported and there have been rare reports of suicidal thoughts. Treatment should begin two and a half weeks before entering the endemic area. Pregnancy should be avoided during and for 3 months after prophylactic use.

Edstein *et al.* (1988) studied two women following the administration of one Lariam tablet (250 mg mefloquine) and deduced that the maximum amount of drug ingested by an infant would be 0.14 mg per kg, assuming a daily milk ingestion of 1 litre, compared with a weekly dose of 62.5 mg for a child weighing under 16 kg. It is highly plasma protein bound and has a relative infant dose quoted as 0.1 to 0.2% (Hale 2012 online access).

The BNF states that although it is present in breastmilk the risk to the infant is minimal. Although all antimalarials are present in breastmilk, the amounts reached are inadequate to provide adequate prophylaxis and the infant should receive its own medication.

Compatible with use during breastfeeding.

References

Edstein MD, Veenendaal JR, Hyslop R, Excretion of mefloquine in human breastmilk, *Chemotherapy (Basel)*, 1988;34:165–9.

Anthelmintics

> **Anthelmintic of choice in a mother during breastfeeding based on evidence of benefit and safety for the baby:**
>
> **Mebendazole**

Mebendazole

Brand name: *Ovex®, Vermox®, Pripsen tablets®*
US brands: *Vermox®*
Australian brands: *Vermox®*

Mebendazole is poorly absorbed from the gastro-intestinal tract. It undergoes extensive first-pass metabolism and is highly protein bound, so low levels are likely to reach breastmilk. Side effects are generally gastro-intestinal with tummy cramps and diarrhoea reported. It is marketed as Ovex®, Pripsen tablets® and Vermox® and is widely used to treat children over two years of age. Ovex® and Pripsen tablets® are available to purchase OTC. These preparations are not licensed for use during lactation. There is a case report of one mother receiving 100 mg twice daily for three days, beginning on the first day after delivery. The levels in breastmilk was below the level of detection (Kurzel *et al.* 1994).

A mother with a 13-week-old infant noted a dramatic reduction in milk supply after commencing mebendazole 100 mg twice daily. She began therapy after she reported seeing worms passed in her stools and was noticeably tense following this event. Although her supply ceased 7 days after starting medication it seems likely that her distress, together with subsequent formula supplementation, was responsible for the lowered supply rather than the drug intake (Rao 1983).

The distress caused to mothers of not treating worm infections which have been noted is likely to be extreme.

The BNF states that although the manufacturer advises it should be avoided during breastfeeding, the amount secreted into breastmilk is too small to be harmful.

> Compatible with use during breastfeeding as very poorly bio-available.

References

Kurzel RB, Toot PJ, Lambert LV, Mihelcic AS, Mebendazole and post-partum lactation, *N Z Med J*, 1994;107:439.

Rao TS, Does mebendazole inhibit lactation?, *N Z Med J*, 1983;96:589–90. Letter.

Piperazine (?)

Brand name: *Pripsen powder®* (Piperazine with senna)
US brands:
Australian brands:

Piperazine has been taken off the market in some European countries because of general concern about its safety and potential risk of producing the potential carcinogen N-mononitrosopiperazine. However, the CSM recommended that it should remain available as an OTC product (Health and Safety Executive 2001).

Piperazine is reported to be excreted in breastmilk (Leach 1990), but no reports on the amounts have located. According to Leach, the mother should take her dose of the drug immediately following feeding her infant, and then express and discard her milk during the next 8 hours as recommended by the manufacturers. It is readily absorbed from the gastro-intestinal tract. It is given directly to babies down to 3 months of age.

Information in the BNF is that it is present in milk and that the manufacturer advises avoiding breastfeeding for 8 hours after dose (express and discard milk during this time).

> No measure of the amount passing into breastmilk but it is given directly to infants >3 months of age. Use mebendazole as alternative if possible.

References

Health and Safety Executive, Proposed Maximum Exposure Limit for Piperazine and Piperazine Dihydrochloride, Draft regulatory impact assessment, 2001 (www.hse.gov.uk/ria/chemical/piperaz.htm)
Leach FN, Management of threadworm infestation during pregnancy, *Arch Dis Child*, 1990;65:399400.

Endocrine system

Diabetes

Non-insulin-dependent diabetes mellitus has historically been associated with older patients. However, with the increasing epidemic of obesity it is affecting younger people and may be seen in women of childbearing age.

> **Oral hypoglycaemic drug of choice in a mother during breastfeeding based on evidence of benefit and safety for the baby:**
>
> **Metformin**

Sulphonylureas

Brand names: Gliclazide (*Diamicron®*); Glibenclamide (*Daonil®, Euglucon®*); Chlorpropamide; Glimepiride (*Amaryl®*); Glipizide (*Glinese®, Minodiab®*), Tolbutamide.
US brands: Glibenclamide (Glyburide *DiaBeta®*, Glynase®, Micronase®); Glimepiride (*Amaryl®*); Glipizide (*Glucotrol®*)
Australian brands: Gliclazide (*Glyade®, Nidem®, Diamicron®*); Glibenclamide (*Daonil®, Euglucon®*); Glimepiride (*Amaryl®*); Glipizide (*Minodiab®, Melizide®*)

Sulphonylureas are oral anti-diabetic agents. They act by augmenting insulin secretion and are useful only where there is residual beta cell activity. All of them can produce hypoglycaemia. They are used in patients who are not overweight or who are unable to tolerate metformin. In women of childbearing age, metformin would be the preferred drug with evidence of reduced morbidity. Theoretically sulphonylureas may produce hypoglycaemia in breastfed infants and it is recommended that they are not used during lactation (BNF).

> Avoid use during breastfeeding as may produce hypoglycaemia in breastfed infant.

Biguanides

Biguanides have a different mode of action from sulphonylureas. They decrease gluco-neogenesis and increase peripheral utilisation of glucose so there needs to be some residual pancreatic islet cells. It is the drug of choice in overweight patients when lifestyle advice has failed to control symptoms of diabetes.

Metformin

Brand name: *Glucophage®*
US brands: *Glucophage®, Fortamet®, Riomet®*
Australian brands: *Diabex®, Diaformin®, Glucohexal®, Glucophage®, Novomet®*

Metformin produces anorexia, diarrhoea and taste disturbances but has been shown to reduce morbidity and mortality in Type 2 diabetes. Metformin is used when dietary modification alone has not produced glycaemic control. It is not associated with weight gain. Biguanides do not usually lower blood-glucose concentrations in patients without diabetes. In a study in seven breastfeeding women, concentrations of metformin in milk were found to be about a third of those in maternal plasma (Hale *et al.* 2002). Blood samples levels of metformin were undetectable in two babies, and very low levels in the others. Similar results have been found in three other studies. There were no reported adverse effects on the babies in the studies (Gardiner *et al.* 2003; Briggs *et al.* 2005; Eyal *et al.* 2010) or in using it to treat polycystic ovary syndrome (PCOS) (Glueck *et al.* 2006).

Relative infant dose quoted as 0.3 to 0.7% (Hale 2012 online access). The BNF states that it may be used during breastfeeding.

> Compatible with use during breastfeeding from measured levels transferred into breastmilk.

References

Briggs GG, Ambrose PJ, Nageotte MP, Padilla G, Wan S, Excretion of metformin into breast-milk and the effect on nursing infants, *Obstet Gynecol*, 2005;105:1437–41.

Eyal S, Easterling TR, Carr D, Umans JG, Miodovnik M, Hankins GD, Clark SM, Risler L, Wang J, Kelly EJ, Shen DD, Hebert MF, Pharmacokinetics of metformin during pregnancy, *Drug Metab Dispos*, 2010;38:833–40.

Gardiner SJ, Kirkpatrick CM, Begg EJ, Zhang M, Moore MP, Saville DJ, Transfer of metformin into human milk, *Clin Pharmacol Ther*, 2003;73:71–7.

Glueck CJ, Salehi M, Sieve L, Wang P, Growth, motor, and social developemnt in breast and formula-fed infants of metformin-treated women with polycyctic ovary syndrome, *J Pediatr*, 2006;148:628–32.

Hale T, Kristensen J, Hackett L, Kohan R, Ilett K, Transfer of metformin into human milk, *Diabetologia*, 2002;45:1509–14.

Thiazolidinediones

Pioglitazone

Brand name: Actos®
US brands: *Actos*®
Australian brands: *Actos*®

The glitazones are the most recently developed oral anti-diabetic agents designed to increase the body's sensitivity to insulin. They are associated with weight gain in patients, particularly around the central line. They are metabolised by cytochrome P450 and therefore subject to drug interactions. They may be given as monotherapy or added into metformin or sulphonylureas where glucose control has not been achieved. When combined with insulin pioglitazone increases the incidence of heart failure. There is no data on transfer into human milk of pioglitazone. It is present in milk in animal studies (BNF).

> No data on transfer into breastmilk. Avoid if possible.

Insulin

Insulin is used to treat Type 1 diabetes, where there is a total lack of insulin being secreted by the pancreatic beta cells of the Islets of Langerhans, or Type 2 diabetes, which has not been controlled by maximal oral medication. Insulin is also used to control diabetes in pregnancy.

Insulin has very large molecular weight of over 6000. It has no hypoglycaemic effect from oral absorption as it is inactivated in the GI tract. Thus it would not be expected to exert any action on the infant's glycaemic control. However, mothers who have Type 1 diabetes should be encouraged to breastfeed as there is a link between diabetes in an infant and lack of breastmilk (Alves *et al.* 2011). Breastfeeding may lower a woman's insulin requirements by up to 30%. To prevent hypoglycaemic attacks (hypos), mothers may need to increase their carbohydrate intake or decrease their insulin dose (Diabetes UK).

During pregnancy and breastfeeding, insulin requirements may be altered and doses should be assessed frequently by an experienced diabetes physician. The dose of insulin generally needs to be increased in the second and third trimesters of pregnancy. The short-acting insulin analogues, insulin aspart and insulin lispro, are not known to be harmful, and may be used during pregnancy and lactation (BNF).

> Compatible with use during breastfeeding due to poor bio-availability and high molecular weight.

References

Alves JG, Figueiroa JN, Menese J, and Alves GV, Breastfeeding protects against type 1 diabetes mellitus: a case-sibling study, *Breastfeed Med*, 2012;7(1):25–8.
Diabetes UK (http:www.diabetes.org.uk).

Thyroid diseases

Underactive thyroid

A mother with an underactive thyroid needs to take medication to return her levels of levothyroxine to 'normal'. Therapeutic drug monitoring regulates the dose of the drug. It is worth repeating blood levels after delivery, as anecdotally, fluctuations seem common at this time. If the supplementation is too low, prolactin levels will be affected resulting in a poor milk supply. The correct dose gives a mother the level of levothyroxine of a normal breastfeeding mother. Symptoms of an underactive thyroid include gain in bodyweight, dry skin and hair and tiredness.

Levothyroxine

Brand name: *Eltroxin®*
US brands: *Levothroid®, Levoxyl®*
Australian brands: *Eutroxsig®, Oroxine®*

Levothyroxine is secreted in extremely low levels into breastmilk, if at all (Bennett 1988; Oberkotter and Tenore 1983; Sato and Suzuki 1979). It is highly bound to proteins in the maternal plasma. The estimated level to which the baby will be exposed is virtually undetectable. Levels secreted into milk are too low to influence tests for neonatal hypothyroidism according to Martindale (2005). Theoretical infant dose is quoted as 0.6 ng per kg per day.

The BNF states that the amount secreted into breastmilk is too small to affect tests for neonatal hypothyroidism.

Compatible with use during breastfeeding due to high plasma protein binding.

References

Bennett PN (ed.), *Drugs and human lactation*, Amsterdam: Elsevier, 1988.
Oberkotter LV, Tenore A, Separation and radioimmunoassay of T3 and T4 in human breast-milk, *Horm Res*, 1983;17:11–18.
Sato T, Suzuki Y, Presence of triiodothyronine, no detectable thyroxine and reverse triiodothyronine in human milk, *Endocrinol Jpn*, 1979;26:507–13.

Overactive thyroid

A mother with an overactive thyroid gland produces raised levels of levothyroxine and will experience symptoms which may include tachycardia, sweating, heat intolerance and loss of bodyweight. Symptoms are initially controlled by anti-thyroid drugs (carbimazole or propylthiouracil [PTU]) and beta blockers. In some cases the gland is removed surgically or by use of radioactive iodine and levels replaced by synthetic levothyroxine.

Drug of choice in a mother during breastfeeding based on evidence of benefit and safety for the baby:

Individual circumstances should be taken into consideration

Carbimazole ⑦

Brand name: *Neomercazole*®
US brands:
Australian brands: *Neomercazole*®

Carbimazole produces sub-clinical levels in infants exposed to less than 30 mg a day through their mother's breastmilk (Rylance *et al.* 1987). The theoretical infant dose is 6.45 µg per kg per day. If this drug is used, monitoring of the infant's thyroid function periodically is recommended. Relative infant dose quoted as 2.3 to 5.3% (Hale 2012 online access).

The BNF states that the amount present in breastmilk may be sufficient to affect neonatal thyroid function and recommends that the lowest possible dose be used. However, it also states that while carbimazole and PTU are present in breastmilk, this does not preclude breastfeeding as long as neonatal development is closely monitored and the lowest effective dose is used.

Appears to be compatible at doses <30 mg daily but consider monitoring infant's thyroid function periodically.

References

Rylance GW, Woods CG, Donnelly MC, Oliver JS, Alexander WD, Carbimazole and breast-feeding, *Lancet*, 1987;1(8538):928.

Propylthiouracil

PTU has in the past been the drug of choice in a breastfeeding mother as the transfer into breastmilk is lower than that with carbimazole. However, in 2009 the US Food and Drug Administration (FDA) alerted practitioners to an increased risk of hepato-toxicity with PTU use and recommended that all patients should be observed and monitored for signs of liver disease particularly during the first 6 months of treatment. Signs of liver damage, which should be reported to the prescriber immediately are: fatigue, weakness, vague abdominal pain, loss of appetite, itching, easy bruising or yellowing of the eyes or skin.

Carbimazole has been associated with congenital defects and PTU is the drug of choice in the first trimester. However, due to the risk of hepatotoxicity consideration should be given to switching to carbimazole in the second trimester. Both drugs cross the placenta and may lead to development of hypothyroidism in the infant (BNF).

Only small amounts are secreted into breastmilk and reports suggest that levels are too low to produce side effects (Cooper 1987). PTU is extensively plasma protein bound (80%) and has an oral bio-availability of 50 to 75%. At doses of 400 mg, a study of nine women and their babies showed levels of PTU in milk reached only 0.7 mg per ml (Kampmann *et al.* 1980). One of the babies was studied for 5 months during which the mother received 200 to 300 mg of PTU daily – there were no changes the infant thyroid functions. Momotani *et al.*'s (200) study of 11 babies has shown that up to 750 mg produces no changes in babies up until 11 months of age. However, monitoring is recommended as a precaution. Relative infant dose quoted as 1.8% (Hale 2012 online access).

The BNF recommends that although the amount in breastmilk is probably too small to be harmful, the baby's thyroid status should be monitored. However, it also states that while carbimazole and PTU are present in breastmilk, this does not preclude breastfeeding as long as neonatal development is closely monitored and the lowest effective dose is used.

> Compatible with use during breastfeeding due to high plasma protein binding. Be aware of risk of hepatotoxicity.

References

Cooper DS, Antithyroid drugs: to breastfeed or not to breastfeed, *Am J Obstet Gynecol*, 1987;157:234–5.

FDA Alert 2009, Information for Healthcare Professionals – Propylthiouracil-Induced Liver Failure (www.fda.gov/Drugs/DrugSafety/PostmarketDrugSafetyInformationforPatientsand Providers/DrugSafetyInformationforHeathcareProfessionals/ucm162701.htme).

Kampmann JP, Johansen K, Hansen JM, Helweg J, Propylthiouracil in human milk, *Lancet*, 1980;1(8171):736–7.

Momotani N, Yamashita R, Makino F, Noh JY, Ishikawa N, Ito K, Thyroid function in wholly breastfeeding infants whose mothers take high doses of propylthiouracil, *Clin Endocrinol (Oxf)*, 2000;53(2):177–81.

Obstetric conditions

Contraception

> **Oral contraceptive of choice in a mother during breastfeeding based on evidence of benefit and safety for the baby:**
>
> **Progesterone-only pill**

The progesterone (progestin)-only contraceptive pill is generally recommended for breastfeeding women. Progesterone (progestins) should not affect breastmilk supply. However, anecdotally a few women do experience lowering of their supply which does not return to normal with increased feeding frequency. For these mothers a barrier method of contraception may be more appropriate.

Similarly, anecdotally, progesterone depot injections may affect some mothers and babies. If noted a yellow card report should be submitted to the MHRA (http://yellow-card.mhra.gov.uk/). Once injected it is impossible to remove these products so a trial of oral medication may identify those women for whom this is more likely. Contraceptive implants should not be used until at least 6 weeks after delivery when maximum prolactin production has been established.

Parenteral progestogen-only contraceptives

Medroxyprogesterone acetate (*Depo Provera®*) can be used 6 weeks after delivery and repeated every 12 weeks. It is used 5 days after delivery for mothers who do not intend to breastfeed.

Norethisterone enantate (*Noristerat®*) is not advised if the baby has symptoms of severe or persistant jaundice – repeated every 8 weeks.

The etonogestrel-releasing implant (*Implanon®*) was discontinued in 2010 but may still be in place for some women until 2013.

> Compatible with use during breastfeeding for majority of women. May lead to reduced breastmilk supply for some women according to anecdotal reports but not reported in large scal trials.

Oral progestogen-only contraceptive pills (POPs)

UK brand names: Desogestrel (*Cerazette®*); Ethynodiol diacetate (*Femulen®*); Norethisterone (*Micronor®, Noriday®*); Levonorgestrel (*Norgeston®*)

The oral progestogen-only contraceptive pill (POP) needs to be taken at the same time every day continuously – a delay of more than 3 hours may mean contraceptive protection is lost. The POP is generally started a minimum of 3 weeks after delivery but ideally no less than 6 weeks to avoid interfering with milk production. Vomiting and severe diarrhoea can interfere with absorption.

The BNF states that the POP does not affect lactation and that oral POP can be started up to and including day 21 post-partum without the need for additional contraceptive precautions. If started more than 21 days post-partum, additional contraceptive precautions are required for 2 days.

> Compatible with use during breastfeeding for majority of women. May lead to reduced breastmilk supply for some women according to anecdotal reports but not seen in large-scale trials.

Intrauterine progestogen-only contraceptives

Intrauterine progestogen-only contraceptives release levonorgestrel directly into the uterine cavity. The *Mirena®* system is used as a contraceptive method for women with excessively heavy periods. It can be used 6 weeks after delivery and is effective for 5 years. Progestogen-only contraceptives do not affect lactation (BNF).

Simple coils can be used in breastfeeding mothers without complication as no medication is involved.

> Compatible with use during breastfeeding for majority of women. May lead to reduced breastmilk supply for some women according to anecdotal reports but not seen in large-scale trials.

Combined oral contraceptive

Combined oral contraceptives containing oestrogen and progestogen are not recommended for the first 6 months after delivery as they may have a negative impact on breastmilk production (WHO 2010). The BNF recommends not using until baby is weaned or at least 6 months post-partum. Although, in theory, when milk supply is well established it has little effect, anecdotally the oestrogen content seems to reduce supply.

> Avoid use during breastfeeding as may reduce breastmilk supply.

Emergency hormonal contraception

Levonelle® is licensed to be given to women during breastfeeding. The patient information leaflet in the packet assures women that it is safe with continued breastfeeding. It contains a progestogen drug levonorgestrel. The tablet should be taken as soon as possible after unprotected intercourse but can be taken up to 72 hours after. As a progestogen-only contraceptive it has no affect on breastfeeding (BNF).

The longer the interval between intercourse and taking the tablet the greater is the chance that it will not be effective. No contraception has a 100% success rate. If vomiting occurs soon after taking the tablets, medical advice should be sought, as soon as possible.

The next period may be early or late and barrier contraception should be continued until the next period. Levonelle is widely available from a variety of healthcare outlets including pharmacies, accident and emergency departments, family planning clinics as well as GP surgeries.

Should the next period be delayed more than 5 days the mother should seek further medical advice. Levonelle is reported by the manufacturers not to show evidence of teratogenicity even if it fails to prevent pregnancy. However, emergency hormonal contraception should not be used if there is any possibility that the woman is already pregnant.

A copper intrauterine contraceptive can be inserted up to 5 days after intercourse as an alternative method of emergency contraception.

Women who do not wish to expose their baby to any medication may wish to consider how frequently they are breastfeeding and therefore the likelihood of ovulation. She and her partner also need to consider the consequences of a subsequent pregnancy for them.

> Levonorgestrel is safe to use during breastfeeding. No data on ulipristal so avoid.

There is no data on emergency hormonal contraceptive ulipristal (ellaOne®)

References

Family Planning Association (www.fpa.org.uk/helpandadvice/contraception/contraception afterbaby#WoPR).

Suppression of lactation

Use of medicines to suppress lactation routinely is not recommended if it can be adequately treated with simple analgesics and breast support. Dopamine-receptor agonists, such as bromocriptine and cabergoline, inhibit prolactin from the pituitary and hence milk production.

Although routine suppression of lactation is not recommended for mothers who choose not to breastfeed, there are situations such as stillbirth or SID where the mother may be particularly disturbed by her milk production in the absence of an infant to nourish. Some mothers choose to donate milk to the special care unit, others choose to allow the milk to dry up naturally following negative feedback to the brain that milk is not being removed although they may experience temporary engorgement needing analgesia and support.

> **Drug choice in a mother during breastfeeding based on evidence of benefit and safety for the baby:**
>
> **Do not use other than in exceptional cases**

References

Spitz AM, Lee NC, Peterson HB, Treatment for lactation suppression: little progress in one hundred years, *Am J Obstet Gynecol*, 1998;179:1485–90.

Bromocriptine ☹

Brand name: *Parlodel*®
US brands: *Parlodel*®
Australian brands: Bromohexal®, *Parlodel*®

In the USA, the FDA has withdrawn its approval for this indication for the use of bromocriptine following reports of numerous maternal deaths, seizures and strokes (US Food and Drug Administration 1994). It is licensed but not recommended for routine suppression in the UK. It inhibits prolactin secretion for up to 14 hours after a single dose. Only about 30% of the drug is absorbed due to extensive first-pass metabolism by the liver leaving a bio-availability of less than 6%. It is 90 to 96% plasma protein bound. It can cause transient hypotension as well as headaches and vomiting. Bromocriptine is occasionally used for hyper-prolactinaemic patients with pituitary tumours. There is limited evidence of use and continued breastfeeding under these circumstances. There is one report of a mother taking 5 mg per day bromocriptine and continuing to breastfeed (Canales *et al.* 1981). No untoward effects were observed in the infant. Levels of bromcriptine measured in breastmilk were found to be below the level of detection in 14 women who took 2.5 mg on three consecutive days for overproduction of milk (Peters *et al.* 1985). There was no noted effect on the infants but although the serum prolactin levels were decreased for the 3 days of treatment there was a return to control levels by 36 hours after the last dose. However, the milk yield decreased by 25% and persisted for at least 12 days after the last dose.

BNF recommends dose to prevent or suppress lactation 2.5 mg on day 1 (prevention) or daily for 2 to 3 days (suppression); then 2.5 mg twice daily for 14 days. Avoid breastfeeding for 5 days if suppression fails.

> Avoid use during breastfeeding as may reduce or halt milk production.

It should not be used post-partum or in puerperium in women with high blood pressure, coronary artery disease or symptoms (or history) of serious mental disorder; monitor blood pressure carefully (especially during first few days) in post-partum women. Very rarely hypertension, myocardial infarction, seizures or stroke (both sometimes preceded by severe headache or visual disturbances), and mental disorders have been reported in post-partum women given bromocriptine for lactation suppression – caution with antihypertensive therapy and avoid other ergot alkaloids. Discontinue immediately if hypertension, unremitting headache or signs of central nervous system toxicity develop.

A study in HIV-infected women requiring lactation suppression (in order to prevent mother-to-child transmission from breastmilk) found that a combined oral contraceptive was as effective as bromocriptine (Piya-Anant *et al.* 2004).

References

Canales ES, García IC, Ruíz JE, Zárate A, Bromocriptine as prophylactic therapy in prolactin-oma during pregnancy, *Fertil Steril*, 1981;36:524–6.

Peters F, Geisthovel F, Breckwoldt M, Serum prolactin levels in women with excessive milk production. Normalization by transitory prolactin inhibition, *Acta Endocrinol (Copenh)*, 1985;109:463–6.

Piya-Anant M, Worapitaksanond S, Sittichai K, Saechua P, Nomrak A, The combined oral contraceptive pill versus bromocriptine to suppress lactation in puerperium: a randomized double blind study, *J Med Assoc Thai*, 2004;87:670–73.

US Food and Drug Administration, FDA moves to end use of bromocriptine for post-partum breast engorgement, FDA Talk Paper T94-37, 1994.

Cabergoline

Brand name: *Dostinex*®
US brands: *Dostinex*®
Australian brands: *Dostinex*®

Cabergoline is a long-acting synthetic ergot alkaloid that produces a dopamine agonist effect. It is recommended in several European countries to inhibit or suppress physiological lactation post-partum. Standard literature still recommends caution in routine use. There is no data on transfer into breastmilk reported. Side effects are similar to those of bromocriptine – dizziness, nausea, postural hypotension, drowsiness together with some gastro-intestinal disturbances.

The dose to inhibit lactation is 1 mg as a single dose on the first day post-partum, or 0.25 mg every 12 hours for 2 days (Webster 1996).

Avoid breastfeeding if lactation suppression fails (BNF).

Since Dostinex® is a special pack of eight tablets each containing 500 µg, care must be take to clarify the dose regimen. It completely and irreversibly suppresses lactation so the mother should be given every opportunity to consider her decision before taking the tablets.

Avoid use during breastfeeding as may reduce or halt milk production.

References

Webster J, A comparative review of the tolerability profiles of dopamine agonists in the treatment of hyper-prolactinaemia and inhibition of lactation, *Drug Safety*, 1996;14:228–38.

Lactation enhancement

Drug therapy has sometimes been used to enhance lactation, although mechanical stimulation of the nipple remains the primary method.

> **Drug choice in a mother during breastfeeding based on evidence of benefit and safety for the baby:**
>
> **Domperidone**

Metoclopramide

Brand name: *Maxolon*®
US brands: *Reglan*®, *Octamide*®, *Reclomide*®
Australian brands: *Maxolon*®, *Pramin*®

Metoclopramide is a dopamine antagonist which can produce modest increases in breastmilk production but carries a risk of adverse effects including dystonias and depression in the mother. Other reported adverse effects are headache, diarrhoea and dry mouth (Ingram *et al.* 2011).

Kauppila *et al.* (1981) found an increase in prolactin levels and milk supply with doses of 10 and 15 mg daily given to 37 women with inadequate production of breastmilk in a placebo-controlled trial. During the study, one-third of babies needed no further supplementation and 89% of women in the trial group reporting a good effect. No adverse effects were noted in the infants.

Hansen *et al.* (2005) studied 57 women who delivered between 23 and 34 weeks of gestation. Half were randomised to receive 10 mg metoclopramide three times daily throughout the study and half a placebo. Both groups were given the same breastfeeding education and support. Participants were not selected for failed milk supply. At the end of 17 days there was no difference in breastmilk volumes in the two groups or in duration of breastfeeding. The authors therefore concluded that metoclopramide did not improve breastmilk volume or duration of breastfeeding in this population of women. Regardless of therapy received, breastfeeding duration in the study of pre-term mothers was poor with mean duration of 8 weeks. The conclusion might be taken to be that metoclopramide does not improve breastmilk supply where it is already adequate.

Gupta and Gupta (1985) studied 33 women with inadequate or absent lactation. Improved breastmilk output was determined in two-thirds of mothers with no breastmilk and all of those with inadequate milk supply. Improvement persisted after medication stopped. No adverse effects were noted in any of the mothers or their infants.

Seema *et al.* (1997) studied 50 mother and baby pairs who had been readmitted to hospital as result of problems with lactation. Half of the mothers were supplemented with metoclopramide in addition to support from skilled breastfeeding advisors, the other half received support with breastmilk problems but no medication. Forty-six mothers achieved complete relactation and three partial relactation, but there was no difference in whether they received medication or not. The authors concluded that strong professional support by a skilled health worker was of prime importance rather than medication.

Sakha and Behbahan (2008) studied 20 primipara nursing mothers referred to a

Children's Hospital in Iran for counselling about prescription of infant formula. All mothers were reported to have perceived milk insufficiency and all babies had failed to gain appropriate weight, determined by their age and birthweight. They were randomly allocated into two equal groups – one group received metoclopramide 10 mg every 8 hours, and the other a placebo, for a period of 15 days. Eighteen of the 20 newborns studied showed an appropriate weight gain at the end of the study period. However, there was no statistically difference between the two groups (p=0.68). The authors concluded that counselling nursing mothers in breastfeeding skills sustained breastfeeding as effectively as the addition of a galactogogue.

Ingram *et al.* (2011) conducted a double-blind, randomised control trial comparing the effects of metoclopramide and domperidone on the breastmilk production of 80 mothers with infants in a tertiary neonatal intensive care unit. Outcomes measured were breastmilk volume (by expression) for 10 days before medication, 10 days during the active trial and 10 days after medication. Mothers in the domperidone group achieved a mean increase in milk volume of 96.3% with three reporting side effects of headache, diarrhoea, mood swings and feeling dizzy although none dropped out of the trial as a result. Mothers in the metoclopramide groups achieved a mean of 93.7% increase in volume with seven reporting side effects: three of headache, one report each of diarrhoea, mood swings, change in appetite, dry mouth and uncomfortable breasts. A further eight who had ongoing prescriptions for metoclopramide (total 29) reported side effects of which two were of depression and two of mood swings. Only one woman stopped her medication after 5 days due to bad headaches and dry mouth.

Zuppa *et al.* (2010) reviewed information on the use of a variety of substances claimed to act as galactogogues, looking at their safety and efficacy. He recommended that when all treatable causes of poor milk supply and additional help and support had been given metoclopramide could be used but only where domperidone was not available. The Academy of Breastfeeding Medicine (2011) has also developed a revised protocol on the use of galactogogues. It suggests that there are few good quality trials which demonstrate an impact on weight gain following the use of medication.

From these studies it could be concluded that for some women metoclopramide increased previously inadequate milk production. However, the value of good breastfeeding support and education should not be ignored. Adverse effects in the mother can be associated with administration of metoclopramide.

There is no licensed dose of metoclopramide to increase lactation but studies have mostly used 10 mg three times daily for 7 to 14 days followed by a tapering dosage. There are no studies of long-term use.

Relative infant dose quoted as 4.7 to 14.3% (Hale 2012 online access).

The BNF states that a small amount is present in breastmilk and that it should be avoided.

Compatible with use during breastfeeding but can induce extra-pyramidal side effects and depression in the mother. Use of domperidone is a safer alternative.

References

Ingram J, Taylor H, Churchill C, Pike A, Greenwood R, Metoclopramide or domperidone for increasing maternal breastmilk output: a randomised controlled trial, *Arch Dis Child Fetal Neonatal Ed*, 2012;97(4):F241– 5.

Gupta AP, Gupta PK, Metoclopramide as a lactogogue, *Clin Pediatr (Phila)*, 1985;24:269– 72.

Hansen WF, McAndrew S, Harris K, Zimmerman MB, Metoclopramide effect on breastfeeding the preterm infant: a randomized trial, *Obstet Gynecol*, 2005;105:383–9.

Kauppila A, Kivinen S, Ylikorkala O, A dose response relation between improved lactation and metoclopramide, *Lancet*, 1981;1:1175–7.

Sakha R, Behbahan AG, Training for perfect breastfeeding or metoclopramide: which one can promote lactation in nursing mothers?, *Breastfeed Med*, 2008;3:120–23.

Seema, Patwari AK, Satyanarayana L, Relactation: an effective intervention to promote exclusive breastfeeding, *J Trop Pediatr*, 1997;43:213–6.

The Academy of Breastfeeding Medicine Protocol Committee. ABM clinical protocol 9: use of galactogogues in initiating or augmenting the rate of maternal milk secretion, *Breastfeed Med*, 2011;6:41– 9.

Zuppa AA, Sindico P, Orchi C, Carducci C, Cardiello V, Romagnoli C, Safety and efficacy of galactogogues: substances that induce maintain and increase breastmilk production, *J Pharm Pharm Sci*, 2010;13(2):162–74.

Domperidone

Brand name: *Motilium*®
US brands:
Australian brands: *Motilium*®

Domperidone has been reported to increase milk production, may cause fewer adverse central effects than metoclopramide and is not associated with an increased risk of depression in young women.

The drug can cause arrhythmias and torsade de pointes with oral use, especially if taken with drugs that inhibit its metabolism. Recent studies have shown that it increases the cardiac death rate in long-term users, although most were elderly.

The drug is not approved in the USA for any indication. Although in the UK the oral form is available for purchase 'over the counter' from pharmacies although the intravenous formulation has been withdrawn.

DaSilva *et al.* (2001) studied 20 women in a double-blind, placebo-controlled study. He showed a steady increase in milk production over placebo in mothers treated with domperidone 10 mg three times a day. In the trial, mothers received counselling support and were double pumping. The increase in production achieved, fell once the drug was stopped after seven days. The babies in the study were all in a Neurology and Neurosurgery Intensive Care Unit (NNICU) and the mothers were only expressing for feeds to be given via naso-gastric tube. They had been identified as producing a milk supply which did not meet the oral feeding needs of the baby. The increase in milk volume began 48 hours after the drug was initiated and continued to the end of the trial. The study was stopped after 7 days when most mothers began some level of direct breastfeeding at which point it became impractical to measure breastmilk volume. Serum prolactin was higher in the treatment group and only small amounts of drug were identified in the breastmilk with a milk serum ratio of 0.4.

Petraglia *et al.* (1985) reported on two small studies on the use of domperidone and mothers with insufficient breastmilk production. In one study, 15 women were given either domperidone 10 mg three times daily or placebo from day 2 to 5 post-partum. Eight women had a history of defective breastmilk supply in an earlier lactation and were treated from delivery and seven women were diagnosed as having a low milk supply at 2 weeks. Fifteen women with matching histories were treated with placebo. No additional lactation support or information on positioning and attachment was given. In the trial, the mothers were only breastfeeding six or seven times a day – a frequency which would not provide optimal supply in many circumstances. Increased milk production was determined by weighing the infants before and after nursing, a notoriously problematic method, although the authors concluded that the active group had benefited from the drug. At 1 month post-partum, all treated mothers were nursing well, but five of seven untreated mothers had inadequate lactation. No correlation was found between baseline serum prolactin and the increase in prolactin and milk production.

Wan *et al.* (2008) studied seven mothers who had delivered pre-term infants using a double-blind, randomised crossover study. Two dose regimes were trialled – 10 mg or 20 mg three times a day. One mother taking the 20 mg dose withdrew early because of severe abdominal cramps. Two mothers failed to respond to either dose. In four of the mothers there was a significant increase in prolactin level and milk volume with a greater response at the higher dose in three of these women. Side effects noted included abdominal cramping, constipation, dry mouth, depressed mood and headache which were more apparent with the higher dose. Wan *et al.* concluded that if there is no response at a 10 mg dose there is no point in further increasing the dose.

The Academy of Breastfeeding Medicine (2011) has also developed a revised protocol on the use of galactogogues. It suggests that there are few good quality trials which demonstrate an impact on weight gain following the use of medication.

Jones and Breward (2011) examined the available studies in the light of anecdotal evidence of use of domperidone to improve lactation in the UK. They recommended that attention to improved and frequent drainage of the breast was most effective in improving milk volumes. The evidence for the use of domperidone largely stems from use in pre-term infants.

Ingram *et al.* (2011) conducted a double-blind, randomised control trial comparing the effects of metoclopramide and domperidone on the breastmilk production of 80 mothers with infants in a tertiary neonatal intensive care unit. Outcomes measured were breastmilk volume (by expression) for 10 days before medication, 10 days during the active trial and 10 days after medication. Mothers in the domperidone group achieved a mean increase in milk volume of 96.3% with three reporting side effects of headache, diarrhoea, mood swings and feeling dizzy although none dropped out of the trial as a result. Mothers in the metoclopramide groups achieved a mean of 93.7% increase in volume with seven reporting side effects: three of headache, one report each of diarrhoea, mood swings, change in appetite, dry mouth and uncomfortable breasts. Only two mothers requested ongoing domperidone supplies from their GP following the study period. Of those who had repeats of metoclopramide, six who had had domperidone during the trial reported adverse effects. One mother switched from metoclopramide to domperidone having found that she could not cope with the tiredness produced by the metoclopramide.

Zuppa *et al.* (2010) reviewed information on the use of a variety of substances claimed to act as galactogogues, looking at their safety and efficacy. They recommended that when all treatable causes of poor milk supply and additional help and support had been given, domperidone was the drug of choice as a galactogogue. The dose used in studies was 10 mg three times a day.

In December 2011 the manufacturers of domperidone issued a communication to all GPs and pharmacists in the UK warning that some epidemiological studies have shown that domperidone may be associated with an increased risk of serious ventricular arrhythmias or sudden cardiac death in doses in excess of 30 mg (one tablet three times a day). It suggested that domperidone should be used at the lowest effective dose in adults and children and should be avoided in patients who are taking concomitant medication known to cause QT prolongation (such as ketoconazole and erythromycin).

Osadchy *et al.* (2012) conducted a systematic review and meta-analysis on placebo controlled studies on the impact of domperidone 10 mg three times a day. They found three randomised, controlled trials with a total of 78 participants. They showed an increase in breastmilk supply following use of domperidone without any reports of adverse effects on mother or neonate.

Donovan *et al.* (2012) conducted a similar meta-analysis looking at studies to improve supply in mothers who delivered pre-term hospitalised infants. They reported modest improvements in supply and recommend further studies be undertaken.

Relative infant dose quoted as 0.01 to 0.04% (Hale 2012 online access).

> Amount secreted into breastmilk too small to be harmful (BNF).

References

Da Silva OP, Knoppert DC, Angelini MM, Forret PA, Effect of domperidone on milk production in mothers of premature newborns: a randomized, double-blind, placebo-controlled trial, *CMAJ*, 2001;164(1):17–21.

DaSilva OP, Knoppert DC, Domperidone for lactating women, *CMAJ*, 2004;171:725–6.

Donovan TJ, Buchanan K, Medications for increasing milk supply in mothers expressing breastmilk for their preterm hospitalised infants, *Cochrane Database Syst Rev*, 2012;3:CD005544.

FDA warns against women using unapproved drug, domperidone, to increase milk production (7 June 2004). Available online: www.fda.gov/bbs/topics/ANSWERS/2004/ANS01292.html

Jones W, Breward S, Use of domperidone to enhance lactation: what is the evidence?, *Community Pract*, 2011;84:35–7.

McNeil Products Ltd and Winthrop Pharmaceuticals UK Ltd (Trading as Zentiva – a Sanofi company) company communication, 2001.

Osadchy A, Moretti ME, Koren G, Effect of domperidone on insufficient lactation in puerperal women: a systematic review and meta-analysis of randomized controlled trials, *Obstet Gynecol Int*, 2012;2012:642893.

Osborne RJ, Slevin ML, Hunter RW, Hamer J, Cardiotoxicity of intravenous domperidone, *Lancet*, 1985;2(8451):385.

Petraglia F, De Leo V, Sardelli S, Pieroni ML, D'Antona N, Genazzani AR, Domperidone in defective and insufficient lactation, *Eur J Obstet Gynecol Reprod Biol*, 1985;19:281–7.

Roussak JB, Carey P, Parry H, Cardiac arrest after treatment with intravenous domperidone, *BMJ*, 1984;289:1579.

The Academy of Breastfeeding Medicine Protocol Committee. ABM clinical protocol 9: use of galactogogues in initiating or augmenting the rate of maternal milk secretion, *Breastfeed Med*, 2011;6:41–9.

Wan EW, Davey K, Page-Sharp M, Hartmann PE, Simmer K, Ilett KF, Dose-effect study of domperidone as a galactagogue in preterm mothers with insufficient milk supply, and its transfer into milk, *Br J Clin Pharmacol*, 2008;66:283–9.

Zuppa AA, Sindico P, Orchi C, Carducci C, Cardiello V, Romagnoli C, Safety and efficacy of galactogogues: substances that induce maintain and increase breast milk production, *J Pharm Pharm Sci*, 2010;13(2):162–74.

Oxytocin nasal spray

The use of oxytocin nasal spray to promote milk ejection has been recommended in the past but is no longer commercially available. Little evidence of benefit exists.

Fewtell *et al.* (2006) studied 51 mothers delivering pre-term infants and randomised them to use intranasal oxytocin or placebo nasal spray before expressing breastmilk. Although the mothers in the active treatment group reported more milk supply this was not obviously evident when compared to placebo. Of the 51 mothers, 22 were convinced that they were receiving active treatment and requested further supplies or complained of a reduction in milk supply when the spray ran out. Of these mothers 9 (41%) were actually receiving a placebo spray. Only one of the 6 mothers convinced they were using pacebo were receiving active treatment.

> Compatible with use during breastfeeding but no evidence of efficacy from studies and no commercial product available currently.

References

Fewtrell MS, Loh KL, Blake A, Ridout DA, Hawdon J, Randomised, double-blind trial of oxytocin nasal spray in mothers expressing breastmilk for preterm infants, *Arch Dis Child Fetal Neonatal Ed*, 2006;91:F169–74.

Drugs used to induce or augment labour

Oxytocin

Brand name: Syntocinon®
US brands: Pitocin®, *Syntocinon*®
Australian brands: *Syntocinon*®

This is used as an intravenous infusion to induce or augment labour, normally after amniotomy. Oxytocin given in high doses, or to women who are hyper-sensitive to it, may cause uterine hyper-stimulation with hypertonic or tetanic contractions, leading to uterine rupture and soft tissue damage. Careful monitoring of fetal heart rate and uterine motility is essential so that dosage of oxytocin can be adjusted to individual response. It is destroyed orally in the stomach (Martindale 2005).

Compatible with use during breastfeeding.

Dinoprostone

Brand name: *Prostin E2 vaginal gel or vaginal tablets*®
US brands: *Prostin E2 vaginal gel or vaginal tablets*®, *Cervidil*®
Australian brands: *Prostin E2 vaginal gel or vaginal tablets*®, *Cervidil*®

For the induction of labour dinoprostone is used to ripen (soften and dilate) the cervix before the membranes are ruptured and to induce labour at term. When administered orally, dinoprostone has been used to suppress lactation but vaginal preparations are rapidly metabolised and are unlikely to affect lactation (Caminiti *et al.* 1980; Nasi *et al.* 1980).

Compatible with use during breastfeeding.

References

Caminiti F, De Murtas M, Parodo G, Lecca U, Nasi A, Decrease in human plasma prolactin levels by oral prostaglandin E2 in early puerperium, *J Endocrinol*, 1980;87(3):333–7.
Nasi A, De Murtas M, Parodo G, Caminiti F, Inhibition of lactation by prostaglandin E2, *Obstet Gynecol Surv*, 1980;35(10):619–20.

Medical termination of pregnancy

Drugs use to induce medical termination of early pregnancy are unlicensed. The regimen depends on the stage of pregnancy of the woman. Guidelines have been provided by the Royal College of Obstetricians and Gynaecologists 2011 (www.rcog.org.uk/files/rcog-corp/Abortion%20guideline_web_1.pdf) but can vary between providers.

Mifepristone

One study (Saav *et al.* 2010) collected milk samples from 12 women who had had medical termination over 7 days (two given mifepristone 200 mg; ten given mifepristone 600 mg). Maternal serum levels were taken on day 3 and data were used to calculate m/p ratio at that time. Levels of mifepristone in breastmilk were highest in 6 to 9 hours after administration in those women receiving 600 mg (0.063 to 0.913 µmol per litre equivalent to 5.6 µg per litre). Levels in those given 200 mg were below the level of detection at all times (<0.013 µmol/litre). Levels in nine of the women given 600 mg averaged 172 µg per litre on day 1 and 66 µg per litre on day 2. Levels in all ten women were 31 µg per litre on day 3 and levels in four women were 24 µg per litre on day 4. Levels measured in three women were 25 µg per litre on day 5 providing a calculated relative infant dose 0.5 to 1.5%.

The breastmilk levels of mifespristone in the mothers given 200 mg were below the level of detection in all mothers (Saav *et al.* 2010). The usual dose for medical termination being 200 mg there would appear to be no reason to interrupt breastfeeding at all. If the mother vomits and has to take a second dose a period of discontinuation of 6 to 9 hours would seem adequate based on the data from Saav *et al.*'s study. Despite the fact that research is limited in the number of subjects studied, the results confirm the conclusions from the pharmacokinetic data that milk transfer of mifepristone is low.

Hale (2012 online access) states that: 'It may be possible to continue breastfeeding without pause when a 200 mg dose is given to the mother.' Saav *et al.* conclude that: 'The levels of mifepristone in milk are low, especially when using the 200 mg dose. Breastfeeding can be safely continued in an uninterrupted manner during medical abortion of this kind.'

Compatible with use during breastfeeding with a maternal dose of 200 mg and informed discussion with the mother.

References

Can mothers breastfeed after a medical termination of pregnancy? UKMI Q&A 261, 2 March 2011.

Drugs and Lactation Data base (LactMed) http://toxnet.nlm.nih.gov/cgi-bin/sis/htmlgen?LACT, accessed online March 2012.

Hale T, Medications and Mothers' Milk, accessed online March 2012.

Martindale: The Complete Drug Reference, 35th Edition. 2006.

Sääv I, Fiala C, Hämäläinen JM, Heikinheimo O, Gemzell-Danielsson K, Medical abortion in lactating women – low levels of mifepristone in breastmilk, *Acta Obstet Gynecol Scand*, 2010;89(5):618–22.

Misoprostol

Misoprostol is a prostaglandin E1 analogue, (prostaglandin E1 and others appear naturally in breastmilk). Levels in breastmilk are likely to be low based on pharmacokinetic data; high plasma protein binding of 80 to 90% and low m/p ratio 0.05 although it is 100% bio-available. With a half-life of a maximum of 20 to 40 minutes all of the drug will have left the mother's body within 3.3 hours. It has a relative infant dose quoted as 0.07% (Hale 2012 online access).

One study (Abden-Aleem *et al.* 2003) looked at 20 women given 600 µg orally during the first 4 days post-partum and measured levels in colostrum of 12 women during the first 5 hours. The average level was highest after 1 hour (20.9 ng per ml) falling to 17.8 ng per ml after 2 hours, 9.4 ng per ml at 3 hours, 2.8 ng per ml at 4 hours and <1 ng per ml at 5 hours post-dose.

In a study by Vogel *et al.* (2004) the half-life in breastmilk averaged 1.1 hours (at which point the mean levels of misoprostol acid, the active metabolite, were 7.6 pg per ml) following a maternal dose of 200 µg. Breastmilk misoprostol levels were found to rise and decline rapidly in the ten women studied. In two women, the peak level was noted at 2 hours post-dose. At 5 hours the levels of misoprostol acid were 0.2 pg per ml. Vogel suggested that an interval of 4 hours should elapse before breastfeeding when levels are below 1 pg per ml and that infants should be monitored for signs of diarrhoea.

There are no studies on the amount of misoprostol passing into mature milk after oral administration of the drug. Vogel *et al.* (2004) and Abden-Aleem *et al.* (2003) studies took place where the mothers were less than 4 days post-partum. In neither of the studies were the infants breastfed.

The recommendation that a mother discontinue breastfeeding for 4 hours (Vogel *et al.* 2004) is based on the time for the level in milk to fall below 1 pg per ml. UKMI (2011) suggest 5 hours interruption based on pharmacokinetic data. LactMed (2012) suggests that 'because of the low levels of misoprostol in breastmilk, amounts ingested by the infant are small and would not be expected to cause any adverse effects in breastfed infants. No special precautions are required'.

> Based on the limited transfer of misoprostol into breastmilk, breastfeeding could continue without interruption or interrupted for 4 hours to minimise any risk of diarrhoea in the infant.

References

Abdel-Aleem H, Villar J, Gülmezoglu AM, Mostafa SA, Youssef AA, Shokry M, Watzer B, The pharmacokinetics of the prostaglandin E1 analogue misoprostol in plasma and colostrum after post-partum oral administration, *Eur J Obstet Gynecol Reprod Biol*, 2003;108:25–8.

Can mothers breastfeed after a medical termination of pregnancy? UKMI Q&A 261, 2 March 2011.

Drugs and Lactation Data base (LactMed) http://toxnet.nlm.nih.gov/cgi-bin/sis/htmlgen?LACT

Hale T, Medications and Mothers' Milk 2010, March 2012 online access.

Martindale: The Complete Drug Reference, 35th Edition, 2006.

Vogel D, Burkhardt T, Rentsch K, Schweer H, Watzer B, Zimmermann R, Von Mandach U, Misoprostol versus methylergometrine: Pharmacokinetics in human milk, *Am J Obstet Gynecol*, 2004;191:2168–73.

Malignant diseases

Sadly some women who are breastfeeding will develop malignant diseases which need to be treated with surgery, chemotherapy and radiotherapy. The risks of continuing to breastfeed in the presence of cytotoxic drugs are high and it is unlikely to be possible.

However, in these circumstances, the mother may need counselling to come to terms with not just her diagnosis, but also her inability to nurture her child with breastmilk. It would be unhelpful to offer platitudes suggesting that concerns are unimportant.

Nutrition and blood

Vitamins and tonics

Most vitamins and tonics cannot be prescribed by the NHS in the UK so mothers may purchase them from pharmacies or health food stores with little information on safety in lactation. It is a very frequent question to the drugs in breastmilk helpline with many mothers having been told that they cannot take multi-vitamin supplements. This may in part be due to the limitation of vitamins A and D during pregnancy. Recent guidelines (Department of Health 2012; NICE 2008; Scottish Government 2010) are that lactating mothers should take supplements of vitamin D in order to maximise levels in their breastmilk. This advice is based on information on the re-emergence of rickets in the UK, particularly in dark-skinned ethnic groups who do not synthesise sufficient vitamin D from skin exposure to sunlight. Additionally all women who may become pregnant should be taking a supplement of folic acid 400 µg daily to prevent neural tube defects. The majority of the population would only take this if they were considering a pregnancy. In fact, the majority of pregnancies are unplanned so best evidence would suggest that women who are not taking adequate contraceptive measures should take it. This argument is being used to promote addition of folic acid to commonly consumed foods such as bread and flour in addition to breakfast cereals.

Compatible with use during breastfeeding.

References

Department of Health, Vitamin D: advice on supplements for at risk groups (www.dh.gov.uk/en/Publicationsandstatistics/Lettersandcirculars/DH_132509).
NICE PH11, Maternal and Child Nutrition. Promotion of breastfeeding initiation and duration. Evidence into practice briefing, 2008 (www.nice.org.uk/niceMedia/pdf/EAB_Breastfeeding_final_version.pdf).
The Scottish Government, Advice on vitamin D, 2010 (www.scotland.gov.uk/News/Releases/2010/09/17113234).

Vitamin A

This is a fat soluble vitamin which is secreted into breastmilk. Overdose of this vitamin is dangerous so large doses should be avoided in lactation. Natural sources are liver, kidney, dairy produce and eggs as well as carrots and dark green and yellow vegetables. Supplements are normally in fish liver oil capsules which can be taken by breastfeeding mothers in normal doses.

Compatible with use during breastfeeding.

Vitamin B1 (Thiamine)

One study showed that supplementation of the mother did not significantly affect the levels in breastmilk and it is therefore considered compatible with breastfeeding.

Absorption of doses larger than 5 mg is limited and as it is not stored in the body excess is excreted in the urine (Nail *et al.* 1980).

Compatible with use during breastfeeding.

References

Nail PA, Thomas MR, Eakin R, The effect of thiamin and riboflavin supplementation on the level of those vitamins in human breastmilk and urine, *Am J Clin Nutr*, 1980;33:198–204.

Vitamin B2 (Riboflavin)

The small amounts of vitamin B2 present in the diet are absorbed from the gastrointestinal tract by an active process. Dietary insufficiency has been described in strict vegetarians.

Compatible with use during breastfeeding.

Vitamin B12

Hydroxycobalamin supplements do pass into breastmilk but are considered compatible. (Samson and McClelland 1980). Vegan mothers may benefit from supplements.

Compatible with use during breastfeeding.

References

Samson RR, McClelland DBL, Vitamin B12 in human colostrum and milk, *Acta Paediatr Scand*, 1980;69:93–9.

Vitamin B6 (Pyridoxine)

The normal daily requirement for pyridoxine is 1.5 to 2 mg which is found adequately in most diets. Meats, especially chicken, kidney and liver, cereals, eggs, fish and certain vegetables and fruits are good sources of pyridoxine. The upper intake recommended is 100 mg per day and recommended dietary allowance is 2 mg (British Nutrition Foundation 2012). Deficiency is rare but supplements have been recommended to alleviate post-natal depression, pre-menstrual tension but there is no evidence of effectiveness of this treatment over placebo (West 1987) and excessive doses have been reported to cause sensory neuropathy. Pyridoxine transfers into breastmilk and high doses have been reported to suppress prolactin levels although this has not been reproduced in all studies (Marcus 1975; Foukas 1973; de Waal *et al.* 1978; Canales *et al.* 1976). In view of the risks and benefits excessive single vitamin supplements of vitamin B6 are probably best avoided but can be taken as part of a balanced multi-vitamin supplement.

Compatible with use during breastfeeding.

References

British Nutrition Foundation, Nutrient requirements and recommendations, 2012 (www.nutrition.org.uk/nutritionscience/nutrients/vitamins?start=9).

Canales ES, Soria J, Zarate A, Mason M, Molina M, The influence of pyridoxine on prolactin secretion and milk production in women, *Br J Obstet Gynaecol*, 1976;83(5):387–8.

de Waal JM, Steyn AF, Harms JH, Slabber CF, Pannall PR, Failure of pyridoxine to suppress raised serum prolactin levels, *S Afr Med J*, 1978;53(8):293–4.

Foukas MD, An antilactogenic effect of pyridoxine, *J Obstet Gynaecol Br Commonw*, 1973;80(8):718–20.

Marcus RG, Suppression of lactation with high doses of pyridoxine, *S Afr Med J*, 1975;49(52):2155–6.

West CP, The premenstrual syndrome, *Prescribers' J*, 1987;27(2):9–15.

Vitamin C

Ascorbic acid is secreted into breastmilk but supplements increase levels reaching the baby only by modest amounts in well-nourished developed world mothers (Daneel-Otterbech *et al.* 2005). Approximately 100 mg ascorbic acid daily is sufficient to produce adequate breastmilk levels. Humans are unable to produce their own vitamin C and are reliant on dietary sources. Deficiency leads to scurvy. This is characterised by capillary fragility, bleeding (especially from small blood vessels and the gums) and slow healing of wounds. Good sources include blackcurrant, citrus fruits, leafy vegetables, tomatoes, potatoes and green and red peppers. Vitamin C is destroyed during the cooking process and during storage. Levels needed for women are around 40 mg day but almost double this level is required by smokers. Deficiency is rare in adults but may occur in infants – hence the now dated use of rosehip and blackcurrant syrup as a weaning drink, use of which is now been discouraged due to the high sugar content which caused massive dental decay particularly if offered in a bottle of spouted drinking cup.

Compatible with use during breastfeeding.

References

Daneel-Otterbech S, Davidsson L, Hurrell R, Ascorbic acid supplementation and regular consumption of fresh orange juice increase the ascorbic acid content of human milk: studies in European and African lactating women, *Am J Clin Nutr*, 2005;81:1088–93.

Iron supplements

Iron supplements may be necessary if the mother is found to be anaemic at delivery or has suffered a post-partum hemorrhage. Some women find iron supplements cause gastric irritation with constipation or diarrhoea. Iron tablets should ideally be taken with a source of vitamin C e.g. a glass of orange juice with or after food. Tea prevents full absorption.

The body contains about 4 g of iron mostly in the form of haemoglobin. Iron is lost in small amounts from the female body in menstruation and in breastfeeding. No increase in dietary need is recommended during lactation. The reference nutrient intake is 14.8 mg daily. Supplements are generally given as ferrous sulphate, gluconate and fumarate. Modified release preparations are claimed to reduce the incidence of gastro-intestinal irritation. Absorption of iron in breastmilk is facilitated by lactoferrin and is about 50% compared with iron absorption of iron from food by adults, which is 5 to 15%. Levels in formula are of necessity considerably higher as they do not have the advantage of lactoferrin.

It has been recommended that exclusively breastfed infants need additional iron supplements from 4 to 6 months as body stores are depleted. Iron supplements taken by the mother, transfer poorly into breastmilk (oral bio-availability <30%). Their use is not contra-indicated in breastfeeding but should be used to increase maternal levels rather than attempt to influence infant levels.

Compatible with use during breastfeeding.

References

Pisacane A, De Vizia B, Valiante A, Vaccaro F, Russo M, Grillo G, Giustardi A, Iron status in breastfed infants, *J Pediatr*, 1995;127(3):429–31.

Vitamin D supplements

As discussed further in the section on pre-conceptual advice (page 67), the incidence of rickets in children seems to be increasing. Levels of calcium and vitamin D have been found to be low in many teenagers and young women due to dietary restrictions and less exposure to sunlight.

Vitamin D is secreted into breastmilk in limited amounts proportional to mother's levels. Supplementing a mother with even moderate doses of vitamin D does not substantially increase milk levels. In the UK the recommended dose is 10 µg (400 IU per day). (SACN 2007; Baby Friendly Initiative 2011; Department of Health 2012).

Compatible with use during breastfeeding.

References

Baby Friendly Initiative, Statement on vitamin D supplementation for breastfed babies, 2012 (www.unicef.org.uk/BabyFriendly/News-and-Research/News/UNICEF-UK-Baby-Friendly-Initiative-Statement-on-vitamin-D-supplementation-for-breastfed-babies/).
Department of Health Healthy Start, 2012.
Greer FR, Issues in establishing vitamin D recommendations for infants and children, *Am J Clin Nutr*, 2004;80(6 Suppl.):1759S–62S.

Hollis BW, Wagner CL, Vitamin D requirements during lactation: high-dose maternal supplementation as therapy to prevent hypovitaminosis D for both the mother and the nursing infant, *Am J Clin Nutr*, 2004;80(6 Suppl.):1752S–8S.

Rothberg AD, Pettifor JM, Cohen DF, Sonnendecker EW, Ross FP, Maternal-infant vitamin D relationships during breastfeeding, *J Pediatr*, 1982;101(4):500–503.

Scientific Advisory Committee on Nutrition (SACN), Update on Vitamin D, February 2007 www.sacn.gov.uk/pdfs/sacn_07_04.pdf

Folic acid

Any women who might become pregnant should take folic acid 400 µg daily (page 66). This includes breastfeeding women not using contraception or trying to conceive. Supplementation is intended to reduce the risk of neural tube defects in subsequent babies. Folic acid is actively secreted into breastmilk (Cooperman *et al.* 1982). One study of 11 breastfeeding mothers taking 400 µg to 1 mg per day of folic acid daily, the level secreted into breastmilk averaged 45.6 µg per litre (Smith *et al.* 1983). In specific circumstances e.g. epilepsy, diabetes, women who have previously had a baby with spina bifida or mothers not actively using contraception should take 5 mg folic acid daily.

> Compatible with use during breastfeeding.

References

Cooperman JM, Dweck HS, Newman LJ, Garbarino C, Lopez R, The folate in human milk, *Am J Clin Nutr*, 1982;36(4):576–80.

Smith AM, Picciano MF, Deering RH, Folate supplementation during lactation: maternal folate status, human milk folate content, and their relationship to infant folate status, *J Pediatr Gastroenterol Nutr*, 1983;2(4):622–8.

Drugs used to treat musculoskeletal and joint pains

Non-steroidal anti-inflammatories

NSAIDs have analgesic, anti-pyretic and anti-inflammatory activity. They are among the most compatible with use in breastfeeding due to their high plasma protein binding leading to low levels in breastmilk. The commonest adverse effects of NSAIDs are generally GI disturbances, such as discomfort, nausea and diarrhoea but in some patients peptic ulceration and severe GI bleeding may occur. Their use is contra-indicated in patients with a history of peptic ulcer disease or allergy to aspirin. They should be taken with or after food. NSAIDs are frequently given as analgesics in the immediate post-partum period and to relieve the symptoms of non-infective mastitis.

> **Drug of choice in a mother during breastfeeding based on evidence of benefit and safety for the baby:**
>
> **Ibuprofen or diclofenac**

Ibuprofen

Ibuprofen is frequently given directly to babies as an antipyretic and analgesic drug although its use is unlicensed under 3 months or 5 kg. Walter and Dilger (1997) estimated that a breastfed infant would ingest about 0.0008% of the maternal dose, which represents 0.06% of the normal infant dose of 30 mg per kg daily. Despite this, some patient information leaflets still suggest that ibuprofen should not be used during feeding orally or topically. Multiple studies have been published with no adverse effects being reported (Weibert *et al.* 1982; Ito *et al.* 1993). The very high plasma protein binding of ibuprofen (90 to 99%) limits its passage into breastmilk. Relative infant dose quoted as 0.1 to 0.7 % (Hale 2012 online access).

The BNF states that the amount present in breastmilk is too small to be harmful but that some manufacturers recommend that neither the oral or topical forms are used during breastfeeding.

> Compatible with use during breastfeeding due to limited transfer into breastmilk.

References

Ito S, Blajchman A, Stephenson M, Prospective follow-up of adverse reactions in breastfed infants exposed to maternal medication, *Am J Obstet Gynecol*, 1993;168:1393–9.

Townsend RJ, Benedetti TJ, Erickson SH, Cengiz C, Gillespie WR, Gschwend J, Albert KS, Excretion of ibuprofen into breastmilk, *Am J Obstet Gynecol*, 1984;149(2):184–6.

Walter K, Dilger C, Ibuprofen in human milk, *Br J Clin Pharmacol*, 1997;44:211–12.

Weibert RT, Townsend RJ, Kaiser DG, Naylor AJ, Lack of ibuprofen secretion into human milk, *Clin Pharm*, 1982;1:457–8.

Diclofenac

Brand name: *Voltarol*®
US brands: *Voltaren*®
Australian brands: *Voltaren*®, *Clonac*®, *Diclac*®, *Diclohexal*®, *Dinac*®

Research studies are not widely documented as it is used less frequently in the USA than in the UK. However, the lack of reports of adverse effects suggests that there is little cause for concern. It is one of the most widely used drugs in the immediate post-partum period in the UK.

Oral diclofenac is almost completely absorbed but it is subject to first-pass metabolism so less reached the systemic circulation. Its high plasma protein binding (in excess of 99%) limits its passage into breastmilk. It is widely used on post-natal wards. Relative infant dose quoted as 1% (Hale 2012 online access).

The BNF states that the amount present in breastmilk is too small to be harmful.

Compatible with use during breastfeeding due to limited transfer into breastmilk.

Naproxen

Brand name: *Naprosyn®*
US brands: *Naprosyn®, Aleve®, Anaprox®*
Australian brands: *Naprosyn®, Anaprox®, Crysanal®, Proxen®*

Naproxen is more than 99% bound to plasma proteins. Davies and Anderson (1997) reported that although naproxen is excreted into breastmilk, the amount of drug transferred comprises only a small fraction of the maternal exposure. In Jamali and Stevens' study (1983) only 0.26% of the mother's dose was recovered from the infant and adverse effect reports are low. However, this drug has a longer half-life than other NSAIDs, normally being taken only twice a day. The BNF considers that the amount of naproxen distributed into breastmilk is too small to be harmful to a breastfed infant; however, some manufacturers recommend that breastfeeding should be avoided during naproxen therapy, due to licensing considerations rather than potential risk. Relative infant dose quoted as 3.3% (Hale 2012 online access).

The BNF states that the amount in breastmilk is too small to be harmful but that the manufacturer advises use should be avoided.

Compatible with use during breastfeeding due to limited transfer into breastmilk. Ibuprofen or diclofenac preferable if baby is <6 weeks due to longer half-life of naproxen.

References

Davies NM, Anderson KE, Clinical pharmacokinetics of naproxen, *Clin Pharmacokinet*, 1997;32:268–93.
Jamali F, Stevens DRS, Naproxen excretion in milk and its uptake by the infant, *Drug Intell Clin Pharm*, 1983;17:910–11.

Celecoxib

Brand name: *Celebrex®*
US brands: *Celebrex®*
Australian brands: *Celebrex®*

Celecoxib has been reported to cause few adverse events in infants exposed to limited amounts passing through maternal breastmilk.

Knoppert *et al.* (2003) studied one mother who took four doses of oral celecoxib 100 mg post-surgery and did not breastfeed her daughter for 48 hours after taking the last dose. Samples of breastmilk were studied and a concentration of 133 ng per ml at approximately 5 hours after a 100 mg dose and an elimination half-life of 4 to 6.5 hours was determined.

Hale *et al.* (2004) studied three breastfeeding mothers on celecoxib at steady state; milk levels were determined as were plasma levels in two infants aged 17 and 22. The average concentration of celecoxib in milk was 66 µg per litre and the absolute infant dose averaged 9.8 µg per kg per day producing a mean relative infant dose quoted as 0.30%. The authors suggest that the use of celecoxib in breastfeeding mothers at these doses is very unlikely to cause untoward effects in breastfed infants. These results were confirmed by Gardiner *et al.* (2006).

Adverse gastro-intestinal effects of NSAIDs are generally believed to be due to inhibition of cyclo-oxygenase-1 (COX-1). More selective inhibition by COX-2 NSAIDs such as celecoxib may cause less gastric irritation than the non-selective inhibition of the traditional NSAIDs such as ibuprofen and diclofenac. However, COX-2s are believed to be more cardio-toxic and there have been links with myocardial infarction and ischaemia. This action is limited to the patient taking medication. Relative infant dose quoted as 0.3 to 0.7% (Hale 2012 online access).

The BNF states that it is present in the milk of animals studied and that the manufacturer advises that it should be avoided.

> Probably compatible with use during breastfeeding due to limited transfer into breastmilk and lack of adverse reactions reported in limited studies

References

Gardiner SJ, Doogue MP, Zhang M, Begg EJ, Quantification of infant exposure to celecoxib through breastmilk, *Br J Clin Pharmacol*, 2006;61:101–4.

Hale TW, McDonald R, Boger J, Transfer of celecoxib into human milk, *J Hum Lact*, 2004;20(4):397–403.

Knoppert DC, Stempak D, Baruchel S, Koren G, Celecoxib in human milk: a case report, *Pharmacotherapy*, 2003;23(1):97–100.

Eye preparations

> **Drug choice in a mother during breastfeeding based on evidence of benefit and safety for the baby:**
>
> **According to maternal need**

Absorption of eye drops into breastmilk is unlikely in the majority of conditions:

- Local anaesthetic drops e.g. lignocaine (lidocaine);
- Antibacterial eye drops e.g. chloramphenicol, fusidic acid (Fucithalmic®);
- Antiviral eye drops e.g. aciclovir (Zovirax®);
- Corticosteroid eye drops e.g. betamethasone (Betnesol®), prednisolone (Predsol®);
- Ocular lubricants e.g. hypromellose, carbomers.

Compatible with use during breastfeeding due to poor bio-availability.

Beta blocker eye drops

There is concern over the systemic absorption of beta blockers to treat glaucoma and consideration should be given if the baby suffers from asthma or heart disease and the mother alerted to the possibility, even if remote, of adverse reactions.

In a case report of a single mother (Lustgarten and Podos 1983) who used one drop of 0.5% timolol maleate, the authors estimated that use of 0.5% timolol drops in one eye twice daily gave the infant 0.63% of a cardiac dose. No side effects were reported.

Johnson *et al.* (2001) reported on one mother who used eye drops of timolol, dipivifrin, dorzolamide and brimonidine as well as oral acetazolamide. No apnoea or bradycardia was observed in the infant.

Compatible with use during breastfeeding, according to the results of limited studies.

References

Johnson SM, Martinez M, Freedman S, Management of glaucoma in pregnancy and lactation, *Surv Ophthalmol*, 2001;45:449–54.

Lustgarten JS, Podos SM, Topical timolol and the nursing mother, *Arch Ophthalmol*, 1983;101:1381–2.

Ear drops

Drug choice in a mother during breastfeeding based on evidence of benefit and safety for the baby:

According to maternal need

Absorption of eardrops is unlikely to reach clinical significance in breastmilk, as there is virtually no means of absorption into the systemic system from the external ear canal. Eardrops generally include corticosteroids to reduce inflammation, antibiotics to reduce otitis external, antifungals, local anaesthetics for pain and ingredients to soften and remove earwax. Treatment of otitis media with eardrops is generally ineffective and is better treated by simple analgesia and, if necessary, antibiotics. Almond oil, olive oil and sodium bicarbonate solution are all used to soften ear wax.

Examples of drugs: dexamethasone *(Sofradex®, Otomize®)*, gentamicin *(Genticin® and Gentisone HC®)*, *(Otosprorin®)* urea hydrgen peroxide ☺ *(Otex®)*, chlorbutanol *(Cerumol®)*, betamethasone *(Betnesol®)*, hydrocortisone and neomycin *(Neo-cortef®)*, prednisolone *(Predsol®)*, prednisolone and neomycin *(Predsol N®)*. Compatible with use during breastfeeding due to poor bio-availability

Nasal drops

The passage of drugs from nasal drops and sprays into breastmilk is very limited and can be discounted. Drugs delivered by nasal drops include anti-histamines and corticosteroids to treat nasal allergy, nasal decongestants and anti-infective agents to treat nasal *Staphylococci*. They can be used during breast-feeding.

> **Drug choice in a mother during breastfeeding based on evidence of benefit and safety for the baby:**
>
> **According to maternal need**

For example: normal saline, beclometasone (*Beconase®*), budesonide (*Rhinocort®*), fluticasone (*Flixonase®*), mometasone (*Nasonex®*), sodium cromoglycate (*Rynacrom*), ephedrine, xylometazoline (*Otrivine®*), mupirocin nasal cream (*Bactroban®*).

Dental treatment

Dental treatment can be undertaken while a mother is breastfeeding. Anecdotally, mothers report being concerned about the removal of old fillings and the absorption of local anaesthetics into breastmilk and may defer treatment other than in an emergency.

Dental fillings

Use of local anaesthetics or replacement of fillings should not be discouraged just because a mother is breastfeeding. Treatment can continue as normal (Lebedevs *et al.* 1993). However, there are occasions when a new mother may need a filling inserted or replaced. When mercury is removed some will be vaporised by the high-speed drill and a very small amount may be swallowed or inhaled. These amounts are minute and passage into breastmilk is insignificant compared with the background levels of mercury in the environment. The limitation of the consumption of tuna in line with Food Standards Agency guidance is more important on limiting the body burden of mercury and it is very difficult to prove any link between mercury fillings and long-term health problems (Food Standard Agency 2004; Lawson 2006). Preventative dental health to minimise the risk of decay is perhaps the message which is of paramount importance.

> Compatible with breastfeeding.

References

Peter Lawson BDS, FDS, FRCPS personal communication: Amalgam and mercury, 2006.
Food Standards Agency, Advice on tuna consumption, 2004 www.food.gov.uk/news/newsarchive/2004/mar/fish

Lebedevs TH, Wojnar-Horton RE, Yapp P, Roberts MJ, Dusci LJ, Hackett LP, Ilett K, Excretion of lignocaine and its metabolite monoethylglycinexylidide in breastmilk following its use in a dental procedure. A case report, *J Clin Peridontol*, 1993;20:606–8.

Tooth extraction

If a tooth is to be removed, the mother is likely to be offered a local anaesthetic injection or sedation. She may also need pain killers and or antibiotics.

There is no reason to stop breastfeeding after dental anaesthesia.

There are a few anecdotal reports of babies rejecting their mother's milk after she has had dental treatment. There is no apparent scientific reason for this. Feeding when the baby is sleepy may help. It may be that there is a relationship with the fear which some people experience when visiting the dentist that may inhibit let down.

Compatible with breastfeeding.

Mouthwashes

Can be used by a breastfeeding mother as they will not be absorbed into the bloodstream e.g. *Oraldene®*, *Corsodyl®*, chlorhexidine mouthwash (Corsodyl®), benydamine (Difflam®).

Compatible with during breastfeeding due to poor absorption through mucosal membrane of the mouth.

Mouth ulcer

Mouthwashes, gels and liquids e.g. Difflam®, Anbesol®, Orabase®, Medijel® and Rinstead pastilles® can all be used. Some products contain salicylates e.g. Bonjela® and while there is no evidence of risk in using these products during breastfeeding, as they are not recommended for paediatric use it may be prudent to avoid them as there are alternative products available.

Compatible with use during breastfeeding due to poor absorption through mucosal membrane of the mouth.

Tooth-whitening agents

There appears to be no information available on the use of tooth-whitening agents during lactation. While it is unlikely that any significant transfer of the agents used into breastmilk will take place, it is unlikely that urgent treatment is necessary and can be delayed until breastfeeding has finished naturally.

Probably acceptable during breastfeeding due to poor absorption through mucosal membrane of the mouth and rapid breakdown in the bloodstream but no evidence from studies.

Miconazole oral gel (pages 60–5)

The gel is used to treat oral candida in babies. Miconazole has poor bio-availability from the gastro-intestinal tract. Peak plasma concentrations of 1 µg per ml are achieved about 4 hours after a dose of 1 g daily while the oral gel contains only 24 mg per ml. Over 90% is reported to be bound to plasma proteins (Martindale 2007).

Breastfeeding mothers who experience symptoms of oral thrush can carry on breastfeeding as normal during treatment. It is important that nothing which goes into the baby's mouth e.g. dummy is sucked by the mother – anecdotally mothers do this to 'clean' the dummy if it has been stored in a non-sterile environment!

> Compatible with use during breastfeeding due to poor oral bio-availability.

Skin

Topical creams

Absorption of topical creams is generally unlikely to reach clinical significance in breastmilk unless applied to excess or directly to the nipples. Creams applied to the nipples should be applied after a feed. Repeated washing of the nipples may lead to damage due to removal of natural lubricants and should be avoided wherever possible.

The use of creams to heal cracked nipples has not been shown to be effective without additional support with positioning and attachment. However, small amounts of cream applied to a crack will prevent scab formation and the development of deep fissures as the scab is disturbed at each feeding. Products such as Lansinoh®, Kamillosan® and Calendula® have all been recommended. However, excessive application may leave the nipple soggy and more likely to develop thrush in consequence. No pharmaceutical preparation has been shown to heal the damage to the nipple effectively or to reduce pain without correct positioning having been achieved. Even badly damaged nipples heal remarkably quickly under these circumstances.

Application of normal therapeutic amounts of corticosteroids for eczema, moisturisers, aciclovir cream for herpes, anti-fungal and antibacterial creams can be applied to the skin of a breastfeeding mother without concerns over continued breastfeeding since the levels achieved in breastmilk are likely to be substantially less than oral medications known to be compatible with breastfeeding. Use caution with skin-to-skin transfer, especially with high-potency corticosteroids which can damage infants' vulnerable skin.

Emollients

Emollients are preparations that soothe and rehydrate the skin. Use during lactation is highly unlikely to affect breastmilk. Care should be taken if the nipple area is moisturised before a feed that no taste remains to discourage the baby from feeding.

Examples: aqueous cream, *E45®*, *Diprobase®*, *Oilatum®*, *Unguentum M®*, *Balneum®*, *Calmurid®* creams

Compatible with use during breastfeeding due to poor absorption through skin.

Bath preparations

Bath preparations provide hydration to the skin during soaking. Many of these preparations are used for babies suffering from dry skin. No ingredient which can affect breastmilk will be absorbed during use.

Compatible with use during breastfeeding due to poor absorption through skin.

Topical corticosteroids

Application of topical corticosteroids is recommended to treat inflammatory conditions of the skin in particular eczema and dermatitis. Used in normal quantities (i.e. a maximum of 30g or less per week) application is unlikely to lead to systemic absorption. Potent topical corticosteroids such as Dermovate® should be used sparingly for as short a time as possible. Use of less-potent corticosteroid applications to large areas of the body should be kept to a minimum accompanied by frequent application of emollient preparations.

Drug choice in a mother during breastfeeding based on evidence of benefit and safety for the baby:

According to maternal need, lower potency corticosteroids preferable, but no reason to stop breastfeeding if mother needs more potent products in normal amounts, but avoid skin-to-skin contact

Mild corticosteroids: hydrocortisone 0.1 to 2.5%
Moderate-strength corticosteroids: *Betnovate RD®, Eumovate®*
Potent corticosteroids: Betamethasone 0.1%, Betnovate®, Locoid®, *Metosyn®*
Very potent products: Dermovate®, Nerisone Forte®

Compatible with use during breastfeeding in normal amounts due to poor absorption through skin.but avoid skin-to-skin contact with medium to high potency agents.

Eczema

Eczema is treated with a combination of corticosteroid cream and emollient preparations according to patient preference. Severe irritation may necessitate the use of sedating anti-histamines, such as chlorpheniramine. Mothers with eczema may be keen to breastfeed in order to minimise the risk of their child developing a condition which is cosmetically and psychologically difficult to deal with.

Moisturisers, emollients and corticosteroid creams are compatible with use during breastfeeding due to poor absorption through skin but avoid skin-to-skin contact with medium- to high-potency agents.

References

Stoukides C, Topical Medications and Breastfeeding, *J Hum Lact*, 1993;9:185–9.

Psoriasis

Psoriasis is characterised by epidermal thickening and scaling. Mild symptoms respond well to emollient use alone. Emollients remain an essential adjunct to other treatments.

Other preparations used include coal tar, dithranol and analogues of vitamin D such as calcipotriol. Mothers applying these products to their skin should be careful to wash their hands thoroughly before touching the baby and avoid direct skin contact between baby's skin and the area treated. None of these creams is likely to penetrate breastmilk (Stoukides 1993).

Brand preparations: *Dovonex®, Dovobet®, Silkis®, Dithranol®*

Compatible with use during breastfeeding due to poor absorption through skin.

References

Stoukides C, Topical Medications and Breastfeeding, *J Hum Lact*, 1993;9:185–9.

Acne

Acne is common in teenagers but by the mid-twenties most cases have resolved. Mild acne responds well to topical therapy particularly benzoyl peroxide, retinoids or antibacterials. It is unlikely that sufficient amounts of these products could be absorbed through the skin to produce significant levels in breastmilk.

Drug choice in a mother during breastfeeding based on evidence of benefit and safety for the baby:

Topical preparations according to maternal need – avoid oral products during breastfeeding

Brand names:
Benzoyl peroxide products: *Acnecide* (5%)®, *Brevoxyl* (4%)®, *PanOxyl* (5%, 10%)®
Retinoids: tretinoin *(Retin-A®)*, isotretinoin *(Isotrex®)*, adapalene *(Differin®)*
Topical antobiotics: Benzoyl peroxide+erythromycin *(Benzamycin®)*, erythromycin 2% *(Stiemycin®)*, clindamycin 1% *(Dalacin T®)*, erythromycin+zinc acetate *(Zineryt®)*, isotretinoin+erythromycin *(Isotrexin®)*

Benzoyl peroxide is generally considered a first-line choice of topical treatment. Topical antibacterials may be used for inflammatory acne or if there has been response to topical benzoyl peroxide. Moderate acne might be treated with oral antibiotics in non-lactating women. Tetracycline, doxycycline, lymecycline, oxytetracycline or minocycline would normally be used. However, due to the possibility of staining of teeth by long-term use of tetracyclines the risk might outweigh the benefit. Severe acne should be treated on an individual basis after discussion with the mother.

Warts and verrucas

Preparations to treat warts and verrucas are widely available to purchase or be prescribed. There is little likelihood of systemic absorption although care should be taken to cover any areas of dried collodion that might come into contact with sensitive areas of the baby's skin.

Brand names: *Cuplex®*, *Duofilm®*, *Salactol®*, *Glutarol®*

> Compatible with use during breastfeeding due to poor absorption through skin.

Sunscreens

There is no need to restrict use of sunscreen preparations by lactating mothers.

> Compatible with use during breastfeeding.

Topical antibacterials, anti-fungals and anti-virals

Localised bacterial, viral and fungal skin infections can be treated with appropriate topical agents rather than oral preparations. This minimises the chance of the development of resistant micro-organisms. Lactating mothers can use these preparations without concern about systemic absorption affecting breastmilk. If the application is made to the nipple area it should be done after a feed and applied sparingly. Any visible at the next feed should be wiped off gently. Washing of the nipple should be minimised to avoid removal of the natural moisturisers in this area.

> **Drug of choice in a mother during breastfeeding based on evidence of benefit and safety for the baby:**
>
> **According to maternal need**

Antibacterial creams, ointments and gels

Mupirocin (*Bactroban®*), neomycin (*Graneodin®*), silver sulphadiazine (*Flamazine®*), fusidic acid (*Fucidin®*)

> Compatible with use during breastfeeding due to poor absorption through skin.

Antifungal ointments, creams, lotions and paints

Amorolfine (*Loceryl®*), clotrimazole (*Canesten®*), ketoconazole (*Nizoral®*), miconazole (*Daktarin®*), nystatin (*Nystan®*, *Tinaderm M®*), terbinafine (*Lamisil®*), tioconazole (*Trosyl®*)

> Compatible with use during breastfeeding due to poor absorption through skin.

Antiviral cream

Aciclovir

Brand name: *Zovirax®*
US brands: *Zovirax®*
Australian brands: *Zovirax®*

> Compatible with use during breastfeeding due to poor absorption through skin

Head lice treatment

Infection with *Pediculus humanus capitis* (the head louse) is common in many families with older children who are at nursery and school. Head lice may be mechanically removed by meticulous combing of wet hair with a fine-toothed detection comb. Combing needs to be undertaken for at least 30 minutes, at 4-day intervals, for a minimum of two weeks. If combing is not undertaken to this level treatment may not be effective. Conditioner facilitates combing particularly of long hair. Anecdotally, use of tea tree oil is effective but has no evidence from clinical trials.

Treatment with lotions or liquids is preferable to shampoos, which are diluted below an effective therapeutic concentration. Aqueous solutions are recommended for children with eczema or asthma. A mosaic approach is considered advisable, however, whereby the child or adult is treated with a different chemical at each infestation or if a treatment fails. Head lice infestation should be treated using lotion or liquid formulations only if live lice are present. A contact time of 8 to 12 hours or overnight treatment is recommended for lotions and liquids; a 2-hour treatment is not sufficient to kill eggs.

In general, a course of treatment for head lice should be two applications of the product 7 days apart to kill lice emerging from any eggs that survive the first application. All affected household members should be treated simultaneously.

> **Drug choice in a mother during breastfeeding based on evidence of benefit and safety for the baby:**
>
> **According to preference**

Absorption of the products through the skin in sufficient quantities to affect breast-milk is unlikely although there are no research data to support this. If a lactating mother has to treat several children's heads it may be sensible to use rubber gloves to protect her hands and ensure the room is well ventilated.

Malathion

Brand: *Derbac M®*
US brands: *Ovide®*
Australian brands: *Lice Rid®*

Malathion has been widely used to eradicate head lice, crab lice and scabies. It is an organophosphorus insecticide. Some resistance has been reported. It should be used twice at 7-day intervals. Derbac M is an aqueous liquid. Hair should be allowed to dry naturally and the treatment washed off after 12 hours.

> Compatible with use during breastfeeding due to poor absorption through skin.

Permethrin

Brand: *Lyclear®*
US brands: *Acticin®, Elimite®, Nix®*
Australian brands: *Lyclear®, Quellada®, Pyrifoam®*

Less than 2% of permethrin is absorbed after topical application. It is rapidly metabolised in the skin to inactive metabolites. It is therefore acceptable to apply both directly onto infants' skin or to be used by a breastfeeding mother. In Ito *et al.*'s telephone follow-up study, five mothers who used permethrin during breastfeeding reported no adverse reactions in their breastfed infants.

Permethrin is also popular and effective in the treatment of crab lice and scabies (Lyclear Dermal Cream®). According to the BNF it is no longer recommended to treat head lice (BNF). However, the summary of product characteristics (SPC) states that 97 to 99% of individuals with head lice are successfully treated with a single application of Lyclear creme rinse and that residual activity may persist for up to 6 weeks. It is applied after the hair has been washed and left on for 10 minutes before rinsing the hair.

> Compatible with use during breastfeeding due to poor bio-availability through skin.

References

Ito S, Blajchman A, Stephenson M, Eliopoulos C, Koren G, Prospective follow-up of adverse reactions in breastfed infants exposed to maternal medication, *Am J Obstet Gynecol*, 1993;168:1393–9.
Manufacturer's information Lyclear SPC 2012 www.medicines.or.uk
Porto I, Antiparasitic drugs and lactation: focus on anthelmintics, scabicides, and pediculicides, *J Hum Lact*, 2003;19:421–5.

Dimeticone

Brand: *Hedrin*®

Dimeticone is effective in killing head lice (*Pediculus humanus capitis*). It coats the surface of the organism and prevents the excretion of water by the louse. It should be used twice at 7-day intervals. Hedrin is a lotion and should be used away from naked flames and the hair allowed to dry naturally.

Vaccines

Vaccines have low bio-availability and absorption from breastmilk is unlikely in most circumstances other than with live vaccines. Cessation or interruption of breastfeeding is not normally required but individual regimens should be considered especially with yellow fever (Data taken from LactMed website [2012]; Martindale [2005]; Advisory Committee on Immunization Practices [ACIP]; CDC [Kroger 2006]; Advisory Committee on Immunization Practices [2006]). UK data are available in the Department of Health 'The Green Book' available on the internet (Plotkin and Orenstein 2004; Department of Health Green Book 2006).

Although there is a theoretical risk of live vaccine being present in breastmilk, vaccination with common vaccines is not contra-indicated for women who are breastfeeding when there is significant risk of exposure to disease. There is no evidence of risk from vaccinating women who are breastfeeding, with inactivated viral or bacterial vaccines or toxoids (BNF).

References

Advisory Committee on Immunization Practices, *MMWR Recomm Rep*, 2006;55(RR-15):1–48.

Immunisation against infectious disease – 'The Green Book' – 2006 updated edition www.dh.gov.uk/en/Publicationsandstatistics/Publications/ublicationsPolicyAndGuidance/DH_079917

Kroger AT, Atkinson WL, Marcuse EK, Pickering LK, Advisory Committee on Immunization Practices (ACIP) Centers for Disease Control and Prevention (CDC). General recommendations on immunization: recommendations of the Advisory Committee on Immunization Practices (ACIP), *MMWR Recomm Rep*, 2006;55(RR-15):1–48.

Plotkin SA, Orenstein WA, *Vaccines 4th edition*, Philadelphia: WB Saunders, 2004 (cited in Department of Health Green Book chapter 34, 2011).

Measles, mumps and rubella

Rubella vaccine virus can appear in breastmilk and result in infections in some infants (Buimovici-Klein *et al.* 1977). There is no evidence of mumps and measles vaccine viruses being found in breastmilk. Some breastfed infants acquire passive immunity to rubella after maternal vaccination, as do infants of mothers with natural rubella immunity. However, neither group of infants has a decreased response to rubella vaccine administered directly (Krogh *et al.* 1989). The CDC (Kroger *et al.* 2006) state that vaccines given to a nursing mother do not affect the safety of breastfeeding for mothers or infants and that breastfeeding is not a contra-indication to MMR vaccine. Breastfed infants should be vaccinated according to the routine recommended schedules (Plotkin and Orenstein, 2004; Department of Health Green Book 2006).

Compatible with use during breastfeeding.

References

Buimovici-Klein E, Hite RL, Byrne T *et al.* Isolation of rubella virus in milk after pospartum immunization, *J Pediatr*, 1977;91:939–41.

Immunisation against infectious disease – 'The Green Book' – 2006 updated edition www.dh.gov.uk/en/Publicationsandstatistics/Publications/PublicationsPolicyAndGuidance/DH_079917

Kroger AT, Atkinson WL, Marcuse EK, Pickering LK, Advisory Committee on Immunization Practices (ACIP) Centers for Disease Control and Prevention (CDC). General recommendations on immunization: recommendations of the Advisory Committee on Immunization Practices (ACIP), *MMWR Recomm Rep*, 2006;55(RR-15):1–48.

Krogh V, Duffy LC, Wong D, Rosenband M, Riddlesberger KR, Ogra PL, Post-partum immunization with rubella virus vaccine and antibody response in breastfeeding infants, *J Lab Clin Med*, 1989;113(6):695–9.

Plotkin SA, Orenstein WA, *Vaccines 4th edition*, Philadelphia: WB Saunders, 2004 (cited in Department of Health Green Book chapter 34, 2011).

Diphtheria, tetanus and pertussis

One study of previously vaccinated infants found that at 21 to 40 months of age breastfed infants had higher immunoglobulin G (IgG) levels against diphtheria, higher secretory IgA levels in saliva against diphtheria and tetanus and higher fecal IgM against tetanus than formula-fed infants (Hahn-Zoric *et al.* 1990).

Pisicane *et al.* (2010) found that breastfed infants were also less likely to have fever after immunisation than their non-breastfed counterparts. Lopez-Alarcon *et al.* (2002) found they were also less likely to experience loss of appetite and reduced energy intake after routine childhood immunisation than those who are not breastfed. Although baseline calorie intakes were higher in the formula-fed infants mean intakes fell by 12% in the post-immunisation period.

There is no evidence of risk from vaccinating pregnant women or those who are breastfeeding with inactivated viral or bacterial vaccines or toxoids (Kroger 2006; Plotkin and Orenstein 2004; Department of Health Green Book 2006).

Compatible with use during breastfeeding.

References

Hahn-Zoric M, Fulconis F, Minoli I, Moro G, Carlsson B, Böttiger M, Räihä N, Hanson LA, Antibody responses to parenteral and oral vaccines are impaired by conventional and low protein formulas as compared to breastfeeding, *Acta Paediatr Scand*; 1990;1979:1137–42.

Immunisation against infectious disease – 'The Green Book' – 2006 updated edition www.dh.gov.uk/en/Publicationsandstatistics/Publications/PublicationsPolicyAndGuidance/D H_079917

Kroger AT, Atkinson WL, Marcuse EK, Pickering LK, Advisory Committee on Immunization Practices (ACIP) Centers for Disease Control and Prevention (CDC). General recommendations on immunization: recommendations of the Advisory Committee on Immunization Practices (ACIP), *MMWR Recomm Rep*, 2006;55(RR-15):1–48.

López-Alarcón M, Garza C, Habicht JP, Martínez L, Pegueros V, Villalpando S, Breastfeeding attenuates reductions in energy intake induced by a mild immunologic stimulus represented by DPTH immunization: possible roles of interleukin-1beta, tumor necrosis factor-alpha and leptin, *J Nutr*, 2002;132:1293–8.

Pisacane A, Continisio P, Palma O, Cataldo S, De Michele F, Vairo U, Breastfeeding and risk for fever after immunization, *Pediatrics*, 2010;125:e1448–52.

Plotkin SA, Orenstein WA, *Vaccines 4th edition*, Philadelphia: WB Saunders, 2004 (cited in Department of Health Green Book chapter 34, 2011).

Meningococcal vaccination

Immunisation of pregnant or lactating women with meningococcal vaccine increased the specific secretory IgA content of milk (Lakshman *et al*. 2000; Shahid *et al*. 2002). There is no evidence of risk from vaccinating pregnant women or those who are breastfeeding with inactivated virus or bacterial vaccines or toxoids (Granoff *et al*. 2004, Department of Health Green Book 2006).

Compatible with use during breastfeeding.

References

Granoff DM, Feavers IM, Borrow R, Meningococcal vaccines. In: Plotkin SA, Orenstein WA, *Vaccines 4th edition*, Philadelphia: WB Saunders, 2004 (cited in Department of Health Green Book, 959–88, 2011).

Immunisation against infectious disease – 'The Green Book' – 2006 updated edition www.dh.gov.uk/en/Publicationsandstatistics/Publications/PublicationsPolicyAndGuidance/D H_079917

Lakshman R, Seymour L, Akhtar S *et al*. Secretory antibody responses to quadrivalent meningococcal vaccine in lactating mothers, *Clin Infect Dis*, 2000;31(1):321. Abstract 629.

Shahid NS, Steinhoff MC, Roy E, Begum T, Thompson CM, Siber GR, Placental and breast transfer of antibodies after maternal immunization with polysaccharide meningiococcal vaccine: a randomized, controlled evaluation, *Vaccine*, 2002;20:2404–9.

Typhoid vaccination

Recommended as compatible with breastfeeding by the CDC and the American Academy of Pediatrics (AAP). There is no evidence of risk from vaccinating pregnant women or those who are breastfeeding with inactivated viral or bacterial vaccines or toxoids (Kroger 2006; Plotkin and Orenstein 2004; Department of Health Green Book 2006).

Compatible with use during breastfeeding.

References

Immunisation against infectious disease – 'The Green Book' – 2006 updated edition www.dh.gov.uk/en/Publicationsandstatistics/Publications/PublicationsPolicyAndGuidance/DH_079917

Kroger AT, Atkinson WL, Marcuse EK, Pickering LK, Advisory Committee on Immunization Practices (ACIP) Centers for Disease Control and Prevention (CDC). General recommendations on immunization: recommendations of the Advisory Committee on Immunization Practices (ACIP), *MMWR Recomm Rep*, 2006;55(RR-15):1–48.

Plotkin SA, Orenstein WA, *Vaccines 4th edition*, Philadelphia: WB Saunders, 2004 (cited in Department of Health Green Book chapter 34, 2011).

Influenza vaccination

Use of live, attenuated or inactivated vaccine is recommended as compatible with breastfeeding by the CDC and the AAP. There is no evidence of risk from vaccinating pregnant women, or those who are feeding, with inactivated viral or bacterial vaccines or toxoids (Plotkin and Orenstein 2004). Where possible, pregnant women should receive a thiomersal-free influenza vaccine (Department of Health Green Book 2006).

Compatible with use during breastfeeding.

References

Immunisation against infectious disease – 'The Green Book' – 2006 updated edition www.dh.gov.uk/en/Publicationsandstatistics/Publications/publicationsPolicyAndGuidance/DH_079917

Kroger AT, Atkinson WL, Marcuse EK, Pickering LK, Advisory Committee on Immunization Practices (ACIP) Centers for Disease Control and Prevention (CDC). General recommendations on immunization: recommendations of the Advisory Committee on Immunization Practices (ACIP), *MMWR Recomm Rep*, 2006;55(RR-15):1–48.

Plotkin SA, Orenstein WA, *Vaccines 4th edition*, Philadelphia: WB Saunders, 2004 (cited in Department of Health Green Book chapter 34, 2011).

BCG vaccination

BCG vaccination against tuberculosis is recommended as compatible with breastfeeding by CDC and the AAP (Kroger 2006). Although no harmful effects on the foetus have been observed from BCG during pregnancy, it is wise to avoid vaccination, particularly in the first trimester, and wherever possible to delay until after delivery. Breastfeeding is not a contraindication to BCG (Plotkin and Orenstein 2004; Department of Health Green Book 2006).

Compatible with use during breastfeeding.

References

Immunisation against infectious disease – 'The Green Book' – 2006 updated edition www.dh.gov.uk/en/Publicationsandstatistics/Publications/publicationsPolicyAndGuidance/DH_079917

Kroger AT, Atkinson WL, Marcuse EK, Pickering LK, Advisory Committee on Immunization Practices (ACIP) Centers for Disease Control and Prevention (CDC). General recommendations on immunization: recommendations of the Advisory Committee on Immunization Practices (ACIP), *MMWR Recomm Rep*, 2006;55(RR-15):1–48.

Plotkin SA, Orenstein WA, *Vaccines 4th edition*, Philadelphia: WB Saunders, 2004 (cited in Department of Health Green Book chapter 34, 2011).

Pneumococcal vaccines

Some evidence of decreased pneumococcal disease has been found among breastfed infants of vaccinated mothers (Lehmann *et al.* 2003). Pneumococcal-containing vaccines may be given to pregnant women when the need for protection is required without delay. There is no evidence of risk from vaccinating pregnant women or those who are breastfeeding with inactivated viral or bacterial vaccines or toxoids (Kroger 2006; Plotkin and Orenstein 2004; Department of Health Green Book 2006).

Compatible with use during breastfeeding.

References

Immunisation against infectious disease – 'The Green Book' – 2006 updated edition www.dh.gov.ukperen/Publicationsandstatist/PublicationsperPublicationsPolicyAndGuidance/DH_079917

Kroger AT, Atkinson WL, Marcuse EK, Pickering LK, Advisory Committee on Immunization Practices (ACIP) Centers for Disease Control and Prevention (CDC). General recommendations on immunization: recommendations of the Advisory Committee on Immunization Practices (ACIP), *MMWR Recomm Rep*, 2006;55(RR-15):1–48.

Lehmann D, Pomat WS, Riley ID, Alpers MP, Studies of maternal immunisation with pneumococcal polysaccharide vaccine in Papua New Guinea, *Vaccine*, 2003;21:3446–50.

Plotkin SA, Orenstein WA, *Vaccines 4th edition*, Philadelphia: WB Saunders, 2004 (cited in Department of Health Green Book chapter 34, 2011).

Varicella vaccine

Recommended as compatible with breastfeeding by the CDC and the AAP (Kroger 2006). Women who are pregnant should not receive varicella vaccine and pregnancy should be avoided for 3 months following the last dose. Studies have shown that the vaccine virus is not transferred to the infant through breastmilk (Bohlke *et al.* 2003) and therefore breastfeeding women can be vaccinated if indicated (Plotkin and Orenstein 2004; Department of Health Green Book 2006).

Compatible with use during breastfeeding.

References

Bohlke K, Galil K, Jackson LA, Schmid DS, Starkovich P, Loparev VN, Seward JF, Vaccine Safety Data link Team. Post-partum varicella vaccination: is the vaccine virus excreted in breastmilk?, *Obstet Gynecol*, 2003;102 (5 Pt 1):970–7.

Immunisation against infectious disease – 'The Green Book' – 2006 updated edition www.dh.gov.uk/en/Publicationsandstatistics/Publications/publicationsPolicyAndGuidance/DH_079917

Kroger AT, Atkinson WL, Marcuse EK, Pickering LK, Advisory Committee on Immunization Practices (ACIP) Centers for Disease Control and Prevention (CDC). General recommendations on immunization: recommendations of the Advisory Committee on Immunization Practices (ACIP), *MMWR Recomm Rep*, 2006;55(RR-15):1–48.

Plotkin SA, Orenstein WA, *Vaccines 4th edition*, Philadelphia: WB Saunders, 2004 (cited in Department of Health Green Book chapter 34, 2011).

Yellow fever vaccine

Until 2009 no adverse effects to yellow fever vaccine had been reported in infants exposed via breastfeeding. In 2009, the first case of meningoencephalitis caused by the yellow fever vaccine virus transmitted via breastmilk was confirmed.

Traiber *et al.* reported on a 38-day-old infant who was exclusively breastfed by a mother who had received yellow fever vaccination, the baby was discharged when convulsions resolved.

Kuhn *et al.* reported a case study of a previously healthy 5-week-old baby admitted to hospital with a 2-day history of fever and irritability, he subsequently fitted in the emergency department. When the baby was 10 days of age his mother was given travel vaccinations including yellow fever for a holiday to Venezuela. Hospital tests showed symptoms consistent with encephalitis. His symptoms resolved following a 21-day course of aciclovir.

The CDC (Kroger 2006) recommend against vaccinating nursing mothers with yellow fever vaccine before the baby is 6 months of age. However, if travel by the nursing mother to a high-risk yellow fever endemic area cannot be avoided or postponed, the mother may be vaccinated. Exposure to yellow fever vaccine via breastmilk would not increase the risk to an infant who receives the vaccination after the age of 6 months (Plotkin and Orenstein 2004, Department of Health Green Book 2006).

Compatible with use during breastfeeding. Avoid in first 6 months unless essential.

References

Centers for Disease Control and Prevention (CDC), Transmission of yellow fever vaccine virus through breastfeeding – Brazil, 2009, *MMWR Morb Mortal Wkly Rep*, 2010;59:130–32.

Immunisation against infectious disease – 'The Green Book' – 2006 updated edition www.dh.gov.uk/en/Publicationsandstatistics/Publications/publicationsPolicyAndGuidance/DH_079917

Kroger AT, Atkinson WL, Marcuse EK, Pickering LK, Advisory Committee on Immunization Practices (ACIP) Centers for Disease Control and Prevention (CDC). General recommendations on immunization: recommendations of the Advisory Committee on Immunization Practices (ACIP), *MMWR Recomm Rep*, 2006;55(RR-15):1–48.

Kuhn S, Twele-Montecinos L, MacDonald J, Webster P, Law B,Case report: probable transmission of vaccine strain of yellow fever virus to an infant via breastmilk, *CMAJ*, 2011;183(4):E243–5.

Plotkin SA, Orenstein WA, *Vaccines 4th edition*, Philadelphia: WB Saunders, 2004 (cited in Department of Health Green Book chapter 34, 2011).

Staples JE, Gershman M, Fischer M, Centers for Disease Control and Prevention (CDC). Yellow fever vaccine: recommendations of the Advisory Committee on Immunization Practices (ACIP), *MMWR*, 2010;59 (RR-7):1–27.

Traiber C, Amaral PC, Ritter VR, Winge A, Infant meningoencephalitis probably caused by yellow fever vaccine virus transmitted via breastmilk, *J Pediatr (Rio J)*, 2011;87:269–72.

Hepatitis B vaccine

Recommended as compatible with breastfeeding by the CDC and the AAP (Kroger 2006). Breastfed infants of hepatitis B surface antigen positive mothers have a different response in the development of Ig subtypes after vaccination with hepatitis B vaccine than do formula-fed infants. However, breastfeeding does not interfere with the infant's antibody response to hepatitis B vaccine (Azarri *et al.* 1990; Wang *et al.* 2003). There is no evidence of risk from vaccinating pregnant women or those who are breastfeeding with inactivated viral or bacterial vaccines or toxoids (Plotkin and Orenstein 2004; Department of Health Green Book 2006).

Compatible with use during breastfeeding.

References

Azzari C, Resti M, Rossi ME *et al.* Modulation by human milk of IgG subclass response to hepatitis B vaccine in infants, *J Pediatr Gastroenterol Nutr*, 1990;10:310–15.

Immunisation against infectious disease – 'The Green Book' – 2006 updated edition www.dh.gov.uk/en/Publicationsandstatistics/Publications/publicationsPolicyAndGuidance/DH_079917

Kroger AT, Atkinson WL, Marcuse EK, Pickering LK, Advisory Committee on Immunization Practices (ACIP) Centers for Disease Control and Prevention (CDC). General recommendations on immunization: recommendations of the Advisory Committee on Immunization Practices (ACIP), *MMWR Recomm Rep*, 2006;55(RR-15):1–48.

Plotkin SA, Orenstein WA, *Vaccines 4th edition*, Philadelphia: WB Saunders, 2004 (cited in Department of Health Green Book chapter 34, 2011).

Wang JS, Zhu QR, Wang XH, Breastfeeding does not pose any additional risk of immunoprophylaxis failure on infants of HBV carrier mothers, *Int J Clin Pract*, 2003;57(2):100–102.

Hepatitis A vaccine

Recommended as compatible with breastfeeding by the CDC and the AAP (Kroger 2006). There is no evidence of risk from vaccinating pregnant women or those who are breastfeeding with inactivated viral or bacterial vaccines or toxoids (Plotkin and Orenstein 2004; Department of Health Green Book 2006).

Compatible with use during breastfeeding.

References

Immunisation against infectious disease – 'The Green Book' – 2006 updated edition www.dh.gov.uk/en/Publicationsandstatistics/Publications/publicationsPolicyAndGuidance/DH_079917

Kroger AT, Atkinson WL, Marcuse EK, Pickering LK, Advisory Committee on Immunization Practices (ACIP) Centers for Disease Control and Prevention (CDC). General recommendations on immunization: recommendations of the Advisory Committee on Immunization Practices (ACIP), *MMWR Recomm Rep*, 2006;55(RR-15):1–48.

Plotkin SA, Orenstein WA, *Vaccines 4th edition*, Philadelphia: WB Saunders, 2004 (cited in Department of Health Green Book chapter 17, 2011).

Cholera vaccine

Use of oral cholera vaccine to the mother decreased the risk of cholera in their breast-fed infants by 47% in one study (Clemens *et al.* 1990). The authors hypothesised that vaccination of the mothers reduced their transmission of cholera to their infants. There is no evidence of risk from vaccinating pregnant women or those who are breastfeeding with inactivated viral or bacterial vaccines or toxoids (Kroger 2006; Plotkin and Orenstein 2004; Department of Health Green Book 2006).

Compatible with use during breastfeeding.

References

Clemens JD, Sack DA, Chakraborty J, Rao MR, Ahmed F, Harris JR, van Loon F, Khan MR, Yunis M, Huda S, Field trial of oral cholera vaccines in Bangladesh: evaluation of anti-bacterial and anti-toxic breastmilk immunity in response to ingestion of the vaccines, *Vaccine*, 1990;8:469–72.

Immunisation against infectious disease – 'The Green Book' – 2006 updated edition www.dh.gov.uk/en/Publicationsandstatistics/Publications/publicationsPolicyAndGuidance/DH_079917

Kroger AT, Atkinson WL, Marcuse EK, Pickering LK, Advisory Committee on Immunization Practices (ACIP) Centers for Disease Control and Prevention (CDC). General recommendations on immunization: recommendations of the Advisory Committee on Immunization Practices (ACIP), *MMWR Recomm Rep*, 2006;55(RR-15):1–48.

Plotkin SA, Orenstein WA, *Vaccines 4th edition*, Philadelphia: WB Saunders, 2004 (cited in Department of Health Green Book chapter 34, 2011).

Polio vaccine

Two types of poliomyelitis vaccine are available: inactivated poliomyelitis vaccine (for injection in combination with diphtheria vaccine) and live (oral) poliomyelitis vaccine.

Administration of oral poliovirus vaccine to nursing infants is less effective if it is given the neonatal period, due to maternal antibodies in colostrum and breastmilk (WHO 1995; Zaman *et al.* 1991). However, breastfeeding does not interfere with the infant's response to oral polio vaccine, when given at the normal scheduled times (Kim-Farley *et al.* 1982; John *et al.* 1976). There is no evidence of risk from vaccinating pregnant women or those who are breastfeeding with inactivated viral or bacterial vaccines or toxoids according to the CDC and the AAP (Kroger *et al.* 2006) and the Department of Health Green Book (Plotkin and Orenstein 2004; Department of Health Green Book 2006).

Compatible with use during breastfeeding.

References

Immunisation against infectious disease – 'The Green Book' – 2006 updated edition www.dh.gov.uk/en/Publicationsandstatistics/Publications/publicationsPolicyAndGuidance/DH_079917

John TJ, Devarajan LV, Luther L, Vijayarathnam P, Effect of breastfeeding on seroresponse of infants to oral poliovirus vaccination, *Pediatrics*, 1976;57:47–53.

Kim-Farley R, Brink E, Orenstein W, Bart K, Vaccination and breastfeeding, *JAMA*, 1982;248:2451–2. Letter.

Kroger AT, Atkinson WL, Marcuse EK, Pickering LK, Advisory Committee on Immunization Practices (ACIP) Centers for Disease Control and Prevention (CDC). General recommendations on immunization: recommendations of the Advisory Committee on Immunization Practices (ACIP), *MMWR Recomm Rep*, 2006;55(RR-15):1–48.

Plotkin SA, Orenstein WA, *Vaccines 4th edition*, Philadelphia: WB Saunders, 2004 (cited in Department of Health Green Book chapter 34, 2011).

World Health Organization Collaborative Study Group on Oral Poliovirus Vaccine, Factors affecting the immunogenicity of oral poliovirus vaccine: a prospective evaluation in Brazil and the Gambia, *J Infect Dis*, 1995;171:1097–1106.

Zaman S, Carlsson B, Jalil F, Jeansson S, Mellander L, Hanson LA, Specific antibodies to poliovirus type I in breastmilk of unvaccinated mothers before and seven years after start of community-wide vaccination of theirinfants with live, oral poliovirus vaccine, *Acta Paediatr Scand*, 1991;80:1174–82.

Japanese encephalitis vaccine

Recommended as compatible with breastfeeding by the CDC and the AAP (Kroger 2006) and the Department of Health Green Book (2006). There is no evidence of risk from vaccinating pregnant women or those who are breastfeeding with inactivated viral or bacterial vaccines or toxoids (Plotkin and Orenstein 2004).

Compatible with use during breastfeeding.

References

Immunisation against infectious disease – 'The Green Book' – 2006 updated edition www.dh.gov.uk/en/Publicationsandstatistics/Publications/publicationsPolicyAndGuidance/DH_079917

Kroger AT, Atkinson WL, Marcuse EK, Pickering LK, Advisory Committee on Immunization Practices (ACIP) Centers for Disease Control and Prevention (CDC). General recommendations on immunization: recommendations of the Advisory Committee on Immunization Practices (ACIP), *MMWR Recomm Rep*, 2006;55(RR-15):1–48.

Plotkin SA, Orenstein WA, *Vaccines 4th edition*, Philadelphia: WB Saunders, 2004 (cited in Department of Health Green Book chapter 34, 2011).

Anaesthetics

General anaesthetics

After a caesarian delivery a mother is encouraged to breastfeed as soon as she feels able. But many women are concerned that they need to stop breastfeeding in order to have surgery or wait until the baby is older and breastfeeding has stopped. The half-life of most modern anaesthetic agents is short and although some drug is stored in body fat and released over the next few days, little is transferred to the baby. Once the mother is awake enough to be aware of the need to feed the majority of the active drug has left her system and breastfeeding can be undertaken (Lee and Rubin 1993).

Special precaution: premature babies may have difficulty in eliminating the drugs due to poor liver and kidney function. This needs to be considered on an individual basis.

Other considerations:

- If the baby is going to stay in the hospital with the mother are there adequate facilities?
- If the baby is being taken into hospital for feeds, are the ward staff aware in advance to enable suitable privacy for mother and baby bearing in mind that other patients on the ward may be more seriously ill?
- If the mother is planning to express her milk while in hospital is there an electric pump available or does she need to take in her own pump? Are there facilities to store the milk before it is taken home or will it be discarded?
- If the mother is comfortable without expressing, will she need to re-stimulate her supply once she is home again?
- If the surgery is planned in advance does the mother want to build up a supply of frozen milk for the baby to have in her absence? If this is done immediately before the operation she may develop an overabundant supply and run the risk of mastitis.

References

Lee JJ, Rubin AP, Breastfeeding and anaesthesia, *Anaesthesia*, 1993;48:616–25.

Propofol

Propofol is the most widely used intravenous anaesthetic used to induce and maintain anaesthesia in adults and children. It is associated with rapid recovery and less hang-over effect than other drugs.

Nitsun *et al.* (2006) undertook a study of five lactating women who underwent surgery involving general anaesthetic while breastfeeding. The levels of drugs entering breastmilk were deduced to be equivalent to 0.02% of the maternal weight-adjusted dosage. This level they concluded was insufficient to justify the recommendation commonly made to pump and dump breastmilk for 24 hours after anaesthesia. Mothers in the study were noted to have a reduced milk supply following surgery.

Propofol is routinely used in caesarian section surgery without waiting to initiate breastfeeding (Dailland *et al.* 1989).

Mothers are often instructed to pump to clear the milk of the sedating agent but as maternal levels fall, the drug passes back into the maternal bloodstream from breastmilk to be metabolised.

Relative infant dose quoted as 4.4% (Hale 2012 online access). The BNF states that the drug is present in breastmilk but at amounts too small to be harmful.

> Compatible with use during breastfeeding due to short half-life and poor oral bio-availability in the infant.

References

Dailland P, Cockshott ID, Lirzin JD, Jacquinot P, Jorrot JC, Devery J, Harmey JL, Conseiller C, Intravenous propofol during cesarean section: placental transfer, concentrations in breastmilk, and neonatal effects. A preliminary study, *Anesthesiology*, 1989;71:827–34.

Nitsun M, Szokol JW, Saleh HJ, Murphy GS, Vender JS, Luong L, Raikoff K, Avram MJ, Pharmacokinetics of midazolam, propofol, and fentanyl transfer to human breastmilk, *Clin Pharmacol Ther*, 2006;79(6):549–57.

Sedative and perioperative drugs

These drugs are used to reduce fear and anxiety before an operation. Benzodiazepines are widely used for this purpose as they alleviate anxiety at a dose before producing sedation and are particularly useful for short procedures.

Midazolam

Midazolam may be used for short interventions such as endoscopy, dental sedation or pre-anaesthesia. Midazolam usually has a short elimination half-life of about 2 hours. The half-life of midazolam is prolonged in neonates but it is used extensively in procedures on neonates and pre-term infants. Extensive first-pass metabolism results in a low systemic bio-availability after oral doses so levels reaching the infant's bloodstream from breastmilk can be expected to be low.

In a study of 12 women receiving 15 mg daily for up to 6 days as a hypnotic, neither midazolam nor its metabolite could be detected in breastmilk 4 hours after administration and the maximum level measured was 9 ng per ml between 1 and 2 hours after administration. (Matheson *et al.* 1990). Thus breastfeeding can be continued without interruption after use of this short-acting benzodiazepine.

Qureshi *et al.* (2005) recommended waiting for 4 hours after the use of midazolam in endoscopy procedures. However, this may not be necessary where the baby is more than 2 months of age. Koitabashi *et al.* (1997) measured the levels of midazolam and its metabolites in breastmilk following a single 6 mg intravenous dose of midazolam. After 4 hours, levels were undetectable. Lee and Rubin (1993), Sigsett (1994) and Nitsun *et al.* (2006) recommend that mothers can resume breastfeeding as soon as the mother feels recovered enough.

Relative infant dose quoted as 0.6% (Hale 2012 online access).

The BNF states that it is present in breastmilk and that the manufacturer advises interruption of breastfeeding for 24 hours.

References

Koitabashi T, Satoh N, Takino Y, Intravenous midazolam passage into breastmilk, *J Anesth*, 1997;11:242–3.

Lee JJ, Rubin AP, Breast feeding and anaesthesia, *Anaesthesia*, 1993;48:616–25.

Matheson I, Lunde PKM, Bredesen JE, Midazolam and nitrazepam in the maternity ward: milk concentrations and clinical effects, *Br J Clin Pharmacol*, 1990;30:787–93.

Nitsun M, Szokol JW, Saleh HJ, Murphy GS, Vender JS, Luong L, Raikoff K, Avram MJ, Pharmacokinetics of midazolam, propofol, and fentanyl transfer to human breastmilk, *Clin Pharmacol Ther*, 2006;79:549–57.

Qureshi WA, Rajan E, Adler DG, ASGE Guideline: Guidelines for endoscopy in pregnant and lactating women, *Gastrointest Endosc*, 2005;61:357–62.

Spigset O, Anaesthetic agents and excretion in breastmilk, *Acta Anaesthesiol Scand*, 1994;38:94–103.

Local anaesthetics

Local anaesthetics may be used in minor surgery or dental anaesthetics for fillings or extractions. Anaesthesia is maintained very close to the site of the injection and such injections can be used without difficulty during breastfeeding.

Lidocaine

Little of this drug is available for systemic absorption due to its poor bio-availability, so little passes into breastmilk. The compatibility with breastfeeding is confirmed by a case report of a mother undergoing dental work (Lebedevs *et al.* 1993) where the level in milk was measured as 55 to 66 µg per litre and the dose received by the baby calculated as 0.01 mg per kg. The authors concluded that, with the exception of rare allergic reactions, the levels were clinically insignificant and that breastfeeding mothers could receive lidocaine (lignocine) for routine dental procedures without the need to interrupt breastfeeding. These results were confirmed by Giuliani *et al.* (2001) who studied seven women undergoing dental procedures. Relative infant dose quoted as 0.5 to 3.1% (Hale 2012 online access).

The BNF states that the amount in breastmilk is too small to be harmful.

This may be extended to other minor surgical procedures involving local anaesthetic e.g. bupivacaine, levobupivacaine, prilocaine and ropivacaine.

Compatible with use during breastfeeding because it is poorly bio-available.

References

Giuliani M, Grossi GB, Pileri M, Lajolo C, Casparrini G, Could local anesthesia while breastfeeding be harmful to infants?, *J Pediatric Gastroenterol Nutr*, 2001;32:142–4.

Lebedevs TH, Wojnar-Horton RE, Yapp P, Roberts MJ, Dusci LJ, Hackett LP, Ilett K, Excretion of lignocaine and its metabolite monoethylglycinexylidide in breastmilk following its use in a dental procedure. A case report, *J Clin Peridontol*, 1993;20:606–8.

Homeopathic remedies

Homeopathy is based on the principle that 'like treats like' so that symptoms are treated with a remedy which would cause similar symptoms in a healthy person at a 'normal' dose. Homeopathic remedies are highly diluted, which are claimed to be virtually 100% safe. Prescribing a remedy is based on all aspects of a patient's condition including the patient's personality and lifestyle. Homeopathic remedies utilise minute quantities of medication and are used to treat children as well as adults. Although there appears to be little published literature, most practitioners do not appear to deter lactating mothers from using homeopathic remedies.

> Likely to be compatible with use during breastfeeding but consult homeopathic practitioner.

Caffeine

Caffeine occurs naturally in many foods and drinks.

TABLE 7.1 Caffeine content of selected products

Product	Caffeine content (mg)
Coffee (per mug)	
Instant	100
Percolated ground/filter	140
Tea (per mug)	75
One can of energy drink	Up to 80
50 g chocolate bar	
Plain	Up to 50
Milk	Up to 25
Cola drink per 354 ml can	40

Caffeine acts as a stimulant to the heart and central nervous system. Pregnant women are advised to limit caffeine intake to less than 300 mg per day ((NHS Your Health in Pregnancy 2012). Peak levels appear in breastmilk one to two hours after ingestion. Some babies anecdotally appear to be particularly sensitive to caffeine consumed by their mother and appear to be irritable, fussy and restless. While the half-life in adults is 4.9 hours it may be as long as 97.5 hours in neonates, although this decreases to 14 hours by 3 to 5 months. A baby who appears restless may benefit from lowered caffeine intake by the mother but for the average consumption there is little evidence to support restricting intake.

In a case report in an article by Rivera-Calimlim *et al.* (1977), a 6-week-old breast-fed infant was noted to be jittery. His mother drank 4 to 5 cups of coffee and 2 to 3 litre bottles of cola daily as well as occasional tea and cocoa. The baby was gaining weight, but was observed to be trembling and have increased muscle tone. The infant's symptoms decreased 2 weeks after his mother stopped all caffeine-containing beverages.

Ryu *et al.* (1995) studied nine lactating women and their infants for 9 days. For the first 5 days, the women ingested 750 mg of caffeine daily in the form of 5 cups of coffee, and for the next 4 days they ingested no caffeine and avoided coffee and other caffeine-containing products. The concentration of caffeine in samples of milk on day 5 ranged from non-detectable (less than 0.25 µg per ml) to 15.7 µg per ml. No caffeine was detected in milk samples obtained on day 9. The mean concentration of caffeine in the blood of infants on day 5 ranged from non-detectable to 2.8 µg per ml. Caffeine was still detectable in two infants' sera at the end of the study period. The authors estimated that at this caffeine intake, infants would receive 0.6 to 0.8 mg per kg daily.

Muñoz *et al.* (1988) studied two groups of 48 low-income Costa Rican women who either drank coffee or did not, throughout pregnancy and into lactation. She noted that cord blood haemoglobin, infant birthweight and haemoglobin at 1 month of age, and breastmilk concentration of iron was significantly lower in the coffee group, than in the non-coffee group (equivalent to 3 cups of coffee per day). Whether this conclusion is applicable to well-nourished, Caucasian women is unclear.

Santos *et al.* (2012) studied a sub-sample of babies born during 2004 in Brazil looking at infant sleep pattern in the previous 15 days. The aim of the study was to investigate if maternal caffeine consumption during pregnancy and lactation leads to frequent nocturnal awakening among infants at 3 months of age. Of all babies, 13.8% woke more than 3 times a night sufficient to wake the parents. The highest rate was seen in mothers who consumed more than 300 mg caffeine but the results did not reach significance. The conclusion of the authors was that caffeine consumption during pregnancy and by nursing mothers seems not to have consequences on sleep of infants at the age of 3 months.

Women who drink a significant amount of caffeinated drinks who notice that their babies are jittery and restless may find reduction in caffeine consumption leads to resolution of symptoms. This does not mean that all breastfeeding women need to restrict their consumption of tea and coffee.

Relative infant dose quoted as 6 to 25.9% (Hale 2012 online access).

Compatible with use during breastfeeding up to 300 mg per day, but avoid excessive consumption.

References

Muñoz LM, Lonnerdal B, Keen CL, Dewey KG, Coffee consumption as a factor in iron deficiency anemia among pregnant women and their infants in Costa Rica, *Am J Clin Nutr*, 1988;48:645–51.

NHS, Your Health in Pregnancy, 2012.

Rivera-Calimlim L, Drugs in breastmilk, *Drug Ther*, 1977;7:59–6.

Ryu JE, Caffeine in human milk and in serum of breastfed infants, *Dev Pharmacol Ther*, 1985;8:329–37.

Santos IS, Matijasevich A, Domingues MR, Maternal caffeine consumption and infant night-time waking prospective cohort study, *Pediatrics*, 2012;129:860–68.

Conclusion

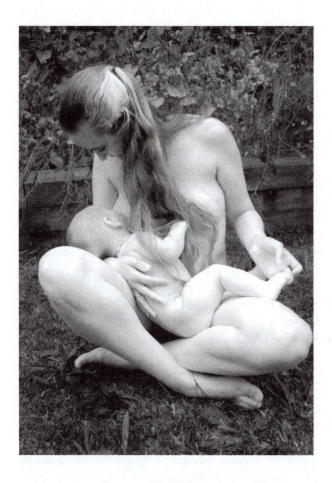

We know that breastfeeding has a multitude of advantages for mother and baby. By having an understanding of how breastfeeding works from a hormonal and physical point of view we are in a better position to intervene with mothers who are experiencing problems. That may be best achieved by signposting them to others with more experience. We can support and encourage the decision to breastfeed. We can empower women who initially choose to breastfeed their baby to continue to do so until they choose to stop breastfeeding and to wean appropriately.

We need to encourage breastfeeding as a social norm in the groups who have in the past chosen to not breastfeed. It has been shown that peer supporters (women in an area who have been given training to support other local mothers) and the availability of breastfeeding drop-in groups encourages women to begin breastfeeding and to continue for longer. Women may report feeling uncomfortable about breastfeeding in public but, in fact, few will ever encounter problems.

The dilemma remains that there is insufficient readily available data, in standard reference books, on the safety of drugs in breastmilk. Prescribing medication during lactation is almost invariably outside of the license application. This does not imply that such use is dangerous, merely that the manufacturers have neither undertaken studies nor been required to add data to the summary of product characteristics.

In order to prescribe, counter-prescribe and dispense prescriptions for mothers who are lactating, we need to exercise professional judgement in assessing the potential risk for any individual mother and baby pair. The decision depends on the age of the baby, the volume of milk being consumed, the mother's need for medication and the potential risk of interrupting breastfeeding even temporarily.

We need to bear in mind the statement from the NICE Maternal and Child Nutrition guidelines (NICE PH11 2008):

- Ensure health professionals and pharmacists who prescribe or dispense drugs to a breastfeeding mother consult supplementary sources.
- Health professionals should discuss the benefits and risks associated with the prescribed medication and encourage the mother to continue breastfeeding, if reasonable to do so. In most cases, it should be possible to identify a suitable medication which is safe to take during breastfeeding by analysing pharmacokinetic and study data.
- Health professionals should recognise that there may be adverse health consequences for both mother and baby if the mother does not breastfeed. They should also recognise that it may not be easy for the mother to stop breastfeeding abruptly – and that it is difficult to reverse.

This book aims to enable healthcare professionals to evaluate safety data and make informed decisions on the best way to treat breastfeeding mothers who need medication and to deal with problems that may relate to the lactation itself. Mothers will be provided with consistent health-promotion messages if we work as a multi-disciplinary team.

Breastfeeding could be said to have the greatest impact on health of any decision we make as parents or advice given as healthcare professionals.

Mimicking human breast milk is virtually impossible. Multiple, expensive medications are needed to relieve the symptoms of asthma, cardiovascular disease, gastro-intestinal conditions and infections. Should we as healthcare professionals not just support but actively promote a process which has so many research based benefits in preventing these conditions?

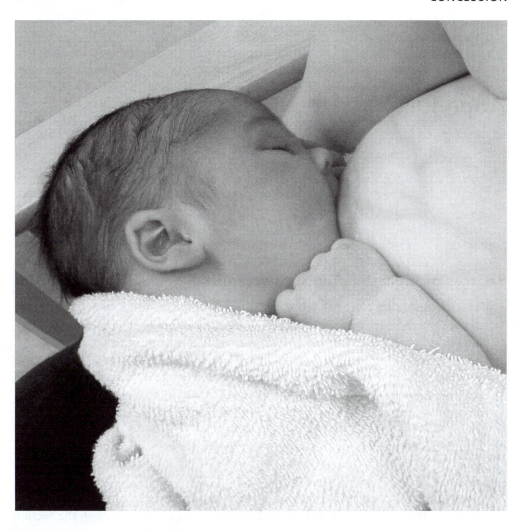

Breastmilk is free at the point of need, available in the right quantity, at the right temperature with the recipient's requirements catered for exactly. What drug could approach that specification?

Promote, Protect and Support Breastfeeding

Appendix

Sources of breastfeeding support in UK

- **The Breastfeeding Network (BfN)** aims to be an independent source of support and information for breastfeeding women and those involved in their care.
Supporterline 0300 100 0210; www.breastfeedingnetwork.org.uk/
- The **National Childbirth Trust (NCT)** is a parental support organisation, which provides accurate, impartial information to enable parents to decide what is best for their family. The NCT also introduces parents to a local network of others to gain practical and emotional support.
Helpline 0300 330 0700; www.nct.org.uk/
- The **Association of Breastfeeding Mothers (ABM)** is a voluntary organisation founded in 1979 by a group of mothers experienced in breastfeeding counselling.
Helpline 0844 122 949; http://abm.me.uk/
- The **National Breastfeeding Helpline** is run in collaboration with the ABM and the BfN. The project is funded by the Department of Health, through the Section 64 grant scheme. Calls are forwarded to the nearest ABM counsellor or BfN supporter. The staff have been trained to provide women with good evidence-based breastfeeding information.
Helpline 0300 100 0212; http://breastfeedingnetwork.org.uk/national-breastfeeding-helpline
- **La Leche League GB** provides friendly mother-to-mother breastfeeding support from pregnancy through to weaning.
Helpline 0845 120 2918; www.laleche.org.uk/index.htm
- **Lactation Consultants of Great Britain (LCGB)** is an association for those with the International Board Certified Lactation Consultant (IBCLC) qualification. It specialises in promoting, protecting and supporting breastfeeding and lactation matters. LCGB is an affiliate member of International Lactation Consultants Association (ILCA).
www.lcgb.org/index.html

Useful websites

LactMed http://toxnet.nlm.nih.gov/cgi-bin/sis/htmlgen?LACT
Motherisk www.motherisk.org/women/index.jsp
InfantRisk www.infantrisk.com/
Medications and Mothers' Milk (paid access) www.medsmilk.com/
Baby Friendly Initiative UK www.unicef.org.uk/
United Kingdom Association for Milk Banking www.ukamb.org/
Best Beginnings www.bestbeginnings.org.uk/
National Electronic Library for Medicines NHS www.nelm.nhs.uk/en
US National Library of Medicine, National Institutes of Health (PubMed)
    www.ncbi.nlm.nih.gov/pubmed

References

Acheson Report 1998 (www.archive.official-documents.co.uk/document/doh/ih/ih.htm).

Ahmed SR, Ellah MAA, Mohamed OA, Eidet HM, Prepregnancy Obesity and Pregnancy Outcome, *Int J Health Sci (Qassim)*, 2009;3(2):203–8.

Akre J, Infant feeding the physiological basis, *Bull World Health Organ*, 1989;67 Suppl.:1–108.

Alexander JA, Cambell MJ, Prevalence of inverted and non protractile nipples in antenatal women who intend to breastfeed, *Breast J*, 1997;6(2):72–8.

Alexander JA, Grant AM, Campbell MJ, Randomised controlled trial of breast shells and Hoffman's exercises for inverted and non-protractile nipples, *BMJ*, 1992;304(6833):1030–32.

Alves JG, Figueiroa JN, Meneses J, Alves GV, Breastfeeding protects against type 1 diabetes mellitus: a case-sibling study, *Breastfeed Med*, 2012;7(1):25–8.

Amir LH, Pirotta M, Raval M, Breastfeeding: Evidence based guidelines for the use of medicines, *Aust Fam Physician*, 2011;40:9.

Anderson PO, Pochop SL, Manoguerra AS, Adverse drug reactions in breastfed infants: less than imagined, *Clin Pediatr (Phila)*, 2003;42(4):325–40.

Aniansson G, Alm B, Andersson B, Håkansson A, Larsson P, Nylén O, Peterson H, Rignér P, Svanborg M, Sabharwal H, A prospective cohort study on breast feeding and otitis media in Swedish infants, *Pediatr Infect Dis J*, 1994;13:183–8.

Arenz S, Ruckeri R, Koletzko B, von Kries R, Breastfeeding and Childhood obesity: a systematic review, *Int J Obes (Lond)*, 2004;28:1247–56.

Australian Institute of Family Studies (AIFS) 2008 (http://www.growingupinaustralia.gov.au/pubs/ar/ar200607/breastfeeding).

Australian National Breastfeeding Strategy 2010–2015 (www.health.gov.au/internet/main/publishing.nsf/Content/aust-breastfeeding-strategy-2010-2015).

Australian National Infant Feeding Survey: Indicator results 2010 (http://aihw.gov.au/media-release-detail/?id=10737420970).

Bachrach VR, Schwarz E, Bachrach LR, Breastfeeding and the risk of hospitalization for respiratory disease in infancy, *Arch Pediatr Adolesc Med*, 2003;157:237–43.

Ball TM, Wright AL, Health care costs of formula-feeding in the first year of life, *Pediatrics,*1999;103:870–76.

Ballard JL, Auer CE, Khoury JC, Ankyloglossia: assessment, incidence, and effect of frenuloplasty on the breastfeeding dyad, *Pediatrics 2002;*110:e63.

Balon AJ, Management of infantile colic, *Am Fam Physician*, 1997;55(1):235–42, 245–6.

Bandolier, Infant colic update, 2004 (www.medicine.ox.ac.uk/bandolier/booth/family/colicup.html)

Bandolier, Treatments for infant colic, 2000 (www.medicine.ox.ac.uk/bandolier/band79/b79-4.html).

Baron JA, Cigarette smoking and prolactin in women, *BMJ*, 1986;293:482.

Barr RG, Colic and gas. In: Walker WA, Durie PR, Hamilton JR, (eds), *Pediatric gastro-intestinal disease: pathophysiology, diagnosis and management*, Philadelphia: Decker, 1991;55–61.

Belch JJ, Shaw B, O'Dowd A, Saniabadi A, Leiberman P, Sturrock RD, Forbes CD, Evening primrose oil (Efamol) in the treatment of Raynaud's phenomenon: A double-blind study, *Throm Haemost*, 1985;54 (2):490–4.

Bolling K, Grant C, Hamlyn B, Thornton A, *Infant Feeding Survey 2005*, Office National Statistics 2007 (www.ic.nhs.uk/pubs/ifs2005).

Breastfeeding Report Card 2011, United States: Outcome Indicators (www.cdc.gov).

Breastfeeding Scotland Bill 2005 (www.legislation.gov.uk/asp/2005/1/content).

British Association for Counselling & Psychotherapy, 2012 (www.bacp.co.uk).

British National Formulary (BNF) Joint Formulary Committee, London: Pharmaceutical Press (www.bnf.org).

British Nutrition Foundation, *Nutrition and Pregnancy*, 2006.

Burr ML, Miskelly FG, Butland BK, Environmental factors and symptoms in infants at high risk of allergy, *J Epidemiol Community Health*, 1989;43:125–32.

Cardelli MB, Raynaud's phenomenon and disease, *Med Clin North Am*, 1989;73(5):1127–41.

CDC National Immunization Survey, 2011 (www.cdc.gov/breastfeeding/data/NIS_data/index.htm).

Centre for Maternal and Child Enquiries, Saving Mothers' Lives Report, 2011 (www.oaa-anaes.ac.uk/assets/_managed/editor/File/Reports/2006-2008%20CEMD.pdf)

Child Health Promotion Programme: Pregnancy and the first five years of life, Department of Health 2008 (www.dh.gov.uk/en/Publicationsandstatistics/Publications/DH_089044).

Clinical Knowledge Summary, Mastitis and breast abscess, 2010 (www.cks.nhs.uk/mastitis_and_breast_abscess#-417660).

Clinical Knowledge Summary, Breastfeeding problems, 2011 (www.cks.nhs.uk/breastfeeding_problems/management/scenario_nipple_soreness_management#-468751?-420413).

CMO update 37 soya milk (infant formula), 2007 (www.dh.gov.uk/en/Publichealth/Nutrition/Nutritionpregnancyearlyyears/DH_127640).

Coates M, Nipple pain related to vasospasm, *J Hum Lact*, 1992;8(3):153.

Codex Alimentarius, COC 2007 Codex standard for infant formula and formulas for special medical purposes intended for infants (www.codexalimentarius.org/).

Cooper A, Structure of the breast in the human female, 1840 (http://jdc.jefferson.edu/cgi/viewcontent.cgi?article=1006&context=cooper).

Croke S, Buist, Hackett LP, Ilett KF, Norman TR, Burrows GD, Olanzapine excretion in human breast milk: estimation of infant exposure, *Int J Neuropsychopharmacol*, 2003;5:243–7.

De Vries TW, Wewerinke ME, de Langen JJ, Near asphyxiation of a neonate due to miconazole oral gel, *Ned Tijschr Geneeskd*, 2006;148:1598–1600.

Department of Health, Alcohol advice, 2011 (www.dh.gov.uk/en/Publichealth/Alcoholmisuse/DH_125368).

Department of Health, Breastfeeding: good practice guidance to the NHS, National Breastfeeding Working Group, 1995.

Department of Health, Folic acid and the prevention of disease: report of the Committee on Medical Aspects of Food and Nutrition Policy, 2000 (www.dh.gov.uk/en/Publicationsandstatistics/Publications/PublicationsPolicyAndGuidance/DH_4005805).

Department of Health, Healthy Lives, Healthy People: Improving outcomes and supporting transparency, 2012 (www.dh.gov.uk/prod_consum_dh/groups/dh_digitalassets/@dh/@en/documents/digitalasset/dh_132360.pdf) P97 added as ref

Department of Health, Infant formula, 2011 (www.dh.gov.uk/en/Publichealth/Nutrition/Nutritionpregnancyearlyyears/DH_127640).

REFERENCES

Department of Health, Nystatin – Prescribing off-label, **2010** (www.dh.gov.uk/en/Healthcare/Medicinespharmacyandindustry/Prescriptions/TheNon-MedicalPrescribingProgramme/Nurseprescribing/DH_4123003#_2)

Department of Health, Risk assessment for venous thromboembolism, 1992 (www.dh.gov.uk/prod_consum_dh/groups/dh_digitalassets/@dh/@en/@ps/documents/digitalasset/dh_113355.pdf 1992).

Department of Health, Smokefree, 2012 (http://smokefree.nhs.uk/smoking-and-pregnancy/just-the-facts/).

Department of Health, Thinking of having a baby: Folic acid – an essential ingredient in making babies, 2004 (www.dh.gov.uk/en/Publicationsandstatistics/Publications/PublicationsPolicyAndGuidance/DH_4081396).

Department of Health, Vitamin D: an essential nutrient for all … but who is at risk of vitamin D deficiency? Important information for healthcare professionals, 2010 (www.nutrition.org.uk/publications/bulletin/nutritionandpregnancy).

DeRosa G, Prolactin secretion after beer, *Lancet*, 1981;2:934.

DiGiacomo RA, Fish oil supplementation in patients with Raynaud's Phenomenon: a double blind, controlled, perspective study, *Am J Med*, 1989;86:158–64.

Dixon M, Khan LR, Treatment of breast infection, *BMJ*, 2011;342:484–9.

Duncan B, Ey J, Holberg CJ, Wright AL, Martinez FD, Taussig LM, Exclusive breast feeding for at least 4 months protects against otitis media, *Pediatrics*, 1993;5:867–72.

Dvorak B, Fituch CC, Williams CS, Hurst NM, Schanler RJ, Increased epidermal growth factor levels in human milk of mothers with extremely premature infants, *Pediatr Res*, 2003;54(1):15–19.

Equality Act 2010 (www.legislation.gov.uk/ukpga/2010/15/contents).

Fewtrell MS, The long term benefits of having been breastfed, *Curr Paed*, 2004;14:97–103.

Food Standards Agency, Folic acid fortification, 2007 (www.food.gov.uk/scotland/scotnut/folic-fortification; www.food.gov.uk/multimedia/pdfs/fsa070604.pdf).

Forsyth S, Nutritional Health Inequalities in children: Do they matter? (www.thpc.scot.nhs.uk/Presentations/Stewart%20Forsyth.pps).

Foster K, Loder D, Cheesborough S, *Infant Feeding Survey 1995*, Social Survey Division of the Office for National Statistics, London: HM Stationery Office, 1997.

Friedman SH, Rosenthal MB, Treatment of perinatal delusional disorder: a case report, *Int J Psychiatry Med*, 2003;33(4):391–4.

Frost BL, Jilling T, Caplan MS, The importance of pro-inflammatory signalling in neonatal NEC, *Semin Perinatol*, 2008;32(2):100–106.

Gardiner SJ, Kristensen JH, Begg EJ, Hackett LP, Wilson DA, Ilett KF, Kohan R, Rampono J, Transfer of olanzapine in to breast milk, calculation of infant drug dose, and effect on breast-fed infants, *Am J Psychiatry*, 2003;160:1428–31.

Garrison C, Nipple Vasospasm, Raynaud's phenomenon and nifedipine, *J Hum Lact*, 2002;18:382.

Garrison MM, Christakis DA, A systematic review of treatments for infant colic, *Pediatrics*, 2000;106(Suppl.):184–90.

Gartner LM, Greer FR, Section on Breastfeeding and Committee on Nutrition. Prevention of Rickets and Vitamin D Deficiency: New Guidelines for Vitamin D Intake (Revised 2008), *Pediatrics*, 2003;111(4):908–10.

Geddes DT, Langton DB, Gollow I, Jacobs LA, Hartmann PE, Simmer K, Frenulotomy for breastfeeding infants with ankyloglossia: effect on milk removal and sucking mechanism as imaged by ultrasound, *Pediatrics*, 2008;122:188–94.

General Recommendations on Immunization: Recommendations From the Advisory Committee on Immunization Practices, *Pediatrics*, 2007;119(5):1008.

Gillman MW, Rifas-Shiman SL, Camargo CA Jr, Berkey CS, Frazier AL, Rockett HR, Field AE, Colditz GA, Risk of overweight among adolescents who were breastfed as infants, *JAMA*, 2001;285:2461–7.

Goldstein DJ, Corbin LA, Wohlreich K, Kwong K, Olanzapine use during breast-feeding, *Schizophr Res*, 2002; 53(3 Suppl. 1):185.

Griffiths DM, Do tongue ties affect breastfeeding?, *J Hum Lact*, 2004;20(4):409–14.

Gunderson EP, Jacobs DR, Chiang V, Lewis CE, Feng J, Quesenberry CP, Stephen Sidney S, Duration of lactation and incidence of the metabolic syndrome in women of reproductive age according to gestational diabetes mellitus status: a 20-Year prospective study in CARDIA (Coronary Artery Risk Development in Young Adults), *Diabetes*, 2010;59(2):495–504.

Hale TW, Hartmann P, Textbook of Human Lactation, Amarillo, Texas: Hale Publishing LP, 2008.

Hale TW, Kristensen JH, Ilett KF, The transfer of medications into human milk. In: Textbook of Human Lactation, Hale TW, Hartmann PE (eds), Amarillo, Texas: Hale Publishing, LP, 2007.

Hale TW, Bateman TL, Finkelman MA, Berens PD, The absence of *Candida albicans* in milk samples of women with clinical symptoms of ductal candidiasis, *Breastfeed Med*, 2009;4(2):57–61.

Hale TW, *Medications and Mothers' Milk 14th Edition*, Hale Publishing LP, 2010.

Hale TW, *Medications and Mothers' Milk 15th Edition*, Hale Publishing LP, 2012.

Hamlyn B, Brooker S, Oleinikova K, Wands S, Infant Feeding 2000, Office National Statistics 2002 (www.dh.gov.uk/en/Publicationsandstatistics/Publications/PublicationsStatistics/DH_4079223).

Healthy Lifestyle in Pregnancy, Folic acid, 2007 (www.food.gov.uk/multimedia/pdfs/health-lifepregnany.pdf).

Healthy lives, healthy people: our strategy for public health in England, 2011 (www.dh.gov.uk/en/Publicationsandstatistics/Publications/PublicationsPolicyAndGuidance/DH_121941).

Healthy People – Improving the Health of Americans, 2020 (www.healthypeople.gov/2020/default.aspx).

Healthy Start 2012 (www.healthystart.nhs.uk).

Healthy weight, healthy lives: a cross-government strategy for England, 2008 (www.dh.gov.uk/en/Publicationsandstatistics/Publications/PublicationsPolicyAndGuidance/DH_082378).

Henderson L, Irving K, Gregory J, Swan G, The National Diet and Nutrition Survey: adults aged 19 to 64 years. Vol 3. Vitamin and mineral intake and urinary analytes, London: HM Stationery Office, 2003:1–160.

Hodinott P, Tappin D, Wright C, Breastfeeding: Clinical Review, *BMJ*, 2008;336:881–7.

Hogan M, Westcott C, Griffiths M, Randomised controlled division of tongue tie infants with breastfeeding problems, *J Paediatric Child Health*, 2005;41(5–6):246–50.

Holmen L, Backe B, Underdiagnosed cause of nipple pain presented on a camera phone, *BMJ*, 2009;339:b2553.

Hoppe JE, Hahn H, Randomized comparison of two nystatin oral gels with miconazole oral gel for treatment of oral thrush in infants, Antimycotics Study Group, *Infection*, 1996;24(2):136–9.

Hoppe JE, Treatment of oropharyngeal candidiasis in immunocompetent infants: a randomised multicenter study of miconazole gel vs. nystatin suspension. The Antifungals Study Group, *Pediatr Infect Dis J*, 1997;16(3):288–93.

Horta BL, Bahl R, Martines JC, Victora CG, Evidence of the long-term effects of breastfeeding, Geneva: WHO, 2007 (http://whqlibdoc.who.int/publications/2007/9789241595230_eng.pdf.).

Host A, Importance of the first meal on the development of cow's milk allergy and intolerance, *Allerg Proc*, 1991;12(4):227–32.

House of Commons Hansard Written Answers 24 June 2009m (www.publications.parliament.uk/pa/cm200809/cmhansrd/cm090624/text/90624w0031.htm).

Howie PW, Forsyth JS, Ogston SA, Clark A, Florey CD, Protective effect of breastfeeding against infection, *Br Med J*, 1990;300:11–16.

REFERENCES

Inch S, Antenatal preparation for breastfeeding in Chalmers *et al*. Effective care in pregnancy and childbirth, Oxford University Press, 1989:335–42.

Inch S, Fisher C, Mastitis: infection or inflammation?, *The Practitioner*, 1995;239:472–6.

Ip S, Chung M, Raman G, Chew P, Magula N, DeVine D, Trikalinos T, Lau J, Breastfeeding and maternal and infant health outcomes in developed countries, Agency for Healthcare Research and Quality (AHRQ), *Evid Rep Technol Assess (Full Rep)*, 2007;(153):1–186.

Ito S, Koren G, Einarson TR, Maternal noncompliance with antibiotics during breastfeeding, *Ann Pharmacother*, 1993;27(1):40–42.

Jack Newman Vasospasm, 2012 (www.drjacknewman.com/help/Vasospasm%20and%20 Raynaud%E2%80%99s%20Phenomenon.asp).

Jamieson L, Educating for successful breastfeeding, *Br J Midwifery*, 1995;3(10):535–9.

Jasper JD, Goel R, Einarson A, Gallo M, Koren G, Effects of framing on teratogenic risk perception in pregnant women, *Lancet*, 2001;358(9289):1237–8.

Jayawickrama HS, Amir LH, Pirotta MV, GPs' decision-making when prescribing medicines for breastfeeding women: Content analysis of a survey, *BMC Res Notes*, 2010;3:82

Johnson B, *Polarity management: identifying and managing unsolvable problems*, Amherst: HRD Press, 1996.

Jones W, *The role of pharmacists in supporting breastfeeding mothers who require medication during lactation*, PhD thesis, University of Portsmouth 2000.

Kanabar D, Randhawa M, Clayton P, Improvement of symptoms in infant colic following reduction of lactose load with lactase, *J Hum Nutr Diet*, 2001;14:359–63.

Kaufman D, Boyle R, Hazen KC, Patrie, JT, Robinson MS, Donowitz LG, Fluconazole prophylaxis against fungal infection in preterm infants, *N Engl J Med*, 2001;345:1660–66.

Kearns GL, McConnell RF Jr, Trang JM, Kluza RB, Appearance of ranitidine in breast milk following multiple dosing, *Clin Pharm*, 1985;4(3):322–4.

Kirchheiner J, Berghofer A, Bolk-Weischedel D, Healthy outcome under olanzapine treatment in a pregnant woman, *Pharmacopsychiatry*, 2000;33:78–80.

Klement E, Cohen RV, Boxman J, Joseph A, Reif S, Breastfeeding and risk of inflammatory bowel disease: a systematic review with meta-analysis, *Am J Clin Nutr*, 2004;80(5):1342–52.

Kramer MS, Guo T, Platt RW, Sevkovskaya Z, Dzikovich I, Collet JP, Shapiro S, Chalmers B, Hodnett E, Vanilovich I, Mezen I, Ducruet T, Shishko G, Bogdanovich N, Infant growth and health outcomes associated with 3 compared with 6 months of exclusive breastfeeding, *Am J Clin Nutr*, 2003;78(2):291–5.

Kwan ML, Buffler PA, Abrams B, Kiley VA, Breastfeeding and the risk of childhood leukaemia. A meta-analysis, *Public Health Rep*, 2004;119:521–35.

LactMed (Drugs and Lactation Database), (http://toxnet.nlm.nih.gov/cgi-bin/sis/htmlgen).

Lagoy CT, Joshi N, Cragan JD, Rasmussen SA, Medication use during pregnancy and lactation: an urgent call for public health action, *J Womens Health (Larchmt)*, 2005;14:104–9.

Lawlor-Smith L, Lawlor-Smith C, Vasospasm of the nipple: a manifestation of Raynaud's Phenomenon: case reports, *BMJ*, 1997;324:644.

Lawrence R, *Breastfeeding: A Guide for the Medical Profession 6th ed.*, St Louis: Mosby, 2005.

Leppert J, Aberg H, Levin K, Ringqvist I, Jonason T, The concentration of magnesium in erythrocytes in female patients with primary Raynaud's phenomenon; fluctuation with the time of year, *Angiology*, 1994;45:283–8.

Li R, Fein SB, Grummer-Strawn LM, Do infants fed from bottles lack self-regulation of milk intake compared with directly breastfed infants?, *Pediatrics*, 2010;125(6):e1386–93.

Liu B, Jorm L, Banks E, Parity, Breastfeeding and the Subsequent Risk of maternal Type 2 diabetes, *Diabetes Care*, 2010;33(6):1239–41.

Livingstone VH, Willis CE, Berkowitz J, *Staphylococcus aureus* and sore nipples, *Can Fam Physician*, 1996;42:654–9.

Lucas A, Brooke OG, Morley R, Cole TJ, Bamford MF, Early diet of preterm infants and development of allergic or atopic disease: Randomised prospective study, *BMJ*, 1990;300:837–40.

Lucassen PL, Assendelft WJ, Gubbels JW, van Eijk JT, Douwes AC, Infantile colic: crying time reduction with a whey hydrolysate: A double-blind, randomized, placebo-controlled trial, *Pediatrics*, 2000;106(6):1349–54.

Lucassen PLBJ, Assendelft WJJ, Gubbels JW, van Eijk JTM, van Geldrop WJ, Knuistingh Neven A, Effectiveness of treatments for infantile colic: systematic review, *BMJ*, 1998;316:1563–9.

Marild S, Hansson S, Jodal U, Odén A, Svedberg K, Protective effect of breastfeeding against urinary tract infection, *Acta Paediatr*, 2004;93(2):164–8.

Martin RM, Gunnell D, Smith GD, Breastfeeding in infancy and blood pressure in later life: systematic review and meta-analysis, *Am J Epidemiology*, 2005;161:15–26.

Martindale: the Complete Drug Reference 35th edition, London: Pharmaceutical Press, 2007.

Mayer EJ, Hamman RF, Gay EC, Lezotte DC, Savitz DA, Klingensmith GJ, Reduced risk of IDDM among breast-fed children. The Colorado IDDM Registry, *Diabetes*, 1988;37:1625–32.

McFadden A, Toole G, Exploring women's views of breastfeeding: a focus group study within an area with high levels of socio-economic deprivation, *Matern Child Nutr*, 2006;2:156–68.

McFadden A, Renfrew MJ, Dykes F, Burt S, Assessing learning needs for breastfeeding: setting the scene, *Matern Child Nutr*, 2006;2(4):196–203.

McGavock H, *How Drugs Work: Basic Pharmacology for Healthcare Professionals*, *revised edition*, Radcliffe Publishing Ltd, 2005.

McVea KL, Turner PD, Peppler DK, The role of breastfeeding in sudden infant death syndrome, *J Hum Lact*, 2000;16(1):13–20.

Metcalf TJ, Irons TG, Sher LD, Young PC, Simethicone in the treatment of infant colic: a randomized, placebo-controlled, multicenter trial, *Pediatrics*, 1994;94:29–34.

Mohrbacher N, Stock J, LA Leche League International, *The Breastfeeding Answer Book 3rd edition*, La Leche League International Book, 2000.

National Breastfeeding Helpline (www.breastfeedingnetwork.org.uk/national-breastfeeding-helpline*)*.

National Childbirth Trust, What's in a nappy?, *(www.nctshop.co.uk/professional/NCT-Information-sheet-Whats-in-a-nappy/productinfo/3213/)*.

NHS Choices, Why do I need folic acid?, 2011 (www.nhs.uk/chq/Pages/913.aspx?CategoryID=54&SubCategoryID=129).

NHS Choices, Can I drink Alcohol if I'm pregnant?, 2010 (www.nhs.uk/chq/Pages/2270.aspx?CategoryID=54&SubCategoryID=130). add after DOH 2011 under alcohol in pregnancy section

NHS Payment by Results 2010–11 National Tariff Information (http://data.gov.uk/dataset/payment-by-results-2010-11-national-tariff-information).

NHS The Information Centre, Infant Feeding Survey 2010: Early Results, 2011 (www.ic.nhs.uk/webfiles/publications/003_Health_Lifestyles/IFS_2010_early_results/IFS_2010_headline_report_tables2.pdf).

NICE Division of ankyloglossia (tongue-tie) for breastfeeding (IPG 149), 2005 (http://guidance.nice.org.uk/IPG149/PublicInfo/pdf/English).

NICE Postnatal Care Guidelines, 2006 (http://guidance.nice.org.uk/CG37/CostReport/doc/English).

NICE Postnatal Care Guidelines CG37 2006 (www.nice.org.uk guideline 37).

NICE Maternal and Child Nutrition, Improving the nutrition of pregnant and breastfeeding mothers and children in low-income households, 2008 (www.guidance.nice.org.uk/PH11).

NICE PH11 Maternal and Child Nutrition, Promotion of breastfeeding initiation and duration. Evidence into practice briefing, 2008 (www.nice.org.uk/niceMedia/pdf/EAB_Breastfeeding_final_version.pdf).

NICE PH27, Weight management before, during and after pregnancy, 2010 (www.nice.org.uk/PH27).

NICE CG 62 Antenatal care: Routine care for the healthy pregnant woman, 2008 http://guidance.nice.org.uk/CG62/NiceGuidance/pdf/English).

REFERENCES

NICE Donor Breastmilk Banks CG 93 2010 (http://guidance.nice.org.uk/CG93/Guidance).

NICE Food allergy in children and young people CG 116, 2011 (http://guidance.nice.org.uk/CG116/Guidance).

NICE guideline CG45 Antenatal and post natal mental health (http://guidance.nice.org.uk/CG45).

NICE PH10 Smoking Cessation services 2008 (http://guidance.nice.org.uk/PH10/Guidance/pdf/English).

Oddy WH, Holt PG, Sly PD, Read AW, Landau LI, Stanley FJ, Kendall GE, Burton PR, Association between breastfeeding and asthma in 6 year old children: findings of a prospective birth cohort study, *BMJ*, 1999;319:815?19.

Off to the Best Start, 2007 (www.nhs.uk/start4life/Documents/PDFs/off-to-the-best-start.pdf).

Owen CG, Martin RM, Whincup PH, Davey-Smith G, Gillman MW, Cook DG, The effect of breastfeeding on mean body mass index throughout life: a quantitative review of published and unpublished observational evidence, *Am J Clin Nutr*, 2005;82:1298–1307.

Owen CG, Whincup PH, Odoki K, Gilg JA, Cook DG, Infant feeding and blood cholesterol: a study in adolescents and a systematic review, *Pediatrics*, 2002;110:597–608.

Park HS, Yoon CH, Kim HJ, The prevalence of congenital inverted nipples, *Aesth Plast Surgery*, 1999;23:144–6. under nipples P24

Patient.co.uk, Pregnancy and alcohol, 2012 (www.patient.co.uk/health/Pregnancy-and-Alcohol.htm).

Paton LM, Alexander JL, Nowson CA, Margerison C, Frame MG, Kaymakci B, Wark JD, Pregnancy and lactation have no long-term deleterious effect on measures of bone mineral in healthy women: a twin study, *Am J Clin Nut*, 2003;77:707–14.

Pearce SHS, Cheetham TD, Diagnosis and management of vitamin D deficiency, *BMJ*, 2010;340:b5664.

Pisacane A, Graziano L, Zona G, Breastfeeding and urinary tract infection, *J Pediatr*, 1992;120:87–9.

Polatti F, Capuzzo E, Viazzo F, Colleoni R, Klersy C, Bone mineral changes during and after lactation, *Obstet Gynecol*, 1999;94:52–6.

Public Health Collaborating Centre on Maternal and Child Nutrition, Promotion of breastfeeding initiation and duration. Evidence into practice briefing, 2006 (www.nice.org.uk/niceMedia/pdf/EAB_Breastfeeding_final_version.pdf).

Quigley MA, Kelly YJ, Sacker AS, Breastfeeding and hospitalization for diarrheal and respiratory infection in the United Kingdom millennium cohort study, *Pediatrics*, 2007;119;e837–e842.

Ramsay DT, Kent JC, Hartmann RA, Hartmann PE, Anatomy of the lactating human breast redefined with ultrasound imaging, *J Anat*, 2005;206(6):525.

Rebhan B, Kohlhuber M, Schwegler U, Fromme H, Abou-Dakn, Koletzko BV, Breastfeeding duration and exclusivity associated with infants' health and growth: data from a prospective cohort study in Bavaria, Germany, *Acta Paediatr*, 2009;98:974–80.

Reijneveld SA, Brugman E, Hirasing RA, Infantile colic: maternal smoking as potential risk factor, *Arch Dis Child*, 2000;83(4):302–3.

Renfrew MJ, McFadden A, Dykes F, Wallace LM, Abbott S, Burt S, Anderson JK, Addressing the learning deficit in breastfeeding strategies for change, *Matern Child Nutr*, 2006;2(4):239–44.

Renfrew MJ, Ansell P, Macleod KL, Formula feed preparation: helping reduce the risks; a systematic review, *Arch Dis Child*, 2003;88:855–8.

Rigg LA, Lein A, Yen SSC, Pattern of increase in circulation prolactin levels during human gestation, *Am.J Obstet Gynecol*, 1977;129:454–6.

Riordan JM, Auerbach KG, *Breastfeeding and Human Lactation 4th ed.*, Sudbury: Jones and Bartlett, 2004.

Riordan JM, The cost of not breastfeeding: a commentary, *J Hum Lact*, 1997;13(2):93–7.

Rothenbacher D, Weyermann M, Beermann C, Brenner H, Breastfeeding, soluble CD14 concentration in breast milk and risk of atopic dermatitis and asthma in early childhood: birth cohort study, *Clin Exp Allergy*, 2005;35:1014–21.

Royal College of Midwives, *Successful Breastfeeding*, Philadelphia: Churchill Livingstone, 2001.

Saarinen UM, Kajosaari M, Breastfeeding as prophylaxis against atopic disease: prospective follow-up study until 17 years old, *Lancet*, 1995;346:1065–9.

SACN Coma Report, *Weaning and the Weaning Diet*, 1994.

SACN Infant Formula and Follow-on Formula Draft Regulations, 2007 (Response to consultation www.sacn.gov.uk/reports_position_statements/position_statements/infant_formula_and_follow-on_formula_draft_regulations_-_september_2007.html).

SACN report on Vitamin D deficiency in children, 2003. (www.sacn.gov.uk/pdfs/smcn_03_02.pdf).

Sadauskaite-Kuehne V, Ludvigsson J, Padaiga Z, Jasinskiene E, Samuelsson U, Longer breastfeeding is an independent protective factor against development of type 1 diabetes mellitus in childhood, *Diabetes Metab Res Rev*, 2004;20(2):150–57.

Schaefer C, Peters P, Miller RK (Eds), *Drugs during pregnancy and lactation: treatment options and risk assessment, 2nd edn*, Oxford: Academic Press, 2007.

Schirm E, Schwagermann MP, Tobi H, Jong-van den Berg LTW, Drug use during breastfeeding. A survey from the Netherlands, *Eur J Clin Nutr*, 2004;58:386–90.

Shealy KR, Scanlon KS, Labiner-Wolfe J, Fein SB, Grummer-Strawn LM, Characteristics of breastfeeding practices among US Mothers, *Paediatrics*, 2008;122:S50–55.

Smith WO, Hammarsten JF, Eliel LP, The clinical expression of magnesium deficiency, *JAMA*, 1960;174:77–8.

St James-Roberts I, Persistent infant crying, *Arch Dis Child*, 1991;66:653–5.

Stoliar OA, Pelley RP, Klaus MH, Kaniecki-Green E, Carpenter CCJ, Secretory IgA against enterotoxins in breast-milk, *Lancet*, 1976;307(7972):1258–61.

Stuebe A, The risks of not breastfeeding for mothers and infants, *Rev Obstet Gynecol*, 2009;2(4):222–31.

The Breastfeeding Network (www.breastfeedingnetwork.org.uk).

The Breastfeeding Network, Treatments for colic, 2002 (www.breastfeedingnetwork.org.uk/pdfs/Colic.pdf).

The Breastfeeding Network, Breastfeeding and thrush, 2009a www.breastfeedingnetwork.org.uk/information/thrush.php).

The Breastfeeding Network, Differential diagnosis of nipple pain, 2009b (www.breastfeedingnetwork.org.uk/pdfs/DiffDiagnosisOfNipplePain.pdf).

Thomsen AC, Espersen T, Maigaard S, Course and treatment of milk stasis, non-infectious inflammation of the breast and infectious mastitis, *Am J Obstet Gynecol*, 1984;149(5):492–5.

Turlapaty P, Altura BM, Magnesium deficiency produces spasms of coronary arteries; relationship to etiology of sudden death ischemic heart disease, *Science*, 1980;208:198–200.

UNICEF Baby Friendly Initiative Statement on Vitamin D supplementation for breastfed babies, 2012 (www.unicef.org.uk/BabyFriendly/News-and-Research/News/UNICEF-UK-Baby-Friendly-Initiative-Statement-on-vitamin-D-supplementation-for-breastfed-babies).

United Kingdom Association of Milk Banks (www.UKAMB.org

van Rossem L, Oenema A, Steegers EA, Moll HA, Jaddoe VW, Hofman A, Mackenbach JP, Raat H, Are starting and continuing breastfeeding related to educational background?, *Pediatrics*, 2009;123(6):e1017–27.

Virtanen SM, Räsänen L, Aro A, Lindström J, Sippola H, Lounamaa R, Toivanen L, Tuomilehto J, Åkerblom HK, Infant feeding in children 7 years of age with newly diagnosed IDDM, *Diabetes Care*, 1991;14:415–17.

von Kries R, Koletzko B, Sauerwald T, von Mutius E, Barnert D, Grunert V, von Voss H, Breastfeeding and obesity: cross sectional study, *BMJ*, 1999;319:147–50.

Walker M, Breastfeeding Management for the Clinician, Using the Evidence, Sudbury: Jones and Bartlett, 2006.

REFERENCES

Ware MR, DeVane CL, Imipramine treatment of panic disorder during pregnancy, *J Clin Psychiatry*, 1990;51:482–4.

Wessel MA, Cobb JC, Jackson EB, Harris GS, Detwiler AC, Paroxysmal fussing in infancy, sometimes called 'colic,' *Pediatrics*, 1954;14:421–34.

WHO, Mastitis causes and management, 2000 (www.who.int/reproductive-health/docs/mastitis.pdf).

WHO, Report of the expert consultation on the optimal duration of exclusive breastfeeding, 2001 (www.who.int/nutrition/publications/optimal_duration_of_exc_bfeeding_report_eng.pdf).

WHO, Nutrient adequacy of exclusive breastfeeding for the term infant during the first 6 months of life, 2002 (www.who.int/nutrition/publications/infantfeeding/9241562110/en/index.html).

WHO, Guidelines for the safe preparation, storage and handling of powdered infant formula, 2007 (www.who.int/foodsafety/publications/micro/pif_guidelines.pdf).

WHO, Infant and young child feeding fact sheet 342, 2010 (www.who.int/mediacentre/factsheets/fs342/en/).

WHO Health Topics, Breastfeeding, 2012 (www.who.int/topics/breastfeeding/en/)

Williams AF, Is breastfeeding beneficial in the UK? Statement of the Standing Committee on Nutrition of the British Paediatric Association, *Arch Dis Child*, 1994;71:376–80.

Williams AF, Early enteral feeding of the preterm infant, *Arch Dis Child Fetal Neonatal Ed*, 2000;83:F219–F220.

Williams AF, Vitamin D in pregnancy: an old problem still to be solved?, *Arch Dis Child*, 2007;92:740–41.

Williams J, Watkin-Jones R, Dicyclomine: worrying symptoms associated with its use in some small babies, *BMJ*, 1984;288:901.

Wilson AC, Forsyth JS, Greene SA, Irvine L, Hau C, Howie PW, Relation of infant diet to childhood health: seven year follow-up of cohort of children in Dundee infant feeding study, *BMJ*, 1998;316:21–5.

Woolridge MW, Fisher C, Colic, 'overfeeding', and symptoms of lactose malabsorption in the breast-fed baby: a possible artifact of feed management, *Lancet*, 1988;ii:382–4.

Zavaleta N, Iron and lactoferrin in milk of anaemic mothers given iron supplements, *Nutr Res*, 2005;15(5):681–90.

Index